KU-504-595

A PRACTICAL GUIDE FOR MEDICAL TEACHERS

Edited by

John A. Dent MMEd MD ILTM FRCS(Ed)
Reader and Honorary Consultant in Orthopaedic and Trauma Surgery,
Ninewells Hospital and Medical School, University of Dundee, Dundee, UK

Ronald M. Harden *OBE* MD FRCP(Glas) FRCPC FRCS(Ed)
Professor of Medical Education, University of Dundee, Dundee, UK;
Director of Education, The International Virtual Medical School

SECOND EDITION

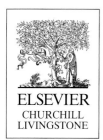

ELSEVIER
CHURCHILL
LIVINGSTONE

EDINBURGH LONDON NEW YORK OXFORD PHILADELPHIA ST LOUIS SYDNEY TORONTO 2005

ELSEVIER
CHURCHILL
LIVINGSTONE

© 2005, Elsevier Limited. All rights reserved.

The right of John A. Dent and Ronald M. Harden to be identified as authors of this work has been asserted by them in accordance with the Copyright, Designs and Patents Act 1988

No part of this publication may be reproduced, stored in a retrieval system, or transmitted in any form or by any means, electronic, mechanical, photocopying, recording or otherwise, without either the prior permission of the publishers or a licence permitting restricted copying in the United Kingdom issued by the Copyright Licensing Agency, 90 Tottenham Court Road, London W1T 4LP. Permissions may be sought directly from Elsevier's Health Sciences Rights Department in Philadelphia, USA: phone: (+1) 215 238 7869, fax: (+1) 215 238 2239, e-mail: healthpermissions@elsevier.com. You may also complete your request on-line via the Elsevier homepage (http://www.elsevier.com), by selecting 'Customer Support' and then 'Obtaining Permissions'.

First edition 2001
Second edition 2005
  Reprinted 2006

ISBN 0 443 10083 7

British Library Cataloguing in Publication Data
A catalogue record for this book is available from the British Library

Library of Congress Cataloguing in Publication Data
A catalogue record for this book is available from the Library of Congress

ELSEVIER your source for books, journals and multimedia in the health sciences
www.elsevierhealth.com

Working together to grow libraries in developing countries
www.elsevier.com | www.bookaid.org | www.sabre.org
ELSEVIER | BOOK AID International | Sabre Foundation

Note
Medical knowledge is constantly changing. Standard safety precautions must be followed, but as new research and clinical experience broaden our knowledge, changes in treatment and drug therapy may become necessary or appropriate. Readers are advised to check the most current product information provided by the manufacturer of each drug to be administered to verify the recommended dose, the method and duration of administration, and contraindications. It is the responsibility of the practitioner, relying on experience and knowledge of the patient, to determine dosages and the best treatment for each individual patient. Neither the Publisher nor the author assumes any liability for any injury and/or damage to persons or property arising from this publication.

The Publisher

A 061698

W 18

THE LIBRARY
KENT & SUSSEX HOSPITAL
TUNBRIDGE WELLS
KENT TN4 8AT

The publisher's policy is to use **paper manufactured from sustainable forests**

Printed in China

A PRACTICAL GUIDE
FOR MEDICAL TEACHERS

THE LIBRARY
KENT & SUSSEX HOSPITAL
TUNBRIDGE WELLS
KENT TN4 8AT

Prefix
MTW

0104367

The Library, Ed & Trg Centre   KTW
Tunbridge Wells Hospital at Pembury
Tonbridge Rd, Pembury
Kent TN2 4QJ
01892 635884 and 635489

Books must be returned/renewed by the last date shown

3 0 JUL 2008
(ILL / KMD)

ILL / SHS

1 9 JUN 2009

DISCARDED

742.32

Commissioning Editor: Laurence Hunter
Development Editor: Janice Urquhart
Project Manager: Frances Affleck
Designer: Erik Bigland
Illustration Manager: Bruce Hogarth
Illustrator: David Graham

PREFACE

Basic medical scientists, hospital-based clinicians, specialists and doctors working in the community, whether they have a health service or a university appointment, have a legitimate and indeed necessary interest in teaching. Since the first edition of this book was published four years ago, there has been fuller recognition of the need for some level of teaching competence in all physicians and of a professionalism and scholarship in this area. It remains difficult for doctors, whether engaged in clinical practice or research, to keep abreast of contemporary thinking and practice of education in addition to working in their own principal field of interest.

The changes that have taken place in medical practice and the increasing pressures on the doctor, together with the significant developments in medical education, have made it even more difficult for doctors to keep up-to-date with current approaches adopted for curriculum planning, teaching and learning, assessment and educational management. Many however are enthusiastic teachers.

It is the purpose of this book to bridge the gap between the theoretical aspects of medical education and the practical delivery of enthusiastic teaching. It is an attempt to help clinicians, as well as other healthcare teachers, in their understanding of contemporary educational principles, and to provide practical help for them in the delivery of the variety of teaching situations which characterise present day curricula.

Whether medical training will continue to be delivered in the context of a hospital-based medical school or an expanded ambulatory care service, the continued support of an expanded cohort of clinical teachers, familiar with some basic principles and techniques of modern medical education, will be essential. Key concepts and appropriate tips have therefore been presented in a digestible form and in a way which indicates both their immediate relevance and practical implications.

Since the first edition was published there have been a number of significant trends in medical education which have been reflected in the revisions and updating of the text. In addition several new chapters have been added including ones on peer assisted learning, simulators, e-learning and virtual learning environments.

A key thrust in the book as with the first edition, is undergraduate medical education. Many of the principles and approaches described however, are equally applicable in postgraduate and continuing education and new chapters have been added on these topics.

The contributions to *A Practical Guide for Medical Teachers* have been expanded in this edition to provide a wider international perspective and include many of the leading international authorities in medical education. Miriam Friedman Ben-David completed her contribution on Principles of assessment, before her sudden death in July 2004 at the 11th Ottawa Conference. She will be seriously missed in medical education and we are pleased to be able to provide this chapter which covers one of her main areas of interest.

Some readers may wish to review their current practice, others to make changes, but all involved in teaching in the healthcare disciplines will, we hope, benefit from this review of current developments in medical education, its practical tips and references to further reading. We hope that they will be encouraged in their role as medical teachers.

R.M. Harden
J.A. Dent
Dundee, 2005

CONTRIBUTORS

Graceanne Adamo MA
Director, Standardized Patient Program, The George
Washington University School of Medicine, Clinical
Learning and Surgical Skills Center; Adjunct Assistant
Professor, Nurse Practitioner Program, Uniformed
Services University of the Health Sciences, Graduate
School of Nursing, Maryland, USA

Raja C. Bandaranayake MB BS PhD MSEd(SoCal) FRCAS
Chairman, Department of anatomy, College of Medicine
and Medical Sciences, Arabian Gulf University,
Manama, Bahrain

Hugh Barr MPhil
President of the UK Centre for the Advancement
of Interprofessional Education; Editor-in-Chief of
the Journal of Interprofessional Care; Emeritus
Professor of Interprofessional Education, University
of Westminster, London; Visiting Professor in
Interprofessional Education, University of
Greenwich, UK

John Bligh BSc MMEd MD FRCGP
Professor of Clinical Education, Associate Dean and
Director of the Institute of Clinical Education,
Peninsula Medical School, Plymouth, UK; Editor in
Chief, Medical Education

Mark G. Brennan BA MA AKC DHMSA FCollP FRSH
Lecturer in Medical and Dental Education, University
of Wales College of Medicine, Cardiff; Senior Lecturer
in Medical Ethics, Royal College of Surgeons in
Ireland, Dublin

Julie Brice BA(Hons) PGCE
Editor's Assistant, Medical Education, Peninsula
Medical School, Plymouth, UK

Suzanne Cholerton BSc PhD
Director of Medical Studies, Faculty of Medical
Sciences, University of Newcastle, Newcastle upon
Tyne, UK

Allan D. Cumming MB ChB MD FRCPE
Director of Undergraduate Learning and Teaching,
College of Medicine and Veterinary Medicine,
University of Edinburgh; Consultant Physician, Renal
Medicine, Lothian University Hospitals Trust,
Edinburgh, UK

David Davies BSc PhD
Senior Lecturer, Medical Education Unit, School
of Medicine, University of Birmingham, Birmingham,
UK

Dave A. Davis MD CCFP FCFP
Associate Dean, Continuing Education, Faculty of
Medicine; Professor, Department of Health Policy,
Management and Evaluation, and Department of Family
and Community Medicine, University of Toronto,
Toronto, Canada

Margery H. Davis MB ChB MRCP
Head, Centre for Medical Education, University of
Dundee, Dundee, UK

John A. Dent MMedEd MD ILTM FRCSEd
Reader and Honorary Consultant in Orthopaedic and
Trauma Surgery, Ninewells Hospital and Medical
School, University of Dundee, Dundee, UK

David Dewhurst BSc PhD
Assistant Principal (e-learning and e-health), and
Director of Learning Technology, College of Medicine
and Veterinary Medicine, University of Edinburgh,
Edinburgh, UK

Rachel Ellaway BSc
eLearning Manager, Learning Technology Section,
College of Medicine and Veterinary Medicine,
University of Edinburgh, Edinburgh, UK

Charles D. Forbes MB ChB DSc MD FRCP
Professor of Medicine, University of Dundee,
Ninewells Hospital and Medical School, Dundee,
UK

Miriam Friedman Ben-David (Deceased)
Joanne Goldman MSc
Knowledge Translation Program, Continuing Education,
Faculty of Medicine, University of Toronto, Toronto,
Canada

Paul Glasziou MB BS FRACGP PhD
Reader in Primary Care and Director, Centre for
Evidence Based Medicine, University of Oxford,
Oxford, UK

Ronald M. Harden MD FRCP(Glas) FRCPC FRCSEd
Professor of Medical Education, University of Dundee,
Dundee, UK; Director of Education, The International
Virtual Medical School

Carl Heneghan BM BCh BA(Hons)
Academic General Practice Registrar, Department
of Primary Health Care, Oxford University and Centre
for Evidence Based Practice, Oxford, UK

E. Anne Hesketh BSc(Hons) DipEd
Senior Education Development Officer, Education
Development Unit (Scottish Council for Postgraduate
Medical and Dental Education), University of Dundee,
Dundee, UK

Susan Humphry-Murto MD FRCPC MEd
Assistant Professor, University of Ottawa, Ottawa;
Executive Secretary of the Objective Structured
Clinical Examination Committee, Medical Council
of Canada, Canada

Reg Jordan BSc PhD HonMRCP
Professor of Medical Education; Dean of Undergraduate
Studies, Faculty of Medical Sciences, University of
Newcastle; Director, Learning and Teaching Support
Network Subject Centre for Medicine, Dentistry and
Veterinary Medicine, University of Newcastle,
Newcastle upon Tyne, UK

Jean S. Ker BSc(Hons) MB ChB DRCOG DFFP MRCGP
Lecturer in Medical Education and General Practitioner,
Faculty of Medicine, Dentistry and Nursing, University
of Dundee, Dundee, UK

Jennifer M. Laidlaw DipEdTech MMedEd
Assistant Director, Education Development
Unit (Scottish Council for Postgraduate Medical
and Dental Education), University of Dundee, Dundee,
UK

Sam Leinster BSc MD FRCS(Ed & Eng) ILTM
Dean, School of Medicine, Health and Policy,
University of East Anglia, Norwich, UK

Sean McAleer BSc DPhil
Senior Lecturer in Medical Education, Centre for
Medical Education, University of Dundee, Dundee, UK

P. McCrorie BSc PhD
Head of Medical and Healthcare Education, Director
of the Graduate Entry Programme, St George's Hospital
Medical School, London, UK

I. Chris McManus MA MD PhD FRCP
Professor of Psychology and Medical Education,
University College London, London, UK

Marion E. T. McMurdo MB ChB MD
Professor in Ageing and Health, Department
of Medicine, University of Dundee, Ninewells Hospital
and Medical School, Dundee, UK

Meredith Marks MD MEd
Assistant Dean, Professional Affairs, University
of Ottawa, Ottawa, Canada

Stewart Mennin PhD
Assistant Dean, Educational Development and
Research; Professor Department of Cell Biology and
Physiology, School of Medicine, University of New
Mexico, Albuquerque, USA

Elizabeth Mitchell BA
Lecturer in Primary Care Informatics, Tayside Centre
for General Practice, University of Dundee, Dundee,
UK

John Norcini PhD
President and CEO, Foundation for Advancement
of International Medical Education and Research
(FAIMER), Philadelphia, USA

Nivritti Patil MBE MB BS MS FRCSEd FCHK FHKAM(Surgery)
Associate Professor in Surgery and Assistant Dean
(Education and Student Affairs), Faculty of Medicine,
The University of Hong Kong, Hong Kong

Laure Perrier Med MLIS
Continuing Education, Faculty of Medicine, University
of Toronto, Toronto, Canada

Gominda G. Ponnamperuma MB BS DipPsych MMedEd
Lecturer in Medical Education, Faculty of Medicine,
University of Colombo, Sri Lanka

David Prideaux Dip T BA(Hons) Med PhD
Head, Department of Medical Education, School
of Medicine; Associate Head, Faculty of Health
Sciences (Teaching and Learning), Flinders University,
Adelaide, Australia

Sarah Rennie MB ChB BMSc(Hons) MRCS(Ed)
Surgical Registrar, Department of Surgery, Dunedin
Hospital, Dunedin, New Zealand

Michael T. Ross MRCGP MB ChB BSc DRCOG
Coordinator of PPD and Clinical Lecturer in Primary
Care, Medical Teaching Organisation, The University
of Edinburgh Medical School, Edinburgh, UK

Joy R. Rudland BSc(Hons) MPhil DipMedEd DipAdEd
Director of Educational Development and Support,
Faculty of Medicine, University of Otago, Dunedin,
New Zealand

Lambert W. T. Schuwirth MD PhD
Assistant Professor, Department of Educational
Development and Research, Faculty of Medicine,
University of Maastricht, Maastricht, The Netherlands

Ann Jervie Sefton AO BSc(Med) MB BS PhD DSc
Emeritus Professor; Former Associate Dean, Faculties
of Medicine and Dentistry, University of Sydney,
Australia

Stephen R. Smith MD MPH
Professor of Family Medicine, Associate Dean
for Medical Education, Brown Medical School,
Providence, RI, USA

David Snadden MB ChB MCISc MD FRCGP FRCP(Edin)
Professor, Northern Medical Program, University
of Northern British Columbia and Department of Family
Practice, University of British Columbia, Canada

Yvonne Steinert PhD
Professor of Family Medicine; Associate Dean for
Faculty Development and Associate Director of the
Centre for Medical Education, Faculty of Medicine,
McGill University, Montreal, Canada

Alistair Stewart MSc PhD
Educational Consultant, Centre for Medical Education,
University of Dundee, Dundee, UK

Frank Sullivan PhD FRCP(Glas) FRCP(Edin) FRCGP
NHS Tayside Professor of Research and
Development in GP and Primary Care, Community
Health Sciences Division, University of Dundee,
Dundee, UK

Cees P. M. van der Vleuten PhD
Professor of Education, Department of Educational
Development and Research, Faculty of Medicine,
University of Maastricht, Maastricht, The Netherlands

Miles D. Witham BM BCh MRCP
Clinical Lecturer in Ageing and Health, Section
of Ageing and Health, University of Dundee, Ninewells
Hospital and Medical School, Dundee, UK

P. Worley MB BS PhD FACRRM DObstRANZCOG FRACGP
Director, Flinders University Rural Clinical School,
Flinders, Australia

Amitai Ziv MD MHA
Deputy Director, Chaim Sheba Medical Center;
Director, Risk Management;, Director, Israel Center
for Medical Simulation (MSR), Israel

CONTENTS

SECTION 1
CURRICULUM DEVELOPMENT

Chapter 1
New horizons in medical education

J. A. Dent, R. M. Harden

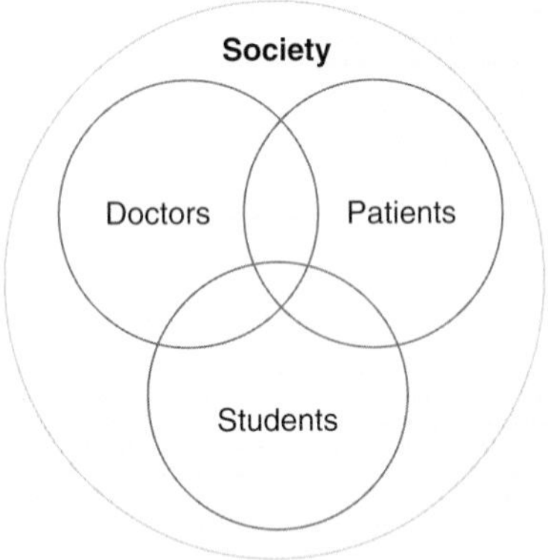

Fig. 1.1 Interaction of key areas

What were the challenges?

When the first edition of this book was published, medical schools in the UK were responding to a variety of challenges to medical education from four broad areas (Dent & Harden 2001):

- patients as consumers
- society in general
- practising doctors
- medical students (Fig. 1.1).

These challenges occurred as a result of changes in:

- patients' expectations
- healthcare delivery
- medical knowledge
- doctors' availability and workload
- students' requirements.

Changes in patients' expectations

As a result of a move to a more open society with ready internet and media access to medical information, patients have become well-informed about health and disease and about the choice of treatment available. Many no longer wish to be the passive recipients of medical opinion but prefer to share in decision making and expect courteous communication and appropriate attitudes from their medical practitioners. Doctors can no longer expect to practise in an authoritarian or paternalistic manner but must adopt a more patient-centred approach to patient care.

While health promotion and disease prevention are seen by some as a priority, there is a universal demand that disease and illness are treated with the most advanced methods of healthcare available irrespective of cost. While in many instances this is possible, some patients have become less tolerant of real or perceived deficiencies in healthcare delivery and, rather than being quiescent, have become increasingly litigious.

Society also expects accountability from anyone perceived as being in a position of privilege or responsibility. The efficiency of a treatment must be known and its cost-effectiveness proven. It is increasingly expected that medicine should be evidence-based. Accountability is looked for in both undergraduate and postgraduate training where funding and regulatory bodies, as well as students and trainees, expect value for money and evidence of self-governance.

Change in healthcare delivery

The style of practice for most doctors has changed. In the community large group practices have replaced the individual, well-known and often admired family physician, while in hospital shift systems have replaced the constantly available junior doctor so compromising continuity of in-patient care to some extent. In these environments the ability to work as a member of a team becomes an important issue and an increased awareness of a multiprofessional approach to healthcare is required to foster cooperation with colleagues from other disciplines.

Stereotyping has become inappropriate in modern medical practice. Professional boundaries are now less rigid. The role of the nurse-practitioner has developed and extended role practitioners in other disciplines are seen to be providing initial assessment and routine management. In the UK the creation of Ambulatory Diagnostic and Treatment Centres (ADTCs) underlines the shift of healthcare delivery towards community settings and away from traditional in-patient practice.

Changes in medical knowledge

Traditionally the medical course was structured as a progression from the basic sciences to the clinical sciences with little attempt at integration. The exponential growth of medical knowledge and the greatly increased content of the scientific aspect of the curriculum has made the selection of appropriate core content and the integration of basic and clinical sciences important aspects of curricular design. New subjects and material have been added to the curriculum but there has been a reluctance to remove older topics, possibly limiting the ability of the course to develop as expected.

There have been changes too in the pattern of disease seen in practice with an ageing population leading to an increase in problems associated with degenerative conditions and chronic ill-health.

Changes in doctors' availability and workload

Individual doctors, although they may seek to be more approachable, may be now less readily accessible to patients than before as contemporary attitudes to work, leisure and restricted hours of duty are adopted.

At work the pressures to deliver a clinical service, engage in research activity and provide accountable training opportunities for trainees have made it more difficult for senior staff to focus on teaching. At the same time junior doctors, now engaged in faster training programmes, with protected time for research and postgraduate training, may have fewer opportunities to take part in undergraduate teaching and be less experienced themselves in clinical procedures.

"Both doctors and patients can experience difficulties when dealing with someone from a different ethnic group......A lack of shared culture means differences in beliefs and expectations, as well as more obvious language issues. Future doctors are expected 'to be more aware and respond sensibly to the culturally determined expectations of their patients' "

Gill & Green 1996

"It has been realised for many years that an undergraduate course such as this suffers from the chronic disorder 'curriculopathy' "

Guilbert 1985

"There is no denying the striking differences between the bright, interesting 18-year-olds seen at interview and the weary, disillusioned, unquestioning absorbers of information seen during the clinical years"

Fraser 1991

Medical education must respond to the context in which it operates (Towle 1998):
- Teach scientific behaviour as well as scientific facts
- Promote the use of information technology
- Adapt to the changing doctor–patient relationship
- Help future doctors to shape and adapt to change
- Promote multiprofessional teamworking and care
- Help future doctors handle broader responsibilities
- Reflect the changing patterns of disease and heathcare delivery
- Involve health service employers and users.

Changes in students' requirements

It has been said that medical courses contribute to the disillusionment and demoralisation of students by deadening their initial enthusiasm for medicine and failing to prepare them adequately for the diversity of problems which they will encounter as professionals (Godfrey 1991). Students' expectations of both the quality and administration of undergraduate teaching are higher than in the past and course review and monitoring are becoming established activities in medical schools.

In many countries there has been a dramatic increase in the number of students admitted to study medicine. In England and Wales alone there has been a 40 percent increase in recent years.

Today's students come from a wider range of social, ethnic and economic backgrounds than previously and with a greater variety of personal and academic achievements. A number will be postgraduates and some schools who previously admitted students directly from school now have an exclusively postgraduate intake. A sizeable group of students will be studying in a language and culture that is not their own which may give rise to difficulties in learning communication skills and in practising aspects of physical examination.

All of these changes place increasing demands on medical education and on the medical teacher.

What was the response to these challenges?

Medical schools and training bodies have responded to these challenges in a number of ways:

- the development of new curricula incorporating new curriculum themes and different educational strategies
- the introduction of new learning situations and the use of new tools and aids to leaning
- the introduction of new methods of assessment
- a realisation of the importance of staff development structures.

A new curriculum

Features common to many of the new curriculum initiatives have included a decrease in the amount of factual knowledge presented, the fostering of adult learning styles, the provision of opportunities for student choices and the early introduction of clinical experience.

New educational strategies

A variety of educational strategies appropriate for adult learning have been adopted in place of 'spoon-feeding': self-directed learning (SDL), problem-based learning (PBL), integrated learning, task-based learning (Harden et al 2000) and multiprofessional learning being examples.

However, facilitating student learning in these ways may prove more difficult than traditional teaching and, in addition, have considerable implications for staffing and other resources. Although methods of changing the style of teaching are becoming better known, not all have found general acceptance. Unfamiliarity with new techniques and mistrust of change often conspire to slow down implementation (Dent & Harden 2001)

New curriculum models

Communication skills, attitudinal and ethical issues, preparation for practice, teamwork and evidence-based practice have all found a place in revised curricula.

This should help new doctors in their relationships with patients and with changing approaches to healthcare delivery, in which problem solving is the doctor's role but decision making is a joint activity between doctor and patient (Towle 1998).

In the UK, the General Medical Council (GMC) has indicated the need for a medical course which will produce doctors with appropriate attitudes to medicine and learning that will fit them for a lifetime of professional self-education (GMC 1993). Courses emphasising self-directed learning, problem solving and the development of critical thought serve students better than courses that demand only passive learning and factual recall.

Examples of different curricular models which may coexist include:

- outcome-based education (Harden et al 1999)
- problem-based learning (Harden & Davis 1998)
- task-based learning (Harden et al 2000)
- core and student-selected components (Harden & Davis 1995)
- an integrated systems-based approach (Harden 2000)
- a spiral curriculum (Harden et al 1997).

New learning situations

While lectures and bedside teaching retain a place, new learning situations have been introduced. There has been an increase in opportunities for independent learning and in small-group teaching events. Bedside teaching may be more difficult to provide than previously, but new opportunities have been sought in clinical skills centres, ambulatory care, day surgery units (Dent 2003) and primary care settings, illustrating that traditional professional skills may be learned in contemporary healthcare situations.

New tools and aids

The use of study guides is well established and the use of computer-assisted learning programmes and the internet has increased. The importance of information technology as a tool for accessing information and lifelong learning has been appreciated (Cox et al 1992). Videos and self-videoing have been used especially to teach clinical skills, consultation techniques and to explore issues of attitude and behaviour. The role of simulators and simulations is now well recognised for training in aspects of physical examination and practical procedures at both undergraduate and postgraduate levels.

New methods of assessment

An integrated curriculum requires an integrated approach to assessment such as the objective structured clinical exam (OSCE) which can test

"With advance planning many traditional clinical activities can be structured to provide highly effective learning without extensive demands on consultant time"

Eaton & Cottrell 1998

performance and competence in a wide diversity of settings. The OSCE, well established in undergraduate programmes, has now found a place in a variety of postgraduate examinations. Extended matching items (EMIs) are beginning to replace shorter multiple choice questions.

The concept of formative assessment has become part of the development of student learning, while portfolio assessment (Friedman et al 2001) and work-based assessment have been introduced as ways of examining a student's sustained performance in a variety of outcomes and locations.

Staff development structures

Finally it has been realised that little can be accomplished in the field of curriculum change without appropriate staff development opportunities. It is not particularly easy to implement these effectively but as curriculum innovations may be stressful it is likely that provision of support for staff in the process of curriculum change will be necessary.

Where do we go next?

The changes of the new curricula of the 1990s are by now well established, but many challenges still remain. As we take a fresh look at current trends in medical education we can see several key issues of particular current importance:

- outcome-based education
- cost-effectiveness of approaches to teaching and learning
- the introduction of new learning technologies
- choice of educational strategies
- approaches to assessment
- staff development and professionalism in medical education
- best evidence medical education
- ambulatory care teaching.

Outcome-based education – what sort of doctor is needed?

The answer is probably a doctor with less knowledge but more abilities. These will include appropriate attitudes, problem-solving skills and use of information technology. Doctors will have an appreciation of a wider variety of possible solutions to healthcare problems including complementary and alternative medicine (CAM), and will have the ability to work as part of a multiprofessional team and to relate to colleagues, patients and employers.

Increasing emphasis will be placed on these and other expected learning outcomes and on the need for the agreed learning outcomes to influence decisions about the curriculum and the teaching and learning and assessment processes.

Cost-effectiveness – how can the curriculum be delivered within the available budget?

At a time of financial constraints the demands made on medical educators will continue to increase. This may entail a fundamental reappraisal

Twelve tips for PAL:
1. Ensure that the organisation is student-led
2. Consider the content of the tutorials
3. Make tutor selection voluntary
4. Train the tutor
5. Reward the tutors
6. Consider which students (tutees) should attend the sessions
7. Consider the timing of peer learning
8. Restrict the duration of the sessions
9. Make the environment conducive to learning
10. Ensure that the medical school supports the peer scheme
11. Evaluate the peer learning scheme
12. Consider when and how to use peer learning.

Wadoodi & Crosby 2002

of the roles expected of the medical teacher with the possible unbundling of teaching responsibilities.

The newly implemented consultant contracts in the UK have recognised the amount of teaching time expected of a consultant and may facilitate consultant input into teaching programmes.

Peer-assisted learning (PAL) programmes have been introduced with appropriate briefing of student tutors, and have been reported to be beneficial to both tutors and tutees (Wadoodi & Crosby 2002). Finally, faculty ownership and administration of resources may lead to the best use being made of expensive equipment and teaching space.

New learning technologies – what can be done differently?

Enormous developments have taken place in information technology and e-learning. As discussed in chapter 24 on e-learning and chapter 22 on virtual learning environments, this may result in dramatic changes in medical education by the end of this decade. The newly established International Virtual Medical School (IVIMEDS) which is a consortium of 37 leading international medical schools is an example of what can be achieved when new learning technologies are combined with innovative educational thinking.

Choice of educational approach – what is the best strategy?

In the past, educators have been preoccupied with identifying and implementing what they believe to be the 'best' educational strategy. There has been a failure to recognise that there is no simple 'best' approach. This will vary with the student, the learning context and the topic being studied.

There is no single best curriculum. Students with different learning styles will prefer different curricular models. Some will make their applications to medical school on the basis of the curriculum style on offer. It is likely, however, that we will see a move to more flexible learning opportunities with an adaptive curriculum in which the different learning needs of individual students are recognised and the programme is tailored to meet these needs.

Assessment – what is the best assessment instrument?

We will see a continuing development and sophistication in approaches to assessment. A range of approaches including new instruments such as portfolio assessment will be used to assess the important new expected learning outcomes. Computers too will have a greater role. Work-based assessment will be increasingly important.

Standard-setting procedures have been on the assessment agenda in recent years. These will become more important and will be applied to new approaches to assessment.

Staff development – can excellence in teaching be fostered?

An amateur role for a medical teacher is no longer sustainable. Competence in teaching is a requirement for all doctors and professionalism and scholarship in medical education are expected. Training and

"E is for everything – e-learning?"
2001 Harden & Davis

"IVIMEDS is a "metacampus" comprising a partnership of medical schools and institutions worldwide. It will draw on the innovative and established curriculum and assessment practices of partner institutions so ensuring maximum benefit from new educational technologies."
IVIMEDS

"The aim of the [IVIMEDS] project is to provide an effective means of sharing digital learning resources among partner institutions."
IVIMEDS

staff development programmes are now widely available at different levels by both face-to-face and distance learning.

Programmes have also been established for recognising and rewarding academic performance (Williams et al 2003)

Best evidence medical education – can you justify your teaching decisions and activities?

While the difficulties of a move to 'evidence-based teaching' are recognised, the principles of best evidence medical education (BEME Collaboration) have now been widely accepted. Best evidence medical education has been defined as the implementation of teachers, in their practice, of methods and approaches to education based on the best evidence available.

Ambulatory care teaching – will this be important?

Almost certainly the trend away from in-patient teaching will continue and increasing opportunities will be sought in ambulatory care venues.

Summary

Over the last few years medical schools have been faced with a variety of challenges from patients, society, doctors and students. They have responded in several ways which have included the development of new curricula, the introduction of new learning situations, the introduction of new methods of assessment and a realisation of the importance of staff development. Many effective and interesting innovations have been forthcoming.

However, as we take a fresh look at medical education we now see several new trends of particular importance:

- outcome-based education
- cost-effectiveness of approaches to teaching and learning
- the introduction of new learning technologies
- choice of educational strategies
- approaches to assessment
- staff development and professionalism in medical education
- best evidence medical education
- ambulatory care teaching

These topics are expanded in subsequent chapters.

"The BEME Collaboration is a group of individuals or institutions who are committed to the promotion of Best Evidence Medical Education through:

- *the dissemination of information which allows medical teachers, institutions and all concerned with medical education to make decisions on the basis of the best evidence available*
- *the production of appropriate systematic reviews of medical education which reflect the best evidence available and meet the needs of the user, and*
- *the creation of a culture of best evidence medical education amongst individual teachers, institutions and national bodies."*

BEME Collaboration

References

BEME [Best Evidence Medical Education] Collaboration
http://www.bemecollaboration.org

Cox J J, Dawson J K, Hobbs K E F 1992 The electronic revolution and how to exploit it. British Journal of Surgery 79:1004–1010

Davis MH, Harden RM 2001 E is for everything – e-learning? Medical Teacher 23:441–444

Dent J A 2003 Twelve tips for developing a clinical teaching programme in a day surgery unit. Medical Teacher 25:364–367

Dent J A, Harden R M 2001 (eds) A practical guide for medical teachers, 1st edition. Edinburgh, Churchill Livingstone

Eaton D M, Cottrell D 1998 Maximising the effectiveness of undergraduate teaching in the clinical setting. Archives of Diseases in Childhood 79:365–367

Fraser R C 1991 Undergraduate medical education: present state and future needs. BMJ 303:41–43

Friedman Ben David M, Davis M H, Harden R M et al 2001 AMEE Guide No 24: Portfolios as a method of student assessment. Medical Teacher 23:535–551

Gill P S, Green P 1996 Learning for a multicultural society. British Journal of General Practice 46:704–705

GMC 1993 Tomorrow's doctors. London, General Medical Council

Godfrey R 1991 All change? Lancet 338:297–299

Guilbert J J 1985 Les maladies du curriculum. Revue d'Éducation Médicale 4:13–16

Harden RM, Crosby J, Davis M H et al 2000 Task-based learning: the answer to integration and problem-based learning in the clinical years. Medical Education 34:391–397

Harden R M 2000 The integration ladder: a tool for curriculum planning and evaluation, Medical Education 34(7):551–557

Harden R M, Davis M H 1995 The core curriculum with options or special study modules. Medical Teacher 17:125–148

Harden R M, Davis M H 1998 The continuum of problem-based learning. Medical Teacher 20(4):317–322

Harden R M, Davis M H, Crosby J 1997 The new Dundee curriculum: a whole that is greater than the sum of the parts. Medical Education 31:264–291

Harden R M, Crosby J R, Davis M H 1999 An introduction to outcome-based education. Medical Teacher 21:7–14

IVIMEDS (International Virtual Medical School) http://www.ivimeds.org

Towle A 1998 Continuing medical education: changes in health care and continuing medical education for the 21st century. BMJ 316:301–304

Wadoodi A, Crosby J R 2002 Twelve tips for peer assisted learning: a classic concept revisited. Medical Teacher 24:241–244

Williams R G, Dunnington G L, Folse J R 2003 The impact of a program for systematically recognizing and rewarding academic performance. Academic Medicine 78:156–166

Chapter 2

Curriculum planning and development

R. M. Harden

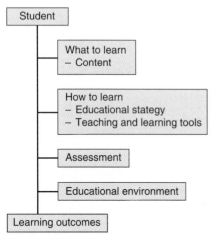

"Curriculum is in the air. No matter what the problem in medical education, curriculum is looked to as the solution"

Davidoff 1996

Fig. 2.1   A wider view of a curriculum

The ten main headings in this chapter provide a useful checklist for planning and evaluating a curriculum.

Introduction

Curriculum planning and development is very much on today's agenda for undergraduate, postgraduate and continuing medical education.

The days are now past when the teacher produced a curriculum like a magician produced a rabbit out of a hat, when the lecturer taught whatever attracted his or her interest and when the students' clinical training was limited to the patients who happened to present during a clinical attachment. It is now accepted that careful planning is necessary if the programme of teaching and learning is to be successful.

What is a curriculum?

A curriculum is more than just a syllabus or a statement of content. A curriculum is about what should happen in a teaching programme – about the intention of the teachers and about the way they make this happen. This extended vision of a curriculum is illustrated in Figure 2.1.

Curriculum planning can be considered in ten steps (Harden 1986b). They have been used as headings to divide this chapter and are reviewed here in the context of the trends in medical education.

Identifying the need

The relevance or appropriateness of educational programmes has been questioned. It has been argued that there is often a mismatch between what is expected of the young doctor and the competencies gained from the training programme.

The need has been recognised to emphasise not only sickness salvaging, organic pathology and crisis care, but also health promotion and preventative medicine. Aspects of medical care which have not been adequately addressed in the past include:

- communication skills
- health promotion and disease prevention
- clinical procedures such as cardiopulmonary resuscitation
- professionalism, including the development of attitudes and an understanding of ethical principles.

A range of approaches can be used to identify the curriculum needs (Dunn et al 1985):

- The 'wise men' approach. Senior teachers and senior practitioners from different specialty backgrounds reach a consensus.
- Consultation with the stakeholders. The views of members of the public, patients, government and other professions are sought.
- A study of errors in practice. Areas are identified where the curriculum is likely to be deficient.
- Critical-incident studies. Individuals are asked to describe key medical incidents in their experience which represent good or bad practice.
- Task analysis. The work undertaken by a doctor is studied.
- Study of star performers. Doctors recognised as 'star performers' are studied to identify their special qualities or competencies.

Establishing the learning outcomes

Since the work of Bloom, Mager and others in the 1960s and 1970s, the value of setting out the aims and objectives of a training programme has been accepted. In practice however, lists of aims and objectives are often used only as window dressing. They are ignored in planning and implementing the curriculum. There are a number of reasons for this:

- The list of objectives is extensive, time-consuming to produce and of only limited assistance in decisions about the curriculum.
- The commonly accepted classification – knowledge, skills and attitudes – does not reflect clinical practice. Most clinical competencies incorporate all three domains.

Despite these problems, the underlying principle has much to recommend it. Indeed, one of the big ideas in medical education today is the move to the use of learning outcomes as the driver in curriculum planning. An outcome-based approach to education is discussed in Chapter 14.

In outcome-based education (Harden et al 1999)

- The learning outcomes are defined
- The outcomes inform decisions about the curriculum.

There is a move away from a process model of curriculum planning, where what matter are the teaching and learning experiences and methods, to a product model, where what matter are the learning outcomes and the product and where there is increasing clarity of focus for learning.

Agreeing the content

The content of a textbook is outlined in the contents pages and in the index. The content of a curriculum is found in the syllabus, in the

"Needs assessment is a central part of a systematic approach to developing educational projects"

Levine et al 1984

Remember that if you don't know where you are going, you can't know how to get there.

If you go from this book with only one idea it should be the concept of outcome-based education.

"In line with current educational theory and research, we have adopted an outcomes-based model"

Rubin & Franchi-Christopher 2002.

"A move from the 'How' and 'When' to the 'What' and 'Whether' "

Spady 1994

"I've seen many schools that purport to emphasise communication skills, appropriate attitudes and health promotion In their curriculum. In looking inside these schools, however, it didn't take long to see that their business was actively teaching content in medicine, surgery and other disciplines – with the noble aims listed above receiving little direct attention"

Senior teacher

handouts relating to the topics covered in lectures and in students' study guides. Traditionally there has been an emphasis in the curriculum on knowledge, and this has been reflected in the assessment. There is now increased recognition of skills and attitudes as important domains.

The content of the curriculum can be analysed from a number of perspectives:

- subjects or disciplines (in a traditional curriculum)
- body systems, e.g. the cardiovascular system (in an integrated curriculum)
- the life cycle, e.g. childhood, adulthood, old age
- problems or tasks (in a problem-based or task-based curriculum)
- learning outcomes (in an outcome-based curriculum).

These approaches are not mutually exclusive. Grids can be prepared which look at the content of a curriculum from two or more of these perspectives.

No account of curriculum content would be complete without reference to the concept of the hidden curriculum. The 'declared' curriculum is the curriculum as set out in the institution's documents. The 'taught' curriculum is what happens in practice. The 'learned' curriculum is what is learned by the student. The 'hidden' curriculum is the informal learning in which students engage and which is unrelated to what is taught (see Fig. 2.2).

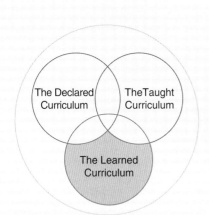

Fig. 2.2 The hidden curriculum (shaded area)

Organising the content

One assumption in a traditional medical curriculum is that students should first master the basic sciences, including anatomy, physiology and biochemistry, and then the applied sciences, including pathology, microbiology and epidemiology. Once they have achieved this they move on to a study of clinical medicine. A common criticism of this approach is that students may not see the relevance to their future career as doctors of what is taught. Once they have passed the examinations in the basic sciences, students tend to forget or ignore what they have learned.

It has been advocated that the curriculum should be turned on its head, with students starting to think like a doctor from the day they enter medical school. In a vertically integrated curriculum, students are introduced to clinical medicine alongside the basic sciences in the early years of the programme. The students continue to look at the basic sciences as applied to clinical medicine in the later years.

A spiral curriculum (see Fig. 2.3) offers a useful approach to the organisation of content (Harden & Stamper 1999). In a spiral curriculum:

- there is iterative revisiting of topics throughout the course
- topics are revisited at numerous levels of difficulty
- new learning is related to previous learning
- the competence of students increases with each visit to a topic.

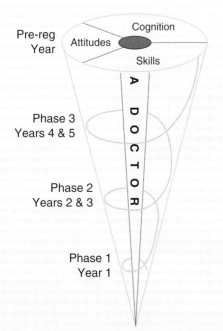

Fig. 2.3 A spiral curriculum

Deciding the educational strategy

Much discussion and controversy in medical education has related to education strategies. Should the curriculum be integrated or discipline-based? What is the role of problem-based learning? How much of the curriculum should be based in the community? The SPICES model for curriculum planning (Fig. 2.4) offers a useful tool to consider these strategies (Harden et al 1984). The model:

- represents each strategy as a continuum, thus avoiding the polarising of opinion
- acknowledges that schools vary in their approach to different strategies
- is useful in planning a new curriculum and in evaluating and changing an existing one.

Student-centred learning

In student-centred learning, what matters is what the student learns rather than what is taught. Students are given more responsibility for their own education. This is discussed further in chapter 15, Independent learning.

Problem-based learning (PBL)/task-based learning (TBL)

PBL is a seductive approach to medical education as described in chapter 16. Eleven steps can be recognised in the PBL continuum between information-orientated and task-based learning (Harden & Davis 1998).

In TBL the learning is focused round a series of tasks which the doctor may be expected to do (Harden et al 1996). Examples are the management of a patient with abdominal pain and the management of the unconscious patient. TBL is a useful approach to integration and PBL in clinical clerkships (Harden et al 2000).

Integration and interprofessional teaching

Integrated teaching is a feature of many curricula (General Medical Council 2002). It is discussed further in Chapter 17. Eleven steps on a continuum between discipline-based and integrated teaching have been described (Harden 2000a). There is also a move to interprofessional teaching where students look at a subject from the perspective of other professions as well as their own (Harden 1998).

Community-based

There are strong educational and logistical arguments for placing less emphasis on a hospital-based programme and more emphasis on the community as a context for student learning (Boaden & Bligh 1999). Many curricula are now community-orientated with students spending 10% or more of their time in the community.

Electives

Elective programmes are now firmly established and valued by staff and students in many medical schools. They have moved from being a fringe

Student-centred	—	Teacher-centred
Problem-based	—	Information-oriented
Integrated or interprofessional	—	Subject or discipline-based
Community-based	—	Hospital-based
Elective-driven	—	Uniform
Systematic	—	Opportunistic

Fig. 2.4 SPICES model of educational strategies

In planning a curriculum ask teachers to identify where they think they are at present on each continuum in the SPICES model and where they would like to go.

"TBL offers an attractive combination of pragmatism and idealism: pragmatism in the sense that learning with an explicit sense of purpose is seen as an important source of student motivation and satisfaction; idealism in that it is consonant with current theories of education"

Harden et al 1996

"The clinical and basic sciences should be taught in an integrated way throughout the curriculum"

General Medical Council 2002

"The community involves a potential broadening of perspective"

Boaden & Bligh 1999

"The elective is a traditional and much enjoyed part of most medical courses"

Bullimore 1998

Implementing an adaptive curriculum may not be as difficult as you think.

Think of the curriculum as a planned educational experience.

There is no holy grail of instructional wizardry which will provide a solution to all teaching problems. The teacher's toolkit should contain a variety of approaches, each with its strengths and weaknesses.

event to an important educational activity. They can be viewed as one type of student-selected component (SSC) of the curriculum. Electives and SSCs are designed to meet the needs of individual students.

A newer concept is the idea of the adaptive curriculum. This is an approach to curriculum planning where teaching and learning can be adjusted to the varying needs of individual students. Students spend different amounts of time studying a unit depending on their learning needs.

The features of an adaptive curriculum are:

- the learning outcomes are made explicit and the learning experiences are matched to the students' individual needs
- students' mastery of the core is assessed before the end of the course, and at a time when further study of the core can be arranged
- feedback is given to students and further studies are organised to meet the students' needs.

Systematic approach

Factors encouraging a move to a more systematic approach to medical education include:

- the increasing complexities of specialist medical practice
- the need to ensure that all students have had comparable learning experiences
- the move to outcome-based education where the learning experience and curriculum content are planned to correspond to the learning outcomes
- the concept of a core curriculum which includes the competences essential for medical practice.

A range of paper and electronic methods may be used to record encounters students have with patients. Such records are analysed to see if there are gaps or deficiencies in the students' experiences.

Deciding the teaching methods

There is no panacea, no magic answer to teaching. A good teacher is one who makes good use of a range of methods, applying each method for the use to which it is most appropriate. Later chapters of this book describe the tools available in the teacher's toolkit:

- The lecture and whole class teaching remain powerful tools if used properly. They need not be passive.
- Small-group work facilitates interaction between students and makes possible cooperative learning, with students learning from each other. Small-group work is usually an important part of problem-based learning.
- Independent learning can make an important contribution. Students master the area being studied, while at the same time they develop the ability to work on their own and to take responsibility for their own learning.

A significant development in recent years has been e-learning and the application of the new learning technologies (Harden 2000b). Computers may be used as a source of information, as a medium for presentation of interactive patient simulations, and as a method of facilitating and managing learning.

Teaching and learning experiences can be rated in terms of:

- authenticity, with theoretical approaches at one end of the spectrum and real-life ones at the other
- formality, with different levels of formality and informality.

Teaching situations can be located in each quadrant of the formality/authenticity grid (see Fig. 2.5).

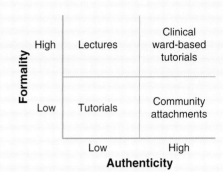

Fig. 2.5 Teaching situations

Preparing the assessment

Assessment is a key component of the curriculum. The significant effect that examinations have on student learning is well documented.

Issues that should be addressed in assessment include:

- What should be assessed?
  — The outcome model provides a useful framework.
- How should it be assessed?
  — Which methods should be used?
  — How can one determine whether students have achieved the appropriate level of competence?
- What are the aims of the assessment process?
  — To pass or fail the student, to grade the student, to provide the student and teacher with feedback or to motivate the student?
- When should students be assessed?
  — At the beginning of the course to assess what they already know or can do, during the course or at the end of the course?
- Who should assess the student?
  — The teacher, other teachers in the same institution, teachers from other institutions, a national board or the students themselves?

These issues are addressed in more detail in later chapters.

Communication about the curriculum

Failure in communication between teacher and student is a common problem in medical education (see Fig. 2.6). Teachers have the responsibility to ensure that students have a clear understanding of:

- what they should be learning – the learning outcomes
- the range of learning experiences and opportunities available
- how and when they can access these most efficiently and effectively
- how they can match the available learning experiences to their own needs
- whether they have mastered the topic or not, and if not, what further studies and experience are required.

"I believe that teaching without testing is like cooking without tasting"

Ian Lang, former Scottish Secretary

"Systems of assessment should be adapted to the new style curriculum, should encourage appropriate learning skills and should reduce emphasis on the uncritical acquisition of facts"

General Medical Council 1993

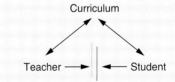

Fig. 2.6 Failure in communication

Failure to keep staff and students informed about the curriculum is a recipe for failure.

"The establishing of this climate is almost certainly the most important single task of the medical teacher"

Genn & Harden 1986

"The educational climate is the soul and spirit of the medical curriculum"

Genn 2001

The style of management must be designed to suit the institution within which it has to operate.

"Medical school deans should identify and designate an interdisciplinary and interdepartmental organisation of faculty members"

American Association of Medical Colleges 1984

Communication can be improved in a number of ways:

- the provision of clear curriculum documentation with learning outcomes, timetables and annotated lists of learning resources included
- the use of study guides as a method of communication with the student
- the development of a curriculum map which identifies the areas to be studied and relates these to the courses where they are most appropriately learned.

Promoting an appropriate educational environment

The educational environment or 'climate' is a key aspect of the curriculum. It is less tangible than the content studied, the teaching methods used or the examinations. It is none the less of equal importance. There is little point in developing a curriculum whose aim is to orientate the student to medicine in the community and to health promotion, if the students perceive that what is valued by the senior teachers is hospital practice, curative medicine and research. In the same way it is difficult to develop in students a spirit of teamwork and collaboration if the environment in the medical school is a competitive rather than a collaborative one.

Tools to assess this educational environment or climate in medicine have not been readily available (Genn & Harden 1986). Roff et al (1997) have described the Dundee Ready Education Environment Measure (DREEM) which can be used for this purpose.

Managing the curriculum

Curriculum management has become more important in the context of:

- increasing complexity of the curriculum
- integrated and interdisciplinary teaching
- increasing pressures on staff with regard to their clinical duties, teaching responsibilities and research commitments
- shortage of resources to support teaching
- rapid changes taking place in medical education and medical practice
- increasing demands for accountability.

In the context of undergraduate medical schools it is likely that:

- responsibilities and resources for teaching will be at a faculty rather than departmental level
- an undergraduate medical education committee will be responsible for planning and implementing the curriculum
- a teaching dean or director of undergraduate medical education will be appointed who has a commitment to curriculum development and implementation
- staff will be appointed with particular expertise in curriculum planning, teaching methods and assessment to support work on the curriculum

- time and contributions made by staff to teaching will be recognised
- a staff development programme will be a requirement for all staff
- an independent group will have responsibility for academic standards and quality assurance.

A number of approaches to curriculum development management can be recognised (Harden 1986a).

- The architect approach. The emphasis is on the plans with a clear statement of expected learning outcomes.
- The mechanic approach. The emphasis is on the teaching methods and educational strategies. There is more concern about how the curriculum is working rather than where it is going. The educational strategy may itself become the goal of the curriculum rather than a means to an end.
- The cookbook approach. Consideration is given to the details of the content and how much of each component or ingredient is included. The emphasis is on the individual components rather than on the overall curriculum where the whole should be greater than the sum of the parts.
- The railway timetable approach. The emphasis is on the timetable, what courses are held and when, and the duration of each course. This simplistic view of curriculum planning ignores many of the real challenges facing medical education.

A final word: don't expect to get the curriculum right first time. The curriculum will continue to evolve and will need to change in response to changes in medicine (see chapter 1, New horizons in medical education).

Summary

The development of a teaching programme can no longer be left to chance. A curriculum must be carefully planned. Ten questions have been identified which need to be addressed:

1. the need the training programme is intended to fulfil
2. the expected student learning outcomes
3. the content to be included
4. the organisation of the content including the sequence in which it is to be covered
5. the educational strategies to be adopted – integrated teaching is an example
6. the teaching methods to be used, including large-group teaching, small-group teaching and the use of e-learning and the other new learning technologies
7. assessment of the students' progress and of the teaching programme
8. communication about the curriculum to all the stakeholders including the students
9. the educational environment
10. management of the curriculum.

For the curriculum to be successful a mixture of approaches is required, with the emphasis varying at different times in the development of the curriculum.

"A little known fact is that the Apollo moon missions were on course less than 1% of the time. The mission was composed of almost constant mid-course corrections"

Belasco 1996

References

Association of American Medical Colleges 1984 Physicians for the 21st century: Report of the Project Panel on the General Professional Education of the Physicians and College Preparation for Medicine. Journal of Medical Education 59 Part 2:1–208

Belasco J A 1996 In: Simon J, Parker R A dictionary of business quotations. Hutchinson, London

Boaden N, Bligh J 1999 Community-based medical education: towards a shared agenda for learning. Oxford University Press, New York

Bullimore D W 1998 Study skills and tomorrow's doctors. Saunders, Edinburgh

Davidoff F 1996 Who has seen a blood sugar? Reflections on medical education. American College of Physicians, Philadelphia, Pennsylvania, p 46

Dunn W R, Hamilton D D, Harden R M 1985 Techniques of identifying competencies needed by doctors. Medical Teacher 7(1):15–25

General Medical Council 1993, 2002 Tomorrow's doctors: recommendations on undergraduate medical education. General Medical Council, London

Genn J M 2001 AMEE Medical Education Guide no. 23. Curriculum, environment, climate, quality and change in medical education – a unifying perspective. AMEE, Dundee

Genn J, Harden R M 1986 What is medical education here really like? Suggestions for action research studies of climates of medical education environments. Medical Teacher 8(2):111–124

Harden R M 1986a Approaches to curriculum planning. ASME Medical Education Booklet no 21. Medical Education 20:458–466

Harden R M 1986b Ten questions to ask when planning a course or curriculum. Medical Education 20:356–365

Harden R M 1998 Effective multi-professional education: a three-dimensional perspective. Medical Teacher 20(5):402–408

Harden R M 2000a The integration ladder: a tool for curriculum planning and evaluation. Medical Education 34:551–557

Harden R M 2000b Evolution or revolution and the future of medical education: replacing the oak tree. Medical Teacher 22(5):435–442

Harden R M, Davis M H 1998 The continuum of problem-based learning. Medical Teacher 20(4):301–306

Harden R M, Stamper N 1999 What is a spiral curriculum? Medical Teacher 21(2):141–143

Harden R M, Sowden S, Dunn W R 1984 Some educational strategies in curriculum development: the SPICES model. Medical Education 18:284–297

Harden R M, Laidlaw J M, Ker J S, Mitchell H E 1996 AMEE Medical Education Guide no. 7. Task-based learning: an educational strategy for undergraduate, postgraduate and continuing medical education, part 1 & 2. Medical Teacher 18(1):7–13 and 18(2):91–98

Harden R M, Crosby J R, Davis M H 1999 An introduction to outcome-based education. Medical Teacher 21(1):7–14

Harden R M, Crosby J R, Davis M H et al 2000 Task-based learning: the answer to integration and problem-based learning in the clinical years. Medical Education 34:391–397

Levine H G, Cordes D L, Moore Jr D E, Rennington F C 1984 In: Green J S, Grosswald S J, Suter E, Walthall D B (eds) Continuing education for the health professions. Jossey Bass, San Francisco

Roff S, McAleer S, Warden R M, Al Qahtani M et al 1997 Development and validation of the Dundee Ready Education Environment Measure (DREEM). Medical Teacher 19(4):295–299

Rubin P, Franchi-Christopher D 2002 New edition of tomorrow's doctors. Medical Teacher 24(4):268–269

Spady W G 1994 Outcome-based education: critical issues and answers. American Association of Schools Administrators, Arlington, Virginia

Chapter 3
The undergraduate curriculum

S. Leinster

Planning is an essential part of any good educational intervention. The overall plan of a whole programme is usually referred to as the curriculum. There is often confusion between the terms 'curriculum' and 'syllabus'. The syllabus refers to the content of the course whereas the curriculum encompasses learning methods, assessment methods, resources and timetabling in addition to content. Traditionally, much effort has gone into identifying the content and the learning methods have been assumed. As the awareness of different learning approaches has grown, the temptation has been to concentrate on learning methods to the relative detriment of content. Medical schools are labelled by their predominant teaching methods, for example as problem-based, systems-based, community based or traditional. However, medical education is a preparation for practice rather than a purely intellectual exercise and it is arguable that there must be a minimum essential content. If an effective curriculum is to be created, all areas must receive careful attention (Table 3.1).

Defining the content

Aims and objectives

Curriculum planning must begin with identifying the aims and objectives of the programme. There is a temptation to assume that there is a shared understanding of the aims of the programme but unless the meaning of

Table 3.1	The scope of curriculum planning
Content	What knowledge, skills and attitudes should the course cover? What are the learning outcomes of the course?
Delivery	How will the learning be delivered? What teaching or learning methods will be used?
Assessment	How will the students' learning be tested?
Structure	How will the content be organised? How will learning and teaching be scheduled?
Resources	What staff, learning materials, equipment and accommodation is needed?
Evaluation	How will the organisers know that the course has been effective in delivering the learning outcomes?

The curriculum needs to define the learning outcome, the setting in which it should be performed and the standard to which it should be performed.

The core curriculum should reflect the consensus views of specialists and generalists. Specialists should not be permitted to determine the core curriculum in their own discipline.

the aims is made explicit misunderstandings will arise. The terms that are employed must be defined and must be specific. It is unhelpful to have the stated aim of 'producing a good doctor'. This begs the question of how a good doctor is to be defined.

In the past there has been an assumption that being a good doctor meant having a large amount of knowledge. The assessment system tended to concentrate on the recall of facts and the student with the most recall was adjudged the best student. Clinical examinations took place but even in the clinical examination much of the judgement of performance was based on how much the student knew rather than what they were able to do. While there is a correlation between knowledge and clinical performance the two are not identical. It is now recognised that the ability to apply knowledge appropriately is the important measure. The emphasis should be on 'what can the student do?' rather than 'what does the student know?'

Core material

Development is an intrinsic part of medicine. Knowledge has grown rapidly in the last 50 years, new skills have become a routine part of practice and old skills have become redundant. By the end of the 1980s it had become obvious that medical undergraduate courses were overloaded with facts. In the first edition of *Tomorrow's Doctors* (GMC 1993) the General Medical Council recommended that the factual content of the course should be reduced. This was to be achieved by the identification of a core of knowledge, skills and attitudes that all students had to learn. This core, it was suggested, should occupy about two-thirds of the course with the balance being made up of student-selected studies. This raised the problem of how the core should be identified.

There are a number of possible solutions. Some specialties could be considered optional. There are problems with this as some common or important conditions may fall within the province of 'optional' specialties. The opposite approach is to ask each specialty to identify its own core material. This gives rise to practical problems as the core identified in this way is too large to fit into a standard undergraduate programme. An approach that has been adopted by a number of medical schools is the identification of index cases or presentations that are based on the different ways in which the population comes into contact with healthcare professionals. The core knowledge that students need within each discipline is determined by what they need to know in order to understand and manage these core clinical problems. The cases may be identified from published health statistics or may be based on consensus among experienced practitioners. The list may vary from school to school depending on the patterns of practice around that school but there is considerable overlap between the lists, suggesting that a realistic core is being identified (Bligh 1995, Mandin et al 1995, O'Neill 1999).

Learning outcomes

The core defines the scope of the curriculum. The next step is to define what it is that the student needs to learn about the core. The most effective way to do this is to define learning outcomes for the course. These clearly express what the student will be able to do at the end of the course. When an entire course of 4–6 years is being considered the outcomes will, necessarily, be very broad. As smaller and smaller components of the course are considered the outcomes become more and more focused and specific. The detailed outcomes for each component should map on to the overall outcomes (Simpson et al 2002).

Domains of learning

The Quality Assurance Agency recognises four domains in higher education in which outcomes should be defined: knowledge and understanding, generic skills, cognitive skills, and subject-specific skills (QAA 2004). In medical education a fifth domain is important, that of attitudes and professional development.

Within the knowledge and skills domains there is a hierarchy of outcomes which map on to the 'cognitive process' dimension in Bloom's revised taxonomy (Table 3.2; Krathwohl 2001). The attainment of each level assumes the attainment of the lower levels. The level which the students are expected to attain is specified by the descriptors used in the outcome. It is generally accepted that an adequate curriculum will be defined in terms of the higher levels of the taxonomy; there are few situations where remembering would be regarded as an adequate outcome.

Table 3.2 Cognitive processes in Bloom's revised taxonomy for knowledge and descriptors of outcome

Bloom's taxonomy	Meaning	Outcome descriptors
Remember	Retrieving relevant material from long-term memory	recognise, recall
Understand	Determining the meaning of instructional messages, including oral, written, and graphic communications	interpret, exemplify, classify, summarise, infer, compare, explain
Apply	Carrying out or using a procedure in a given situation	execute, implement
Analyse	Breaking material into its constituent parts and detecting how the parts relate to one another and to an overall structure or purpose	differentiate, organise, attribute
Evaluate	Making judgements based on criteria and standards	check, critique
Create	Putting elements together to form a novel, coherent whole or make an original product	generate, plan, produce

(Krathwohl 2001)

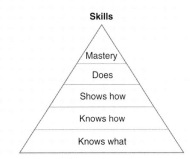

Fig. 3.1 Miller's skills triangle

The specificity of the learning outcome depends on the component of the course to which it applies. For the whole course, the learning outcome on prescription might be 'Write safe prescriptions for different types of drugs' (GMC 2003). For an individual teaching session on the control of pain in chronic musculoskeletal disease it might be 'Write a safe prescription for a common nonsteroidal anti-inflammatory drug in an elderly patient.'

The learning methods to be employed should be determined by the desired outcomes.

Although Bloom recognised the psychomotor domain in addition to the cognitive and affective domains, he did not produce a taxonomy for it. However, a similar grid can be produced that can be used to define the learning outcomes in relation to skills that the student must acquire. This grid is commonly expressed in the form of Miller's triangle (Fig. 3.1) with the outcome levels ranging from 'knows how' through to 'mastery'.

The curriculum planner must specify which skills are necessary and to what level each should be displayed.

Further elements of learning outcomes

So far, we have considered learning outcomes in terms of what the student can do. It is equally important to define the conditions in which the student can be expected to perform the task. Students qualifying from a medical school in the UK are required by law to start work in a closely supervised environment as preregistration house officers. It is reasonable to define some of their learning outcomes as the ability to perform the task under close supervision. However, some tasks (such as emergency resuscitation) require the doctor to act independently as they may be the first on the scene. The learning outcomes for resuscitation should specify that the student will perform competently without direct supervision. The conditions may also include the setting in which the student should be able to perform. The ability to manage a patient with a specific illness in a hospital ward may be different from the ability to manage the same condition in the community or presenting as an emergency in the Accident and Emergency Department.

A third element is the standard to which the student will fulfil the learning outcome. This is the most difficult part of setting learning outcomes and the area where there is the most controversy. *Tomorrow's Doctors* (GMC 2003) specifies learning outcomes such as 'Be able to perform clinical and practical skills safely'. There is still enormous scope for debate on how this should be interpreted.

In practical terms this decision is taken by defining the nature and standard of the assessments that are set.

Delivery of the curriculum

In parallel with determining the content of the curriculum, decisions must be taken about how it will be delivered. While there is debate over which learning methods are the most effective and efficient, there are some established principles that should be taken into account. It is clear that knowledge is applied most effectively when it is learnt in the context in which it is to be applied. It is also accepted that active learning is more effective than passive learning (Schmidt 1983). However, a wide range of learning methods can meet these conditions.

Both traditional lecture-based courses and courses based on small-group, problem-based learning produce effective medical practitioners (Schmidt et al 1996). The evidence for any difference in knowledge outcomes between traditional and problem-based courses is weak. However, there are differences in other outcomes (Albanese & Xakellis 2001,

O'Neill et al 2003). The choice of methods for a given curriculum will depend on the range of outcomes that have been chosen. It is important that the outcomes determine the methods and not the other way round. In general, the use of a mixture of methods is likely to be more efficient than a doctrinaire adherence to a single method.

Assessment

Whatever the stated aims and objectives of the course, the students' perceptions of what is important will be determined by what is assessed and how the assessment is carried out (Newble & Jaeger 1983). The assessment policy and the detailed methods should form an important part of the curriculum planning process. A good case can be made for beginning the planning process by planning the assessment before planning the teaching. Certainly, the assessment should not be an afterthought.

Outcomes are defined in terms of actions. It follows that an outcome is valid only if the action can be observed and therefore assessed. Although 'knowledge' and 'understanding' are major levels in Bloom's taxonomy, 'know' and 'understand' are not useful terms as outcomes. The outcome descriptors in Table 3.2 are much more useful as they define how the outcome could be tested. Thus knowledge can be tested by asking the student to recall something and understanding can be tested by asking the student to explain or compare something.

The outcomes relating to skills are measured against Miller's classification. While the highest level of outcome is 'mastery' the highest level that it is practicable to assess is 'showing how'. Some argue that examinations conducted using simulated patients are equivalent to 'doing' but they do not measure how the candidate behaves when not being observed. For undergraduate training this is probably adequate, but for postgraduate training and continuing education it is not. Evidence that an individual has attained mastery or even that he or she regularly 'does' the relevant skill can only be inferred indirectly from such things as clinical records and audits (see chapter 36, Work-based assessment).

Outcomes relating to attitudes are even more difficult to assess. The use of self-reporting questionnaires may be biased by students giving the 'correct' or 'expected' answer rather than revealing what they really feel. Observed behaviour can act as a surrogate for attitude. For this reason, attitudinal outcomes may be written in terms of observed behaviour

Curriculum structure

The organisation of students' learning is an important part of planning. Traditionally, teaching was organised according to disciplinary boundaries. There was usually a very marked divide between the subjects that were considered to be clinical and those that were preclinical. This made it very difficult to teach material in context and led to compartmentalisation of knowledge, as illustrated in (Fig. 3.2).

Both horizontal and vertical integration are needed.

Planning the assessment should be an integral part of planning the curriculum.

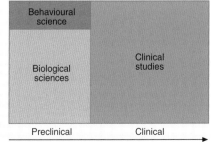

Fig. 3.2 The traditional curriculum

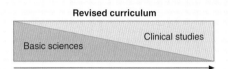

Fig. 3.3 The 'inverted triangles' curriculum model

Integrated curriculum

Professional development
Population sciences
Behavioural sciences
Biological sciences
Clinical studies
Clinical and communication skills

Fig. 3.4 The total integration model

The curriculum should have a logical and transparent structure.

Horizontal integration has been achieved by replacing discipline-based teaching with system-based teaching. The focus has been moved from subjects such as anatomy or physiology to body systems such as the cardiovascular system or the digestive system. All of the relevant basic science is taught at the same time. This can take place with a preclinical/clinical divide or can be combined with vertical integration.

Vertical integration implies that clinical methods and science are taught at the same time as the basic science. This may be organised on the basis of body systems or as a number of 'vertical themes' that run through all the years of the curriculum. Often these vertical themes are related to generic professional skills and attitudes that are pertinent to all areas of medical practice such as clinical or communication skills. The commonest form of vertical integration involves the early introduction of clinical contact in the course. As time goes on, the amount of clinical contact increases and the amount of basic science reduces. This has been described as an 'inverted triangles' curriculum (Fig. 3.3).

Some schools have gone further and have equal proportions of basic science and clinical contact throughout the course (Fig. 3.4).

Whatever the formal structure of the course, integration can only take place at the level of the students' experience of learning. Different approaches to achieving integration have been used with varying degrees of success. The most basic approach is to schedule within the same time frame lectures on the same system from the different disciplines. While this is relatively simple, any integration is largely a matter of chance. For integration to occur, the scope and content of the lectures must be coordinated by an overseeing committee. Attempts have been made to have totally integrated lectures delivered by two or more individuals from different disciplines. These can be very effective if sufficient effort is put into planning and preparation. They do not work if the teachers prepare independently and meet up only to deliver the session.

Case-based curricula attempt to overcome the problems of integration by focusing learning around a series of clinical cases. As the students develop an understanding of the range of material relevant to the case so they are led to integrate this knowledge for themselves.

Ordering

An important part of curriculum planning is determination of the order in which the learning outcomes will be delivered. There is no absolutely correct order but there should be a transparent logic behind the arrangement. This will enable students to appreciate the relevance of particular learning outcomes and diminish the tendency to learn inefficiently by rote just because the topic has been placed in the curriculum and will be assessed.

An effective structure will avoid needless duplication of material but will allow revisiting and reinforcement. Topics are first introduced at a simple level. Later in the course they will be studied in more depth and breadth. A common approach is to start with normality then move on to abnormality. Subjects may be revisited on several occasions. Harden and colleagues (1997) have described this as a 'spiral curriculum'. This spiral approach can take place within any of the previous models of curricular structure.

Resources

Curriculum planning must consider the resources needed to deliver the curriculum. A lecture-based curriculum will need lecture halls large enough to hold an entire class at one time. Laboratory-based practicals will need teaching laboratory space. A curriculum based on small-group work will need a sufficient number of tutorial rooms.

Clinical placements are often a major constraint on curriculum planning. The number of patients willing to participate in teaching and suitable for the purpose is limited and will inevitably affect the structure of the planned course.

The greatest resource constraint is associated with the teaching staff. PBL and other small-group teaching results in greater staff–student contact time and from this it has been deduced that this form of teaching must be more expensive. On the other hand, many forms of PBL do not use expert tutors and teaching staff can be deployed with greater efficiency as they are not restricted to delivering a comparatively few teaching sessions on their own discipline. Whatever the theoretical considerations, a number of medical schools have introduced PBL without any increase in resources.

Evaluation

Every educational endeavour should be evaluated. Designing the evaluation strategy is an important part of overall curriculum planning. The evaluation should cover outcome as well as process, although evaluation of the latter is easier to achieve. The process evaluation should encompass the views of the students, the teachers and the administrative staff, and should take place in such a way that rapid intervention and correction of faults can take place. Outcome evaluation is by necessity a much slower undertaking. There is likely to be a close relationship between the assessment process and the evaluation of outcomes. It is important that this linkage is prospective and incorporated in the overall design of the curriculum rather than being an afterthought.

The plans for evaluation should be made while the curriculum is being planned.

Finally – who should plan the curriculum?

The question of who should plan the curriculum can be a major source of conflict within a medical school. Traditionally, it has been assumed that subject specialists are the only people who can decide what should be taught within their discipline. As medical knowledge has developed, new disciplines have arisen to claim their place in the curriculum while the content of established disciplines has grown. This led to an overcrowding of the curriculum and the need for students to adopt superficial learning styles in order to cover the material within the time constraints of the course. Centralised curriculum planning can lead to the disengagement of most teachers who may feel that what they are being asked to teach conveys at best an inadequate, and at worst an inaccurate, picture of their discipline. It is important that the teachers who are to deliver the curriculum should feel that they have a stake in it. This is one reason why it is less than ideal to import a curriculum that has been developed elsewhere.

Consensus planning allows the wider community of teachers to be involved. A multidisciplinary group agrees on the content of the curriculum through a process of discussion and compromise. The level at which the content is pitched is more likely to be realistic as the specialists' views are immediately tested against those of their colleagues. The wider community of potential teachers should comment on the results of these discussions. The process of discussion and review should continue until a broad consensus is reached. It is particularly important that generalists should be included in the review process as they are best placed to assess the utility of the decisions.

At this stage it is helpful to have input from the public and from future employers. The roles of health professionals are undergoing rapid change and the competencies expected of a doctor in the future are unpredictable. Medicine exists to meet community needs for healthcare. Discussion with the community will inform the planning.

Summary

Planning is essential for the development of any successful curriculum. The first stage is to define the aims and objectives of the programme. The core content is then specified in terms of learning outcomes. Once the content is defined, the modes of delivery have to be decided. A mixture of methods is likely to be better than adherence on principle to a single approach. Assessment is a major component of the curriculum and the approach to assessment should be developed in parallel with the other aspects of the curriculum. A clear structure should be developed and the necessary resources identified. Finally, evaluation of the curriculum should be planned prospectively.

References

Albanese M A, Xakellis G C 2001 Building collegiality: the real value of problem-based learning Medical Education 35:1143

Bligh J 1995 Identifying the core curriculum: the Liverpool approach. Medical Teacher 17:383–390

General Medical Council 1993 Tomorrow's Doctors, 1st edn. General Medical Council, London

General Medical Council 2003 Tomorrow's Doctors, 2nd edn. General Medical Council, London

Harden R M, Davis M H, Crosby J R 1997 The new Dundee medical curriculum: a whole that is greater than the sum of its parts. Medical Education 31:264–271

Krathwohl D R 2001 In: Anderson L W, Krathwohl D R (eds) A taxonomy for teaching, learning and assessing: a revision of Bloom's taxonomy for educational objectives. Addison Wesley, New York

Mandin H, Harasym P, Eagle C, Watanabe M 1995 Developing a 'clinical presentation' curriculum at the University of Calgary. Academic Medicine 70:186–193

Newble D I, Jaeger K 1983 The effect of assessment and examinations on the learning of medical students. Medical Education 17:165–171

O'Neill P A 1999 The core content of the undergraduate curriculum in Manchester. Medical Education 33: 121–129

O'Neill P A, Jones A, Willis S C, McArdle P J. 2003 Does a new undergraduate curriculum based on *Tomorrow's Doctors* prepare house officers better for their first post? A qualitative study of the views of pre-registration house officers using critical incidents. Medical Education 37:1100–1108

Quality Assurance Agency for Higher Education 2004 http://www.qaa.ac.uk

Schmidt H G 1983 Problem-based learning: rationale and description. Medical Education 17:11–16

Schmidt H G, Machiels-Bongaerts M, Hermans H, ten Cate T J et al 1996 The development of diagnostic competence: comparison of a problem-based, an integrated and a conventional medical curriculum. Academic Medicine 71:658–664

Simpson J G, Furnace J, Crosby J, Cumming A D et al 2002 The Scottish Doctor – learning outcomes for the medical undergraduate in Scotland: a foundation for competent and reflective practitioners. Medical Education 24: 136–143

Chapter 4

The postgraduate curriculum

N. G. Patil

Setting the scene

Attending an international meeting of medical educators were: Dr Washington, a physician from the USA; Mr Darwin, a surgeon from the UK; Dr Ali, a paediatrician from Nigeria; Dr Yang, dean of a medical school in China, and Dr Guru, an obstetrician and gynaecologist from India. All were participating in a 'food for thought' luncheon discussion on the status of postgraduate medical education in their respective countries. Dr Washington and Mr Darwin highlighted their apprehension about the implications of reductions in working hours for the training of residents. Dr Ali and Dr Guru expressed concerns about the overwhelming clinical duties of residents, which hindered their structured educational training, as well as raising the issue of doctors leaving for further specialty training abroad.

Introduction

Postgraduate medical education has become an issue of global significance, appeal and dimensions. While postgraduate educational opportunities in western countries are much sought after by doctors in the rest of the world, many doctors from western nations are equally eager to gain clinical experience working outside their countries. There is also increasing internationalisation of the medical workforce following regional and international free trade agreements such as those implemented by the European Union (EU). The National Advice Centre for Postgraduate Medical Education (NACPME) at the British Council provides information to overseas-qualified doctors on postgraduate medical education and training in the United Kingdom.

In 2003, the World Federation for Medical Education (WFME) published a comprehensive document titled *Postgraduate medical education – WFME global standards for quality improvement*. This publication also provided a timely reminder that in formulating the postgraduate medical curriculum the needs of the country, as well as of the region and the available human and material resources, should be taken into account.

Fundamentals of postgraduate medical education

Postgraduate medical education is an important phase of medical education in which doctors go on to develop their competencies and capabilities following the completion of their basic medical qualification. This phase of training is usually conducted in accordance with specified regulations and rules. Similarly to an apprenticeship, trainee doctors are placed in various clinical settings under the guidance of senior and experienced colleagues such as consultants who take the responsibility for their instruction and supervision (WFME).

Postgraduate medical education initially involves a preregistration year which provides on-the-job training in a protected environment. The aim of this 12-month programme is to ensure that the trainees possess the necessary practical knowledge and skills essential for safe medical practice. Successful completion of this internship allows a graduate to register as a medical practitioner with the relevant medical council or board. Graduates are also entitled to enrol for general practice or family medicine training, specialist and sub- or superspecialist training or for other formalised training programmes for defined expert functions. These are organised by the universities, specialist boards, medical societies and colleges, or institutes for postgraduate medical education. This further training typically lasts for a period of 6 to 8 years.

Thus, as summarised in Figure 4.1, following achievement of a basic medical degree, postgraduate medical education involves an internship (usually 12 months) and basic and higher specialty training for 6–8 years.

Internationally, there are considerable variations in the number of recognised specialties and expert functions in medicine as well as in the organisation, structure, content and requirements of postgraduate medical education. For example, the Hong Kong Academy of Medicine, with its membership of 15 constituent professional colleges, offers postgraduate training in nearly 51 specialties in 2004 (Hong Kong Academy of Medicine). The common curricular approach of all member colleges, of course, centres around the recognised clinical or practical placements, expert supervision, theoretical teaching, research experience, systematic assessments and evaluation of the training programmes.

Career paths

Historically, clinical specialties were the preferred choice in postgraduate medical education of almost all medical graduates. This trend continues to the present day. However, there is a growing interest in postgraduate courses and degrees in specialties such as health administration and medical education and research. The recognition of talent in these areas has been taken seriously and has been consciously addressed by postgraduate medical institutions around the world.

Clinical streams

The two main clinical streams are general practice or family medicine and the hospital–based specialties. The latter may be subcategorised as medical (e.g. general medicine, paediatrics, psychiatry, geriatrics), surgical (e.g. general surgery, orthopaedics, obstetrics and gynaecology) or laboratory-based (e.g. general pathology, microbiology, haematology).

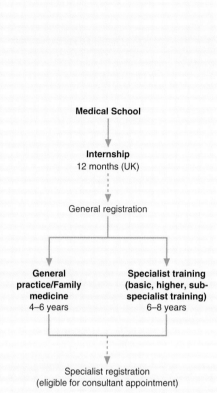

Fig. 4.1

"The role of the GP is changing, but, will remain central to the delivery of patient care in the UK"

Field S 2002

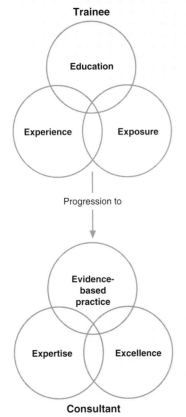

Fig. 4.2

With its emphasis on preventative medicine and primary care, structured training in general practice/family medicine is that of a major specialty with a defined exit outcome and recognized qualifications on par with those of hospital-based careers.

As mentioned, hospital-based postgraduate specialties are primarily divided into medical or surgical streams. However, with the advent of integration, superspecialization and the use of interventional procedures by physicians and clinical radiologists, such divisions are increasingly blurred in terms of teaching and training of practical skills.

Postgraduate medical 'trainees' are usually known as residents, specialist registrars, junior doctors or medical officers. 'Trainers' are recognized as consultants, specialists, senior doctors or supervisors. Most colleges around the world assign an approved or nominated trainer as the educational supervisor for each trainee.

Characteristics of postgraduate education

As shown in Figure 4.2, postgraduate medical training may be summarised as 'education, exposure and experience' leading to 'expertise, evidence-based practice and excellence'.

Postgraduate medicine is a high-stake education and practice. The ultimate goal in postgraduate medical education has to be that the trainees will, progressively, receive the appropriate clinical exposure to gain the necessary experience required in achieving expertise that allows them to provide a high standard of care in their respective fields. Another chief aim of postgraduate medical education is that the trainee eventually becomes the trainer and goes on to participate in the training of their juniors and medical students. The principles of adult learning and the process of structured educational training are both vital in postgraduate medical education with respect to the development of clinical and practical skills. In specialties related to surgery, acquisition of practical or operative skills requires additional attention (Patil et al 2003).

Process of learning

Components of postgraduate medical training include:

- 'see', 'do' and 'learn to teach'
- apprenticeship
- structured educational activities, such as tutorials, journal clubs, clinicopathological conferences (CPCs) etc.
- practice workshops and skills development courses, at basic and advanced levels
- teaching medical and nursing students
- e-learning using online resources.

The time-honoured dictum of 'See, do and teach' is still essential to the acquisition of clinical and practical skills. With advances in simulations, virtual reality and multimedia technology, this principle has now been extended to skills development centres and laboratory-based train-

The use of simulators, multimedia technology and practice-tip workshops is like 'neo-adjuvant' therapy for mastering basic and advanced clinical and practical skills.

ing, where clinical and practical skills are sharpened through repeated practice in a non-threatening atmosphere.

Nuts and bolts of the postgraduate curriculum

Features of a postgraduate training include the following:

- a progressive syllabus that has both formal and informal elements
- a recognized trainer and training unit
- proactive supervision
- balance of clinical duties and educational activities
- protected time for education
- defined exit outcomes.

There has been a marked improvement in provision by the relevant bodies of structured syllabi for most postgraduate medical diploma or degree courses. This is in stark contrast to the days when the syllabus was a 'sea of uncertainty', and trainees felt that the sky was the limit when preparing for their examinations. Nowadays, the various authorities publish, both on their websites and as booklets, clear guidelines on core curriculum and assessment criteria for particular postgraduate specialties (Academy of Medical Royal Colleges, Royal College of Physicians and Surgeons of Canada).

Clinical attachments, also known as residencies in the USA or as specialist registrarships in the UK, and other postgraduate training programmes provide trainees with a comprehensive exposure to all areas of clinical practice. Trainees also actively participate in the teaching of medical students and junior colleagues. This contributes significantly to the enhancement of their clinical maturity.

Clinical training lasts for 6 to 8 years with rotations to a different discipline every 4–6 months. This usually suffices to meet the stipulations of individual colleges with regard to adequate exposure and experience in particular disciplines. The training is further divided into basic and higher specialty training attachments. In most programmes a segment of training, in continuity with clinical attachments or as a dedicated rotation, is devoted to research.

Protected time, to attend structured educational activities such as X-ray meetings or workshops and for individual study, is regarded as mandatory for all trainees. In practice, however, protected time for educational activities may be encroached upon by clinical commitments unless conscientious efforts are made by trainers and departments to make such time truly protected.

Consolidation of core competencies and capabilities

The roles shown in Figure 4.3 demand skills in these areas:

- history taking and consultation
- clinical practice

Conscientious efforts must be made by trainers and departments to make 'protected time' truly protected.

Specific objectives of training

- Medical expert/Clinical decision-maker
- Communicator
- Collaborator
- Manager
- Health advocate
- Scholar
- Professional

Fig. 4.3 Postgraduate training prepares for a variety of roles (Royal College of Physicians and Surgeons of Canada)

- management planning
- decision making and judgement
- communication and informed consent
- team performance
- technical
- critical care
- teaching medical and nursing students and junior colleagues
- professional behaviour
- ethical practice
- education of patients and their families.

Competence is defined as 'the state of being sufficiently capable and properly qualified to do something to a level that is acceptable', and incompetence as the 'lack of ability or skill to do something successfully or as it should be done'.

Undergraduate medical education lays the foundation for core clinical and communication competencies. The enrichment of attributes such as compassion, a caring attitude, effective communication, the ability to think and work under stress, transparency and honesty, and good clinical decision-making skills is achieved through daily clinical practice as part and parcel of patient management. Traditionally, the standard of competence that a specialist aims for is the ability to practise independently as a consultant. The measure of that competence, in general, is assessed on the clinical outcome of his or her patients.

Formative assessment

This is provided in a variety of ways, including:

- presentations at ward rounds and grand rounds
- journal reviews
- performance at practical or surgical procedures
- audit of morbidity and mortality
- review of patient charts
- mock examinations.

In the postgraduate curriculum, formative assessment to assist trainees in monitoring their progress is not structured or appreciated as it is in undergraduate medical education. This is mainly because postgraduates are believed to be mature learners who do not need such close scrutiny. In addition, consultants may consider this commitment as an extra burden in their supervisory roles (Fig. 4.4).

The provision of commentary on the trainee's performance at journal reviews, ward rounds, morbidity and mortality meetings and procedure-related activities is a very useful practical measure. One structured approach that can be used to assess the trainee, the supervisor and the teaching quality of the unit or department is to hold in-house 'mock examinations'; here the strengths and weaknesses of the clinical experience as well as the effectiveness of the educational programme are identified and discussed in a nonthreatening manner. These mock exam-

"Competence – that is, what the doctor knows or is able to do in terms of knowledge, skills, and attitudes.
Capable – that is, able to adapt to change, generate new knowledge, and continue to improve their performance"

Fraser & Greenhalgh 2001

"Compassion, Communication, Care and Competence are essential ingredients of successful clinical practice"

Anonymous

In-house 'mock examinations' are useful for evaluating the effectiveness of the training programme in individual departments or units.

inations also help candidates to prepare for their summative examinations.

Effective modalities for formative assessment of trainees include the Objective Structured Assessment of Technical Skills (OSATS) developed at the University of Toronto (see Performance assessment, chapter 35). This evaluation makes use of an operation-specific checklist involving direct observation of trainees performing various structured tasks. Another useful tool is the Imperial College Surgical Assessment Device (ICSAD), which utilises computer-based assessment techniques to track the number of movements and the total time taken for a trainee to complete a set task (Patil et al 2003).

Interaction between trainer and trainee

The quality of consultant supervision is the single most important factor in determining whether a trainee is satisfied with his/her training post. There are various opportunities for interaction between trainer and trained:

- orientation of trainee prior to commencing the rotation
- interactive clinical supervision
- formative logbook review
- trainee and supervisor consultative meetings at regular intervals
- career counselling
- mentoring.

To ensure a rewarding experience for all parties involved, it is important to ensure that quality standards are consistently met and that individual concerns are satisfactorily addressed (Paice & Ginsburg 2003).

The training logbook that is kept by all trainees constitutes a record of all their training postings, work experience, training activities with clinical supervisors, structured educational programmes attended, certified checklists of knowledge and skills, learning portfolio and other educational activities. The logbook should be reviewed by the appropriate clinical supervisors and mentors on a regular basis. Feedback on the interaction between the trainee and clinical supervisor should also be recorded in the training logbook.

Summative examinations

Postgraduate examinations are conducted by professional bodies such as colleges (e.g. for the Royal Colleges of various specialties in the UK, Australia, New Zealand, Canada and Thailand) or boards (e.g. the specialty boards in the USA), or by universities (e.g. in India, Malaysia and Papua New Guinea), following completion of the stipulated period of clinical experience and training. The award of diploma or degree is usually in the form of a fellowship (e.g. Fellowship of the Royal College of Physicians and Surgeons of Canada), a membership (e.g. Membership of the Royal College of Obstetricians and Gynaecologists), or a master's degree (e.g. Master of Medicine as in Singapore and Sudan, or Master of Surgery as in India).

"Consultant supervision is the single most important factor in determining whether a trainee is satisfied with a training post"

Paice & Ginsburg 2003

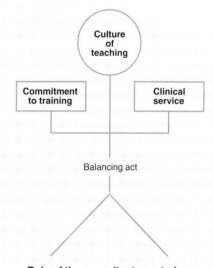

Role of the consultant as a trainer

Fig. 4.4 The role of the consultant as trainer

Examination format

Examinations are of four types:

- Written tests: multiple-choice questions (MCQs), extended matching questions (EMQs), short-answer questions (SAQs) and essays
- vivas
- clinical examinations: short cases, long cases, objective structured clinical examinations (OSCEs)
- logbook evaluation.

Most written tests are now conducted in the form of MCQs and SAQs (see Written assessments, chapter 34). Traditional long essay questions are gradually being reduced or phased out altogether. The majority of examining bodies complement written tests with an oral examination (viva voce) on topics related to applied basic sciences, critical care, evidence-based practice and the logbook (see Work-based assessment, chapter 36).

As for clinical examinations, there is a welcome trend in all specialties to structure these in the format of an objective assessment of the clinical, communication, practical management and procedural skills of each candidate. This is achieved by conducting the examination in an OSCE setting or in a real clinical environment (e.g. wards, ambulatory care units, intensive care units etc) guided by the provision of a check list of items to be tested (see Performance assessment, chapter 35).

Special considerations in training

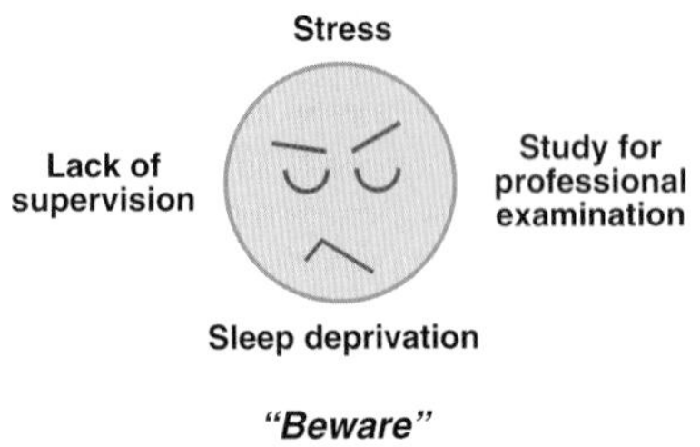

Trainees may be adversely affected by:

- stress
- sleep deprivation
- new environment, disease pattern, language and culture
- preparation for professional examinations
- working hours (Fig. 4.5).

Supervisors need to proactively consider the early recognition of matters that may affect the trainee's performance and the implementation of timely practical solutions to deal with them. Most colleges now offer 'training of the trainers' programmes which address issues related to the special needs of trainees in addition to their educational requirements.

Monitoring and evaluation of training programmes

The requirement for transparency in how specialist competency is evaluated and maintained at an acceptable level has heightened the need for a formal structure to monitor training activities. This monitoring may be undertaken at a global level by colleges, boards, and universities, at a regional level by departments or units or by individuals.

The authority to monitor and evaluate postgraduate medical education programmes usually rests with colleges, boards and universities who in

Fig. 4.5

Stress

Lack of supervision

Study for professional examination

Sleep deprivation

"Beware"

turn must convince the registration authorities that these specialists are 'fit for purpose', that is, they can provide a standard of care of appropriate quality.

The formal structure of the evaluation process operates at various levels, from the educational committees of the colleges to regional directors (e.g. postgraduate deans), to individual specialty programme directors, and nominated college tutors of units or departments. Any deficiency in the implementation of the monitoring procedures or in the performance of supervisors usually results in a warning followed by the withdrawal of recognition from the training unit, the supervisor or both, if no improvement is seen within a stipulated timeframe.

Exit outcomes

For postgraduate training, these include:

- progression to independent responsibility
- recognised postgraduate degree
- Certificate of Completion of Specialist Training (CCST)
- registration as a specialist
- eligibility for appointment as a consultant.

In the UK, the CCST is awarded to those trainees who have satisfactorily completed the designated period of training (6–8 years), have satisfactory appraisals at the end of each year, and who have passed the specialty examination of the appropriate college. The trainee is then recommended by the Specialist Training Authority (soon to be superseded by the Postgraduate Medical Education and Training Board) to the General Medical Council (GMC) for inclusion on its specialist register. Successful registrants are regarded as fully trained and are eligible to apply for a consultant post in the National Health Service (NHS).

Curriculum reforms in the United Kingdom

To bring the British system of specialist training in line with European medical directives, the Calman reforms recommended combining the registrar and senior registrar grades into a unified specialist registrar grade and defining the curriculum and minimum training period for each specialty.

These new arrangements have increased the emphasis on structured teaching and supervised learning and lessened the focus on experiential apprenticeship. Training posts are linked to rotations that deliver a defined curriculum for each specialty. At the beginning of each post, trainees and their supervising consultants have to discuss and agree upon the educational objectives to be achieved. Regular appraisals are mandatory and the supervising consultant must provide feedback on the trainee's progress.

Before the Calman reforms trainees were expected to organise their own training programmes. After the introduction of the reforms the control and responsibility for the organisation of training shifted to the regional committees and advisers.

In specialties such as surgery there is considerable concern that the shortened training period combined with a reduction in working hours does not adequately prepare trainees to fulfil their future role as a consultant. For this reason some form of semi-formal mentoring for newly appointed consultants by senior and more experienced clinicians is under consideration.

Collaborative curricula

Some countries have successfully implemented joint curricula based on similar guidelines and examination procedures. For example, colleges in Hong Kong and the UK regularly hold conjoint fellowship examinations and successful graduates are awarded conjoint fellowship diplomas.

Global initiatives

The issue of mutual recognition of postgraduate programmes for 'registration to practise' across countries is beyond the remit of medical educators because of varying local standards and regional sociopolitical considerations. Steps in the right direction, however, have been taken by organisations such as the World Federation of Medical Education (WFME), which will undoubtedly help to achieve global uniformity and standards in postgraduate medical education.

Education programmes that are gaining prominence in hospital-based postgraduate medical education include: telemedicine or telehealth training aiming to enhance the delivery of healthcare to rural and remote areas; preventative medicine and public health; and cost-effectiveness and cost containment in secondary, tertiary and quaternary services.

"Mrs Smith, if you really wish to have a second opinion, please come back and see me again tomorrow afternoon"

Solo consultant in a remote area

Summary

The journey that lies ahead for new medical graduates who wish to pursue specialty postgraduate training, and for the trainers who have to deliver it successfully, is filled with challenges. The need for reforms in areas including the postgraduate curriculum, the role of trainers, interactive supervision and evidence-based postgraduate medical education has been recognised. The time-honoured saying 'doctor knows best', rephrased today as 'doctor knows best – so does the patient!', is relevant to modern postgraduate medical education.

References

Academy of Medical Royal Colleges www.aomrc.org.uk
Field S 2002 Online. Available: www.rcgp.org.uk/education/presentations
Fraser S W, Greenhalgh T 2001 Coping with complexity: educating for capability. BMJ 323:799–803

Hong Kong Academy of Medicine www.hkam.org.hk
NACPME (National Advice Centre for Postgraduate Medical Education) Online. Available: www.british council.org/governance-health-nacpme.htm
Paice E, Ginsburg R. 2003 Specialist registrar training: what still needs to be improved? Hospital Medicine 64:173–175

Patil NG, Cheng SW, Wong J. 2003 Surgical competence. World Journal of Surgery 27:943–947

Royal College of Physicians and Surgeons of Canada http://rcpsc.medical.org/residency/index.php

WFME (World Federation for Medical Education Online. Available: www.sund.ku.dk/WFME/Activities/ WFME%20Postgraduate.pdf

Chapter 5
Effective continuing professional development

D. Davis, J. Goldman, L. Perrier

Introduction

Consider the two scenarios presented below.

Scenario 1. You have been invited to make a presentation on the broad topic of cardiology at the University of Toronto's 'Saturday at the University' – a large, primary care refresher course run by the University for nearly two decades. In this very popular, lecture-based programme, you have two hours to lecture to over 350 participants. The title of your lecture is 'An Update on Heart Disease: What the Generalist Needs to Know'. You ask the course organiser, 'how can I make this more interesting and informative? How can I possibly fill two hours?'

Scenario 2. You are the coordinator of your hospital's rounds series. You, your department chief, and the hospital's chief executive officer note that rounds attendance has declined in recent years. Even visiting professors' presentations have disappointingly small participation. When you ask your colleagues why this is the case, they claim practice busy-ness, overbooked surgical suites and offices, and other competing interests. You have a feeling that improving rounds, perhaps by improving the quality of the sessions, might be an answer; however you are unsure how to proceed.

These are not uncommon scenarios; many physician-teachers and course organisers are confronted with the challenge of making presentations to colleagues, to other health professional audiences, even to the public and, where there is an element of reflection, have a strong desire to improve this 'product', to make it more effective. From a personal perspective, doing a 'good job' brings the satisfaction of having accomplished a task well. There is however another perspective, sizably different from the case in undergraduate teaching or residency training. Like the work of clinicians themselves, teaching by well-prepared faculty members and speakers (and the effective educational intervention) can bring about practice change and even affect healthcare outcomes (Davis et al 1995) on a more immediate and possibly rewarding basis than undergraduate teaching and residency training. Further, while the steps to improving continuing professional development (CPD) delivery are important, even self-evident in any teaching exercise, they assume far greater importance in the realm of practice. Here, one is engaged in a process of communication with peers – colleagues with their own practice needs, styles and requirements, and, moreover, their own areas of expertise.

This chapter outlines a four-step process to making CPD more effective for the teacher (scenario 1) and the programme provider or organiser (scenario 2). They are captured here as 'knowing' steps:

- know the audience
- know the topic
- know the format
- know the outcome.

Know the audience

It is a truism in CPD that one needs to know one's learners or students: 'Who's the target audience?' is a favourite planning phrase of adult educators. The answer is not so simple, and, apart from needs assessment (the second step in this process) knowing the audience may be the most important step in the process of providing CPD.

Take the first scenario above. In the Canadian context, 'primary care clinicians' can imply many types of practitioners, from semi-autonomous nurse practitioners to independent, self-regulating physicians who may be general practitioners (neither trained in family medicine nor certified by the national body) or family physicians, often with two or more years of specialty training in this complex discipline. In the United States, primary care is more eclectic in its mix; paediatricians, obstetricians, general internists, physician assistants, nurse-practitioners and family physicians (general practitioners) may comprise the audience. As increasing emphasis is placed on interprofessional practice, and with growing recognition of the importance of 'the team', the audience may comprise teams of clinicians, for example professionals engaged in burn care (plastic surgeons, physiatrists, nurses, physical therapists, psychiatrists, etc).

Other audience attributes that may be relevant are methods of payment and types or settings of practice since these affect learners' abilities to maintain or deliver practice competencies. In the second scenario, declining rounds attendance may imply a strict fee-for-service environment, a frequent occurrence in the North American setting, in which time away from practice settings is not reimbursed. In some instances physicians may receive incentives for attending CPD activities. For example, practices enrolled in the Practice Incentives Program in Australia may receive payment for participating in Quality Prescribing Initiative activities (ie. clinical audits, case studies, practice visits) (Health Insurance Commission), and The Continuing Medical Education Program for Rural and Isolated Physicians in Ontario provides financial support for continuing medical education (CME) activities to eligible physicians (Ontario Medical Association).

Fortunately, there are countervailing forces in the form of professional and regulatory guidelines that may compel physicians to attend such

For effective CPD the teacher should:
- Know the audience
- Know the topic
- Know the format
- Know the outcome.

Like clinical practice itself, the well-prepared teacher (and the effective educational intervention) in the CPD environment can bring about practice change and even affect healthcare outcomes (Davis et al 1995) on an immediate and rewarding basis.

'Know the audience' means, among other things, knowing the discipline, training, practice environment and the continuing education or CPD requirements of the physician–learner involved in the event.

Examples of subjective needs assessment tools:
Practice reflection
Diaries or learning/questions logs
Questionnaires
Focus groups
Informal comments.

events. These guidelines suggest a minimum number of hours of formal continuing education or CPD for a wide variety of physician groups. It is useful to know what these are for each jurisdiction and, where possible, to tailor interventions to meet them. For example, in the case of the Royal College of Physicians and Surgeons of Canada, additional CPD 'points' may be gained by asking physicians to perform pre-workshop chart audits, post-lecture structured reading and reflection exercises or personal learning projects resulting from participation in a CPD activity (Royal College of Physicians and Surgeons of Canada).

Know the topic

The consulting cardiologist in scenario 1 might believe, quite correctly, that he or she knows the subject area to be addressed; why else would he or she receive the invitation to make the presentation? Why should the topic of needs assessment even be raised? The answer here however is not about knowledge of the subject area, but knowledge about how to tailor the information to meet needs and expectations at two levels: the practice needs expressed by the learner and the needs of patients or populations. As will be made clear below, this twofold theme reflects and builds on that of a subjective/objective dilemma. This section presents tools, useful in both scenarios, in which CPD providers/teachers can determine the needs of their audiences and their patient populations.

Learning and change in the lives of physicians – a subjective view

Subjective needs are those needs that are identified and expressed by the learner. These needs are based on the learners' abilities to reflect and examine their own knowledge and practices. Examples of subjective needs assessment tools are shown in the Tip opposite.

Subjective needs assessments provide insight into physicians' priority learning areas for which they might be motivated to acquire additional knowledge. On the other hand, although self-assessment may seem straightforward, it has proven more difficult than anticipated (Norman et al 2004), and has been criticised for the neglected aspects of 'self-reporting' (Lockyer 1998).

The work of Fox and his colleagues is enlightening (and possibly humbling) to the CPD provider as it reveals the multiple factors that affect practice changes and the diverse types of practice changes (Fox et al 1989). In this qualitative study, over 300 North American physicians were asked 'What did you change last in your practice? What caused that change? How did you acquire your learning in order to make that change?' Answers to each of these questions may help the CPD provider, whether teacher or organiser, prepare for this audience. First, physicians undertaking any change disclosed that they had an image of what that change was going to look like, for example a surgeon envisaging acquiring a laparoscopic technique. Second, the forces for change were widespread: while some drew from educational and CPD experiences, many more were intrapersonal (e.g. a recent personal experience) or from changing demographics (e.g. ageing or changing populations and patient demands). Third, the changes varied from smaller 'adjustments' or accommodations (e.g. adding a new drug to a therapeutic armamentarium within a class of drugs already known and prescribed) to much larger changes characterised as 'redirections' (e.g., adopting an entirely new way or method of practice). Here, smaller changes might be accomplished with a brief CPD presentation, even a didactic lecture; however, larger changes require a much richer CPD experience, perhaps encompassing a lecture, a highly interactive session such as a hands-on workshop, and possibly refresher or practical experience in the work setting.

The practice gap – the objective view

Objective needs are practice gaps or areas in which we recognise that clinical evidence has not been readily translated into practice. Examples of practice gaps are not difficult to find. For example, despite clear evidence that ACE inhibitors are highly useful in congestive heart failure, nearly one-third of patients do not receive them following hospitalisation (Antonelli et al, 2002, Weil & Tu 2001). Examples of objective needs assessment tools are presented in the Tip.

Each needs assessment strategy enables the collection of different types of information, and has an extensive body of literature on methods and effectiveness. The purpose of the needs assessment should determine the strategies used; a combined approach provides a more comprehensive understanding of the situation (Grant 2002).

Thus the creation of an effective CPD intervention presents, rather than a simple and straightforward process, a tricky minefield. To optimise learning, improve retention of new knowledge and effect practice change, the truly effective CPD provider must weave a path through the learners' trainings and settings, learning styles and experiences, and practice and performance gaps.

Know the format

It is useful to think of the format or educational process in CPD less as a lecture or presentation and more as an intervention. In this manner one broadens the scope of the educational encounter and makes the provider/teacher think more creatively about ways in which he/she can effect performance change in the learner and improve practice outcomes. Green's PRECEED model (Green et al 1980), which incorporates elements that are characterised as predisposing, enabling and reinforcing, helps with this conceptualisation. This chapter has already dealt with much of the preparatory work for the CPD intervention. This section will deal with two key concepts: making the presentation (rounds, lecture, refresher programme, update, or other conference) as effective as possible and enabling the transfer of information back into the practice setting.

Enabling learning: the CPD intervention

Many years ago Miller (1967) described the classical learning experience as 'rows of lecture desks, laden with pitchers of water', with a speaker at

Examples of objective needs assessment tools:
Chart audits
Peer review
Standardised patients to rate task performance
Observation of physician practices
Government publications
Health services reports
Research literature.

"Formal needs assessment can identify only a narrow range of needs and might miss needs not looked for, so breadth and flexibility of needs assessment methods should be embraced"

(Grant 2002)

the front communicating in a one-way manner. Although research regarding formal CPD methods (Davis et al 1999) has moved us forward somewhat, there are still many gaps in the practice of effective CME/CPD. While there are many elements to the theories of adult education (Knowles et al 1998), two key concepts, derived from Steinert & Snell (1999), stand out as crucial to the provision of effective CPD: engagement in the learning experience and relevance to the practice setting or needs of the learner. Interactivity and relevance can be increased by improving lecture delivery methods and by providing case-based material.

Increasing interactivity

Interactivity with one's experiences and setting

Schon (1990) has eloquently written about reflection-in-action as a key element in learning. The effective lecture may begin with or include a suggestion to think about the last case with diabetes that was difficult to manage, the earliest onset of Alzheimer's disease seen by the clinician-learner, or the case that caused the most ethically difficult decision making. One strategy is to ask participants to write down a case, or three questions they have, before the presentation.

Interactivity with learning materials

Handout material is often prized by learners as take-away reminders of lecture notes, slides, references, and management tips. Often however, the lecturer does not use the material during the presentation. This is a deficit which might easily be corrected, for example by providing a multiple choice or similar quiz to be completed before, after or during a lecture, or by developing a small paper case with prompts for diagnosis or management or with blank spaces left for the participant to fill in, for example with points of history, new-start insulin orders, or other clinically relevant material.

Interactivity with the speaker/presenter

The most frequently used and easiest way in which to improve interactivity with the lecturer is the question and answer (Q&A) session. Our first scenario is a real one. 'Saturday at the University' planners found that a large, two hour block of lecture time could be effectively broken up into sequential ten-minute periods of lecture and Q&A (De Buda & Woolf 1990). Other Q&A methods include the audience response system (Miller et al 2003), a computerised vote-counting and rather sophisticated device that polls the audience for responses to projected multiple choice questions and allows the speaker to have an instantaneous read on the uptake of his or her presentation. A somewhat less sophisticated system is one in which participants are given colour-coded cards and asked to hold one up to correspond to a particular answer. This method, while not affording the anonymity of the computerised system, is often deemed just as effective by presenters and as enjoyable by participants. The Tip opposite includes some methods for interactivity with the speaker/presenter.

Saying 'think about a case', may be made a little more powerful by providing time in the lecture to do so.

Methods for interactivity with the speaker or presenter:
Debates
Panels
Written questions
Mandatory question periods.

Interactivity with other learners

The notion of interactivity between learners has been advocated for decades by our adult education colleagues and is the goal of much faculty development activity (Hewson 2000). This type of interactivity builds on the ideas of reflection articulated above and addresses the principles of Knowles and colleagues (1998) and others (Fox et al 1989) about the intelligence and experience of the audience and the notion of translating knowledge into useful practical or tacit intelligence. Based on a relatively large literature (Silver & Rath 2002, Steinert & Snell 1999, Thomson et al 2004a), a brief outline of some methods for promoting interactivity between learners follows:

- *'Buzz groups'* Described by the noise they make in a normally quiet conference or meeting, such methods allow participants to engage neighbouring audience members in conversation about a case presentation, possible diagnoses, personal experiences, etc.
- *'Think-pair-share'* Here the idea builds on practice reflection (a quiet moment for participants to think of a particular case, for example), to discuss it with a neighbouring audience member, then to share it with the larger audience.
- *'Pyramiding' (or 'snowballing')* Here one builds from pairs of participants, to slightly bigger groups of four or six, finally involving the entire audience in a case discussion or similar exercise.
- *'Stand up and be counted'* An interesting device meant to capture diverse viewpoints, this method provides a simple statement such as 'HRT for women over 60 years of age is never indicated'. Placed across one dimension of the lecture hall are the five points often seen in questionnaire design: 'strongly agree–agree–neutral–disagree–strongly disagree', and audience members are asked to position themselves under one of these points. The moderator then moves from group to group (often starting with the 'strongly' groups to determine their perspectives) to explore the reasons for their position, articulating the key concepts for discussion along the way.

Increasing relevance: the clinical scenario

The addition of patient scenarios or vignettes that reflect actual clinical cases, frequently modified to protect patient privacy and to exemplify details of history, diagnosis or management, may enhance the relevance of CPD by promoting reflection and interaction. The Tip opposite provides methods for adding case-based material to presentations.

'Standardised patients', about whom much has been written from the perspectives of teaching undergraduates and residents and assessing competence, are relatively less common in the CPD setting, but are of potential value (Craig 1991, Davis et al 1997, Kantrowitz 1991) (see chapter 8, Clinical skills centre teaching). More ubiquitous and less expensive, the written case is relatively simple to construct, and may be distributed before or during a lecture or presentation to stimulate discussion and problem solving, or can be used as a part of a slide presentation.

Ways to add case-based material to presentations:
Video/audio presentations
Standardised patients, families
Live operating-room links
Real patients
Case materials, e.g., X-rays, ECGs.

"Knowledge is a necessary but not sufficient condition for performance change to occur"

Anonymous

"Knowledge translation involves a complex set of interactions between producers and users of new knowledge. Improved application of research findings occurs when health researchers move beyond a reliance on academic publication as a primary mechanism for disseminating results. Instead, more dynamic mechanisms that engage players whose decision-making would be informed by the research have been shown to increase uptake and application of research"

Canadian Institutes of Health Research

Enabling change and reinforcing learning

In the past few years there has been increasing emphasis on the concept of knowledge translation.

Research has shown that health professionals require information and knowledge that is accessible and can be integrated into their practices, and that desired changes should be supported by appropriate reinforcements (Davis et al 2003). The teacher or course organiser can draw upon the rich literature on reminders, protocols, flow sheets and algorithms for care, more often found in the health services research literature than that related to CPD (Davis et al 2003, Jamtvedt et al 2004, Thomson et al 2004b) to facilitate the translation of knowledge into practice.

Know the outcome

There are many reasons to know the outcomes of CPD activities. These follow the outline provided by Dixon in her landmark article on the evaluation of CPD activities (Dixon 1978) that suggests a relatively linear, though perhaps overly simplistic, model of expected outcomes: perception of the educational activity, competency (knowledge, skill or attitude), performance change, and healthcare outcomes. Other models of change may be equally useful (Miller 1967). In many ways these steps mirror those of needs assessment.

Perception of the learning event

For scenario 1, outcomes may include knowing the audience's perception of the presentation or lecture. The classical 'happiness index' need not however be confined to just an overall rating of quality of presentation; it may expand to incorporate a number of features such as match with learning objectives, use of audiovisual materials, quality of handouts, degree to which interactivity was achieved, relevance, and other topics (Rothman & Sibbald 2002).

Competence

For the purpose of this chapter at least, a consideration of competence includes knowledge, skills and attitudes, the classic triumvirate of this dimension of impact on the learner. Tests for each of these are widely available and may include (Hays et al 2002, Schuwirth & van der Vleuten 2003, Scoles et al 2003, Shaw & Wright 1967, Southgate et al 2001):

- knowledge: multiple choice examinations, true–false tests
- skills: performance simulators (e.g., advanced cardiac life support systems or anaesthesia mannequins), interviews with standardised patients
- attitudes: global rating scores.

Performance change and health care outcome

While it might be difficult to demonstrate performance or healthcare change as the result of a lecture or presentation (as in scenario 1), scenario

2, and other interventions like it, offer an opportunity to demonstrate such outcomes. For scenario 2, a post-intervention questionnaire might ask 'Has the intervention (or series of interventions, like rounds) made any difference to how you practise or to patient outcomes?' Hospital and other records may be scanned for improved length of stay following a series of rounds to decrease complications. Office chart audits may be used to look for an increase in screening measures in primary care. Utilisation data can be employed in a managed care setting to demonstrate decreased utilisation of unnecessary tests.

Summary

This brief chapter has outlined four steps in making the CPD experience more effective – from both the perspective of the individual CPD teacher and the broader viewpoint of the provider/organiser of such experiences. Captured as brief, take home points, they include the following four principles:

- know the audience – its composition, background, practice milieu and, most of all, its expertise
- know the topic – the subject area and the objectives and goals of the session
- know the format – choosing the educational process from a broad and wide range of interactive and relevant methods, adding post-intervention enabling and reinforcing materials and methods
- know the outcome – and wherever possible, measure it.

This last step then becomes, in an attempt to make all such CPD experiences iterative, integral to further planning, and involving the first two steps.

References

Antonelli Incalzi R, Pedone C, Pahor M, et al; Gruppo Italiano di Farmacovigilanza nell'Anziano. 2002. Trends in prescribing ACE-inhibitors for congestive heart failure in elderly people. Aging Clinical and Experimental Research 14(6):516–521.

Canadian Institutes of Health Research. Instituts de Recherche en Santé du Canada. Strategies for knowledge translation in health. Online. Available: http://www.cihr-irsc.gc.ca/e/4143.html. 24 November 2004

Craig J L 1991 The OSCME (Opportunity for Self-Assessment CME). Journal of Continuing Education in the Health Professions 11(1):87–94.

Davis D, O'Brien M A, Freemantle N, et al 1999. Impact of formal continuing medical education: do conferences, workshops, rounds, and other traditional continuing education activities change physician behavior or health care outcomes? JAMA 282(9):867–874

Davis D, Evans M, Jadad A, et al 2003 The case for knowledge translation: shortening the journey from evidence to effect. BMJ 327(7405):33–35

Davis D A, Thomson M A, Oxman A D, Haynes R B 1995 Changing physician performance. A systematic review of the effect of continuing medical education strategies. JAMA;274(9):700–705

Davis P, Russell A S, Skeith K J 1997 The use of standardized patients in the performance of a needs assessment and development of a CME intervention in rheumatology for primary care physicians. Journal of Rheumatology 24(10):1995–1999

De Buda Y, Woolf C R 1990 Saturday at the University: A format for success. Journal of Continuing Education in the Health Professions 10(3):279–284

Dixon J 1978 Evaluation criteria in studies of continuing education in the health professions: A critical review and a suggested strategy. Evaluation and the Health Professions 1:47–65

Fox R D, Mazmanian P E, Putnam R W 1989. Changing and learning in the lives of physicians. Praeger Publications, New York

Grant J 2002 Learning needs assessment: assessing the need. BMJ 324(7330):156–159

Green L W, Kreuter M, Deeds S, Partridge K 1980 Health education planning: A diagnostic approach. Mayfield Press, Palo Alto

Hays R B, Davies H A, Beard J D, et al 2002 Selecting performance assessment methods for experienced physicians. Medical Education 36(10):910–917

Health Insurance Commission. Practice Incentives Program. Online. Available: http://www.hic.gov.au/providers/incentives_allowances/pip.htm 28 June 2004

Hewson M G 2000 A theory-based faculty development program for clinician-educators. Academic Medicine 75(5):498–501

Jamtvedt G, Young J M, Kristoffersen D T, et al 2004 Audit and feedback: effects on professional practice and health care outcomes (Cochrane Review). In The Cochrane Library, Issue 2. John Wiley, Chichester, UK

Kantrowitz M P 1991 Problem-based learning in continuing medical education: some critical issues. Journal of Continuing Education in the Health Professions 11(1):11–18

Knowles M S, Holton E F, Swanson R A, Holton E 1998. The adult learner: the definitive classic in adult education and human resource development. Gulf Publishing, Houston

Lockyer J 1998 Needs assessment: lessons learned. Journal of Continuing Education in the Health Professions 18(3):190–192

Miller G E 1967 Continuing medical education for what? Medical Education 42(4):320–326

Miller R G, Ashar B H, Getz K J 2003 Evaluation of an audience response system for the continuing education of health professionals. Journal of Continuing Education in the Health Professions 23(2):109–115

Norman G R, Shannon S I, Marrin M L 2004 The need for needs assessment in continuing medical education. BMJ 328(7446):999–1001

Ontario Medical Association. CME Program for Rural and Isolated Physicians. Online. Available: http://www.oma.org/cme 28 June 2004

Rothman A I, Sibbald G 2002 Evaluating medical grand rounds. Journal of Continuing Education in the Health Professions 22(2):77–83

Royal College of Physicians and Surgeons of Canada. Guidelines for accredited providers of CPD activities. Online. Available: http://rcpsc.medical.org/maintenance/providers/ 28 June 2004

Schuwirth L W, van der Vleuten C P 2003 The use of clinical simulations in assessment. Medical Education 37 Suppl 1:65–71

Scoles P V, Hawkins R E, LaDuca A 2003 Assessment of clinical skills in medical practice. Journal of Continuing Education in the Health Professions 23(3):182–190

Schon D A 1990 Educating the reflective practitioner: toward a new design for teaching and learning in the professions. Jossey-Bass, San Francisco

Shaw M E, Wright J M 1967 Scales for the measurement of attitudes. McGraw Hill, New York

Silver I, Rath D 2002 Making the formal lecture more interactive. Intercom 15(3):6–8

Southgate L, Hays R B, Norcini J, et al 2001 Setting performance standards for medical practice: a theoretical framework. Medical Education 35(5):474–481

Steinert Y, Snell L S 1999 Interactive lecturing: strategies for increasing participation in large group presentations. Medical Teacher 21(1):37–42

Thomson O'Brien M A, Freemantle N, Oxman A D, et al 2004a Continuing education meetings and workshops: effects on professional practice and health care outcomes (Cochrane Review). In The Cochrane Library, Issue 2. John Wiley, Chichester, UK

Thomson O'Brien M A, Oxman A D, Davis D A, et al 2004b Educational outreach visits: effects on professional practice and health care outcomes (Cochrane Review). In The Cochrane Library, Issue 2. John Wiley, Chichester, UK

Weil E, Tu J V 2001 Quality of congestive heart failure treatment at a Canadian teaching hospital. CMAJ 165(3):284–287

SECTION 2
LEARNING SITUATIONS

Chapter 6
Lectures

J. A. Dent

Introduction

Although lectures are a commonly used method of teaching in tertiary education their role and format can be quite varied. In whatever way they are used it is important that they are delivered in the best possible way to help students learn.

Role

A lecture is usually thought of as a mechanism for imparting factual information but it has the potential to do much more. An opening lecture for a course or block of teaching provides students with a human face for the programme and gives an opportunity to 'paint the big picture' of the topic to the whole class and so stimulate interest and curiosity.

The lecture should have a stated aim and objective. 'Aims' indicate the general direction of the studies that the students are engaged in, for instance, 'To understand how to manage a patient in pain'. 'Objectives' relates to goals which should be attainable either after the lecture or in the near future, for instance, 'After this lecture you should be able to list four drugs which help to control somatic pain and describe their method of action'.

If lectures are outlined in a study guide (see chapter 21) they can be seen in the context of the whole of the course, and their content related to other lectures or to material which will be presented in other learning situations.

Content

Not all course material designated as being 'core' needs to be presented as a lecture and indeed much may be more appropriately presented in other ways. Questions of ethics or patient management lend themselves to learning in small groups, while factual information relating to the pathology or pharmacology of a condition may be more efficiently presented as self-directed learning or computer-assisted learning (CAL) programmes.

Types of lecture session

If lectures are seen as only one of a variety of learning opportunities on a course then they do not need to be used to spoonfeed students with predigested facts (Fig. 6.1); instead they may be used in a variety of more interesting ways:

"An important question for any lecturer to consider when planning a teaching session is, 'How can I help my students to learn during my lecture?' "

Cantillon 2003

"Lecturalgia (painful lecture) is a frequent cause of morbidity for both teachers and learners"

McLaughlin & Mandin 2001

"Lecture; a process by which the notes of a teacher become the notes of a student without passing through the minds of either"

O'Donnell 1997

- Overview – an overview of an entire body system in health and disease can be given in an introductory lecture as a prelude to the whole course. A flavour of the system is given and those aspects designated as being of core importance can be highlighted to be expanded later as the course progresses.
- Core – a series of lectures may be used to present the core content of the course
- Non-core – an occasional lecture may be used to introduce material 'beyond the core'. This may illustrate wider aspects of the topic being studied or include recent research developments.
- Assessment material – the style of assessment material to be used in forthcoming examinations can be introduced and examples worked through with the whole class.
- Patient presentations – these can be used to illustrate general aspects of a case history to the whole class or to discuss the impact of an illness and its management on an individual. The form of the lecture can then be delivered in an interactive style, giving students the opportunity to ask questions and take part in discussions with the patient and the lecturer (Fig. 6.2).
- Shared lecture – two or more lecturers may share the session to present different or multiprofessional approaches or opinions on a topic, e.g. a general practitioner and an orthopaedic surgeon on the management of osteoarthritis.
- Mini-symposium – several participants can take part to demonstrate multiprofessional approaches to the management of a clinical problem.

Components

McLaughlin & Mandin (2001) describe three components of organisation for the main body of the lecture:

- *Selection*
  - For congruence: all the material selected as key points of the lecture should lead towards the realisation of the stated objectives of the lecture.
  - For quantity: limit the content to a maximum of five key points per hour of lecture.
- *Sequencing*
  - Between key points the lecture should proceed in a logical progression.
  - Within key points the use of a variety of examples, illustrations and elaborations will increase the chance of new information being retained. New information is stored in the context in which it is learned, so increasing the variety of contexts illustrating the same key point increases the chance of remembering (encoding specificity).
- *Linking*
  - A summary should be made at the end of the presentation of each key point before progressing to the next.

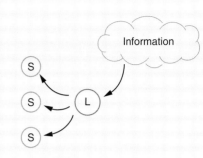

S = Students

L = Lecturer

Fig. 6.1 A didactic lecture

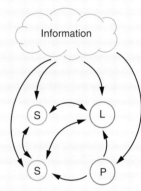

L = Lecturer

S = Students

P = Patient

Fig. 6.2 An interactive lecture

Duration

Studies have shown that students' attention deteriorates after 45 minutes. Lectures should be timed to last no longer than this and should include time for answering questions. Lectures delivered by more than one person can last longer but it should be remembered that students will be in better shape for their next teaching session if they can have a break before it starts!

Format

Lectures are often arranged in three sections:

- introduction
- body
- conclusion

sometimes referred to as 'set, body and close'. This arrangement ensures that the main points of the lecture are clearly identified and repeated. Students are at their most receptive in the first and last few minutes of the lecture so these are the times to emphasise the key points of your lecture.

Introduction

The two checklists given here provide a good reminder of how the first five minutes of a lecture can be best used.

At the outset the lecturer must attract attention and set the mood for the lecture. It is necessary to establish rapport and provide motivation and enthusiasm to inspire the audience to concentrate for the main body of the lecture. An advance organiser provides a statement of the objective of the lecture (e.g. 'At the end of this lecture you should be able to . . .') and indicates the key points which are to be noted on the way. In this way the proposed content of the lecture is outlined so students can arrange their thoughts about what is to come and can pace themselves for the session.

The students' pre-existing knowledge base should be identified. It should be clear to the lecturer and the students where the lecture fits into their previous experiences and prior knowledge. Finally, indicating the usefulness of the content of the lecture for the future will enhance student attention.

Body

The construction of the central portion of the lecture may vary. Brown & Manogue (2001) described:

- *The classical method.* This divides the lecture into sections and subsections (see for example Fig. 6.3). This is easy to plan and take notes from but can soon seem boring.
- *The problem-centred method.* This begins by stating a problem and then argues for and against various solutions (Fig. 6.4).

 Structure your lecture into three parts:
- introduction
- body
- conclusion.

 "Say what you are going to say, say it and say what you have said"

Advice to a young preacher

Ensure that you have arrived at the correct lecture theatre to avoid beginning your lecture with the wrong audience.

'SET' includes:
- Mood
- Motivation
- Utility
- Content
- Knowledge base
- Objectives.
Godolphin & Craig Microteach Programme, University of British Columbia, Canada

A,E,I,O,U
- Attract attention
- Establish rapport
- Identify knowledge base
- Provide advance organiser – objectives and key points
- Indicate usefulness.

This promotes enquiry, cross-referencing and formation of a conclusion.

- *The sequential method* which consists of a series of linked statements which lead to a conclusion as one part logically leads on to the next (Fig. 6.5).

The lecturer should conclude this section by asking for questions so as to clarify any misunderstandings.

Conclusion

Finish the lecture with a review of the objectives and key points which were stated in the introduction. You can then indicate avenues of self-directed learning which the students might now wish to follow but do not introduce new material at this time and do not end your lecture by answering some obscure question.

At the end of your lecture you might like to consider getting feedback on your performance. This might be by informal or brief comments from the students or be part of a faculty peer-review process (Cantillon 2003). In any case the importance of privately reflecting on your teaching session cannot be overemphasized.

Presentation

It is not an exaggeration to think of the lecturer as a performer who has to entertain an audience. It is crucial to the success of your lecture that you maintain the audience's attention. Asking yourself the following questions will make this easier to accomplish:

Where should I stand?

Choose where you are going to position yourself in the lecture theatre and whether you are going to stand, sit or walk around. Do you wish to be behind a podium or table or nearer, and so more able to make contact with, the audience? Wherever you are, be sure you are near the microphone and that it is at the correct height for you, and that you are not obstructing the audience's view of the projector screen.

How should I speak?

Speak clearly, audibly and fluently. Make it clear at the beginning of your lecture whether you expect students to take notes or not. Taking down every word verbatim should be discouraged, but if it is expected that notes are to be taken then a slower pace is necessary and new words should be clearly indicated. If the role of the lecture is to paint a general overview then only the occasional word need be written down and the pace and style of lecture can be quicker and more colloquial.

Changes in pitch and speed make a lecture more engaging and a digression in the form of an anecdote or reference to a current social event may give variety to your lecture and recapture student attention. Do not be afraid to pause to allow students to catch up if you are expecting them to take detailed notes.

If you are unsure of the answer to a question raised, rather than stalling, ask the student to meet you later to discuss it.

Always end your lecture with a summary of the content rather than a discussion of some obscure point raised as question.

Ask yourself, 'What was the take-home message from this lecture?'

"Don't:
Annoy
Bore
Confuse
Distract
Exhaust"

Robert D. Acland, Professor,
Division of Plastic and Reconstructive Surgery,
University of Louisville, USA

It is best to stand or sit to one side of the overhead projector otherwise you will probably be obstructing the view of part of the audience.

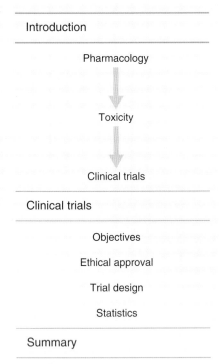

Fig. 6.3 Example of classical method of lecturing (redrawn from Brown & Tomlinson 2001)

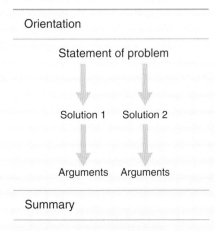

Fig. 6.4 Example of problem-centred method of lecturing (redrawn from Brown and Tomlinson 1979)

It is fatal to read a lecture if student concentration is to be maintained but some notes will help you to keep the main points in view and are invaluable to fall back on if interrupted or diverted.

Finally, if you intend to use any visual aids or other resource make sure to cue these in your notes so that they are not forgotten or brought in at the wrong time.

What should I do?

Maintain eye contact with the audience. Look around various sections of the audience in turn but not repeatedly at any particular student as this can be very disturbing. Do not speak to the walls or the projector! Appropriate use of gestures may enliven your presentation and maintain attention but beware of distracting mannerisms.

In some situations it may be possible to walk around the lecture theatre and speak from different points at the back or towards the middle instead of always from the front. This may be especially helpful when using slides so that you can check that the features illustrated can be seen from the back. However, if the projector is at the back of the room, do not stand next to it but use a remote control so you can be positioned within sight of the audience as they look at the screen.

Beware of dimming the house lights completely as you will lose eye contact with the audience and encourage sleep!

When should I change style?

Student attention diminishes with time. To counteract this a change in delivery style may be useful. This can be used to bring back student attention by asking questions, providing students with opportunities to discuss a problem in small groups or by introducing a short formative assessment (Fig. 6.6). As well as making variations in your pace of delivery you may also wish to vary your style of presentation. At certain points in the lecture it should be possible to stop and ask the audience a question in order to clarify any points which may have been confusing or to check on students' understanding of the material so far. At times asking particular questions to individual students can be used but this may appear threatening so it may be best to ask questions to different areas of the auditorium in turn to help maintain interest. Students can be asked to form small 'buzz groups' where they are sitting to discuss questions and provide answers.

Finally

- Don't – fidget or fiddle with loose change and car keys in your pockets.
- Do – avoid repetitive mannerisms and repetitions such as 'er', 'um' and 'OK'

Resources

Any additional material presented in a lecture must be of good quality or else it will be a distraction.

Illustrations

Traditional photographic slides, digital images or computer-generated illustrations can be used to assist learning and aid concentration. Clinical features, radiographs, results of other investigations or aspects of surgery or other lines of management can be illustrated. Photomicrographs and diagrams or pictures of prosections may be helpful in illustrating basic sciences but line slides and tables should be used cautiously as they are often overcrowded and may be impossible to read. Attention should be paid to the size of the words and the type and colours of font used as when projected some may be illegible from the back of the room (Laidlaw 1987a). Pale print on a dark ground tends to dazzle and be difficult to read as are words written entirely in capital letters. Beware of making individual slides too busy!

Double projection is probably less popular now than it used to be. It requires considerable skill if a meaningful flow of slides is to be constructed. One useful technique is to have text slides in one projector and parallel illustrative material in the other.

Flip charts, blackboards and wipe-clean boards

These are probably less used during lectures than previously. If they are used, the writing must be large and clear to be seen at the back of the room. It is impossible to use any of these without turning your back on audience. Try to avoid speaking to the board!

Handouts

A lesson plan should be available to the students either as a handout or a website. It can be used to indicate:

- Aims and objectives – these terms may often be confused (see above)
- Summary – the main points of the lecture can be listed
- Self-assessment questions – these can be presented during the lecture or in the lesson plan for students to use in their own time to assess their understanding of the topic presented.
- Directions to background reading and other self-directed learning material when appropriate.

The lesson plan may be given at the beginning of a lecture to give an outline of the content.

- Comprehensive handouts avoid the need to take extensive notes but encourage lack of concentration.
- Skeletal handouts which require to be filled in may encourage students to pay more attention.

Other interactive material to promote audience participation may be distributed for use in question and answer sessions during the lecture (Maclean 1991).

Overhead projector or visualiser

These can be used to present previously prepared text or illustrations or, in the case of the visualiser, pages of printed material or three-

"No sleep is so deeply refreshing as that which, during lectures, Morpheus invites us so insistently to enjoy. From the standpoint of physiology it is amazing how quickly the ravages of a short night or a long operating session can be repaired by nodding off for a few seconds at a time"

Medawar 1979

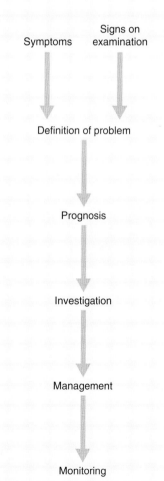

Fig. 6.5 The sequential method (redrawn from Brown & Tomlinson 1979)

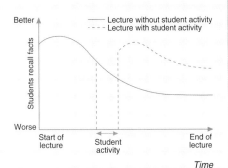

Fig. 6.6 Students' recall of facts is improved when they take part in an activity during a lecture. (Amended and reproduced, with permission from the BMJ Publishing Group, from Cantillon P BMJ 2003;326:437–400)

dimensional objects. Diagrams or tables prepared on acetate sheets for the overhead projector can be built up by removing successive layers of masking or adding successive layers of predrawn or coloured sheets.

Points gathered from interaction with the audience can be written down as they are raised but beware of presenting material which is:

- too small
- too crowded
- too scribbled

(Laidlaw 1987b)

Multimedia presentation

Computer presentations, for example prepared using Microsoft PowerPoint, can avoid the expense of producing slides and be quicker to prepare than overhead projector acetate sheets. New material can even be added during the course of the lecture. It is important to check that everything is working before you start, especially if technical assistance is not available during the lecture. The lecturer must have practised to become familiar with the computer programme to be used. Again attention must be paid to colour, crowding and the type and size of fonts used. The use of additional visuals such as Clip Art or scanned-in photographs help to enliven the presentation (Crosby 1994). Inserting and using video clips during a computerised presentation requires some care, and staff development courses on the use of programmes such as PowerPoint are often available.

Some lecture theatre systems may not have the software to support this type of presentation so beware if visiting an unfamiliar location and allow time to check the system before you start so that you have time to consider an alternative method of presentation.

Some lecture theatre systems allow rapid changes between computer data projection, visualiser and 35mm slides but practice with the system is mandatory to avoid disaster!

Headsets

Radio headsets have been used to receive sounds from a patient or manikin which would normally only be heard by one person. Heart or intrauterine sounds can be transmitted to the whole audience and subsequently discussed.

Video, closed circuit TV and teleconferencing

The lecture can be used to view short sections of previously recorded video or closed circuit TV presentations from another site such as an operating theatre. Interactive teleconferencing from several locations may form part of the event.

Websites and local Intranet

Copies of handouts, illustrations, PowerPoint slides and references to other resource material can subsequently be made available on a website for students to access after the lecture. Directions to additional learning resources can also be given.

Challenges

If you have forgotten your presentation notes or slides it may be necessary, if you cannot restructure the style of your lecture immediately, to apologise and re-schedule your lecture for another day. For the majority of challenges, however, it is simply a matter of keeping calm and not being afraid to stop until the disturbance is over or you have re-found your place in your presentation notes.

Interruptions and technical faults provide a test of the lecturer's skill in holding the floor and it may be wise to work out in advance a strategy for dealing with some of the following before being faced with them. Interruptions may be caused by:

- late arrivals
- uninvited questions
- paging system
- talking on the back row
- students falling asleep
- technical failures may include:
  – no light on the podium
  – projector bulb blows
  – projector remote control fails to function
  – computer crash
  – house lights fail to dim
  – window blackouts are inadequate for projection to be seen.

By always making a point of arriving early to familiarise yourself with the equipment many of these disasters can be avoided.

Feedback

Although everyone thinks they can lecture adequately it is probably true that meaningful, constructive feedback on a lecture will be valuable to all. Feedback may be available from students at the end of a lecture, from colleagues sharing the session or as part of a formal peer-review programme (see chapter 42).

- Students can be asked for verbal feedback or to complete a brief feedback proforma (Cantillon 2003).
- Colleagues may be able to give a constructive objective critique and provide positive advice on content and delivery.
- Personal reflection may be undertaken by privately viewing a video of your own performance.

Videos illustrating examples of good and bad lecturing are available and can be used to stimulate discussion in staff development sessions on how to lecture well.

Summary

In a modern curriculum a lecture is only one of several ways of passing on factual information. As such its role in the context of the entire course

"Some experience of popular lecturing had convinced me that the necessity of making things plain to uninstructed people was one of the very best means of clearing up the obscure corners in one's own mind"

Huxley 1825–95

must be made clear. As well as presenting core material, lectures can also be used to give an overview of the course, present assessment material and make patient presentations which may be a shared activity with multiprofessional participation. However it is used, the lecture should be clearly structured, have defined aims and objectives and be accompanied by an explicit lesson plan. To lecture effectively requires that attention be paid to presentation skills and the use of any visual or technical resources. Even when all is prepared, the lecturer must be able to deal with any unforeseen challenges. Attendance at staff development sessions in lecturing may prove more valuable than originally perceived.

References

Brown G, Manogue M 2001 AMEE Medical Education Guide No 22: Refreshing lecturing: a guide for lecturers

Brown G, Tomlinson D 1979 How to . . . improve lecturing. Medical Teacher 1:128–135

Cantillon P 2003 ABC of learning and teaching in medicine: teaching large groups. BMJ 326:437–440

Crosby J 1994 Twelve tips for effective electronic presentation. Medical Teacher 16:3–8

Huxley T H 1894 Man's place in nature. Also in Gould S J (ed) 2001 Modern Library Science Series. Random House, New York

Laidlaw J M 1987a Twelve tips on preparing 35mm slides. Medical Teacher 9:389–393

Laidlaw J M 1987b Twelve tips for users of the overhead projector. Medical Teacher 9:247–251

MacLean I 1991 Twelve tips on providing handouts. Medical Teacher 13:7–12

McLaughlin K, Mandin H 2001 A schematic approach to diagnosing and resolving lecturalgia. Medical Education 35:1135–1142

Medawar P B 1979 Advice to a young scientist. Harper & Row, New York

O'Donnell M 1997 A sceptic's medical dictionary. BMJ Publishing Group, London

Further reading

Bligh D A 2000 What's the use of lectures? Jossey-Bass, San Francisco

Chapter 7
Learning in small groups

J. R. Rudland

Small-group work is one of a variety of educational methods for promoting student learning. The reason for adopting the small-group approach has to be carefully considered. Other learning situations are detailed in this section of the book and problem-based learning and self-directed learning are covered in Section 3, Educational strategies.

The recent trend to small-group work is indicative of the movement from a teacher-centred approach to education to a more student-centred approach (see Section 1, Curriculum development). However, the reasons for choosing small groups should be dictated by the educational objectives of the session. The organiser of a course or programme has to be clear about the rationale for using small-group work and the outcomes expected of this method. The use of small groups will also be influenced by resource availability, for example, of rooms, facilitators and resource material.

Students tend to learn in different ways and a range of learning situations may ensure appropriate learning for all (Special Needs Opportunity Windows (SNOW)). A mixed approach to the learning situation is often appropriate and may be positively encouraged. The use of both lectures and small groups may be complementary to the learning process.

What is a small group?

Small-group work is characterised by student participation and interaction (Crosby 1996). It is possible to have a small number of students and a tutor and yet participation by the students remains minimal. This may be better called a lecture (albeit for a small number of students). In addition to participation, small-group work is also characterised by group work on a task and reflection on the work completed.

Optimally effective small-group work occurs when there is a small number of students. It is impossible or very difficult to ensure the participation of a large number of students in a group. If the number increases too much, the group may be split into two. The number of students in a group does not conform to any hard and fast rule. Some experienced tutors may be able to facilitate many students whereas an inexperienced tutor may feel more comfortable with fewer students. Numbers in small groups are, however, frequently fixed by curriculum demands and the generation of grouping based on a yearly intake. A tutor may not be able to dictate the preferred size of a group.

Why would you use a lecture and why a small group?

The size of a small group is less important than the characteristics of the group.

"When adults teach and learn in one another's company, they find themselves engaging in a challenging, passionate, and creative activity"

Brookfield 1986

"With undergraduate medical education currently carrying a health warning because of the stress and anxiety exhibited by students and young graduates, any educational process that promotes enjoyment of learning without loss of basic knowledge must be a good thing"

Bligh 1995

Think – how do you learn?

Why small groups?

There are advantages to using small-group teaching over larger class activities or independent learning. Small-group teaching:

- Familiarises students with an adult approach to learning, a generic skill they will need for the rest of their professional lives.
- Encourages students to take responsibility for their own learning. Teacher-centred models of learning tend not to encourage students to do this.
- Promotes deeper understanding of material. Small-group work allows students to bring to the group their own prior learning and perceptions (or misconceptions) of material previously learnt. Learning can then develop from this point.
- Encourages problem-solving skills.
- Encourages participation. The nature of social interactions means that they are usually more enjoyable than solitary pursuits. The element of enjoyment and its influence on motivation may encourage students to learn.
- Develops
  - interpersonal skills
  - communication skills
  - social teamworking skills
  - presentation skills.
- Encourages an awareness of different views on issues and has the potential to encourage an attitude of tolerance.

Personal understanding of an educational issue can be attained in a number of ways but small groups make it possible to turn such understanding into a 'coherent, rational and professionally defensible position that can be clearly articulated' (Walker 1998).

Notwithstanding these advantages, small-group work should only be adopted when it is the most efficient approach to achieve these benefits or objectives. It should not be considered to be universally appropriate for learning. The expertise of the tutor might be regarded as a potential problem. The role of the tutor can be crucial to the success of any small-group work. Staff may be more familiar with traditional modes of teaching and may need training in the specific role of a small-group tutor. The logistics of running small groups may be difficult as more teachers, more rooms and more resource material may be required. The preparation of resource material to support small groups is also an important part of the process and requires considerable time and expertise.

What kind of small-group session?

In the context of a medical undergraduate curriculum a variety of small group sessions may be relevant. At one end of the spectrum is the structured, teacher-centred, tutorial group, usually focusing on an identified task (Entwistle & Thompson 1992) and often pursuing a series of conclusions (a differential diagnosis perhaps or a patient management plan). At the other end is the unstructured, student-centred, discussion/dialogue group (Christensen 1991), the principal purpose of which is to exchange views on a topic and promote reflection (attitudes to patient care perhaps or interpersonal communication). Between these two extremes all manner of group structures and functions exist, limited only by the imagination and creativity of the course organisers and individual tutors. Examples include:

- seminars
- workshops
- clinical skills sessions
- communication skills sessions
- problem-based learning tutorials
- clinical teaching sessions
  - ward-based
  - ambulatory care/ outpatient-based
  - community-based

The majority of these types of small-group sessions are dealt with in detail elsewhere in this book. The main focus of the present chapter is those elements that are common to all small-group, student-centred activities. The text can, of course, only serve as an introduction to actual practice in a variety of settings.

All such activities must complement the institution's overall curricular strategy, address specific course objectives and enhance the educational programme. The sessions should be seen to be an integral component of the course content and relate appropriately to the other learning opportunities on offer. For example, the week's work may be framed around a patient problem. The lectures and small-group work, both theoretical and practical, contribute to an understanding of the patient's problem. Key to the success of small-group work is the tutor, working either alone or in collaboration with a co-tutor.

What is the role of the tutor?

Traditional tutorial role
In the case of the traditional tutorial group, the tutor normally states the objectives of the session (usually known to the participants beforehand), initiates the process, invites learner input (often prepared), promotes discussion and brings the session to an appropriate close. Throughout the session the tutor 'leads from the front' (often literally) and is clearly in control. This format is familiar to most medical teachers and is one in which the tutor's effectiveness is derived from a combination of innate ability, content expertise, teaching experience and personal enthusiasm. Such learning groups are of undoubted value in selected circumstances. The range of discussion, however, may be relatively narrow, the contribution to self-learning limited and interaction between learners at best patchy.

"Leaders can model . . . manual, intellectual and communication skills, and learners can safely rehearse and refine these capabilities"

Westberg & Jason 1996

"I will hand on precepts, lectures and all other learning . . . to those pupils duly apprenticed and sworn"

Hippocratic Oath c.460–377 BC

"over two-thirds of academic and clinical staff had received no formal training in teaching skills"

Preston-Whyte et al 1999

The clinician as role model exerts a potent influence – for good or bad.

Facilitative tutorial role

Increasingly, small-group learning signifies a process in which the learners together provide much of the initiative, explore options, test hypotheses, develop solutions, elaborate ongoing actions (including clinical investigations and treatment) and review outcomes. Role-playing and the performance of practical procedures may be an integral part of such sessions.

The role of the tutor in these circumstances varies according to the stage of academic development of the learners, their familiarity with the process, their maturity as a group, and the frequency and duration of the tutorials. If the small-group session is one of a linked series, say within an 'organ/system/problem-based' course, continuity of contact with a single tutor or pair of tutors has much to recommend it. This is often seen to be a problem for busy clinical teachers, but experience shows that where teaching responsibilities are taken seriously at institutional and individual level, appropriate solutions can usually be found which do not adversely affect the teacher's other functions.

Requirements of a tutor

Preparation

Tutors need to be properly briefed on the specific objectives of the small-group session. Tutor guides containing this kind of information are a feature of modern educational programmes.

If tutors are new to small-group learning then they need to acquire some basic expertise. Appropriate staff development programmes should be available to meet the needs of aspiring teachers. These may take the form of specific courses or 'on the job' training and may include the opportunity to join experienced tutors at work (Hekelman et al 1994). Evidence suggests that the basic skills of small-group facilitation may be acquired in 12 to 24 hours of experiential training. Studies have also shown that while content expertise may be useful in small-group teaching, facilitation skills are essential. This is particularly so in the early years when learners stand to derive the greatest benefit from acquiring the skills and habit of independent self-learning.

A few practical points remain. Tutors should be the first to appear at the appointed hour, not the last. Preferably, they should make a point of turning up before the session starts in order to check the venue, the seating and the resources, to troubleshoot and to set an example.

Group dynamics – conduct of a small-group session

The success of small-group learning may be judged by the extent to which trust is created and collaboration fostered. This is critical in the case of a linked series of tutorials but should be aspired to in all instances.

The opening few minutes of the small-group session can make or mar the entire session. In 'one-off' situations or early in a series the tutor will wish to set the scene, state the objectives and devise with the students some basic ground rules. It may also be advantageous to consider the expectations of the students regarding their role and the role of the tutor in the small-group setting, and how these roles may change as the learners become increasingly competent at handling their own affairs. Ultimately the tutor may merge with the group to the extent that an observer might have difficulty distinguishing tutor from learner (see Fig. 7.1). This is the greatest challenge for the traditional teacher who is likely to be initially uncomfortable with the thought of losing control.

Issues of importance during the group work include:

- participation of all group members (may require control of dominant students and encouragement of quieter ones; a co-tutor may be particularly helpful in this regard)
- critical thinking (assimilation, interpretation and synthesis of information)
- articulation of thoughts/views (an essential generic skill)
- learner interaction (enhancement of understanding, growth of mutual respect and promotion of teamworking)
- review of objectives ('keeping on track')
- intermittent summary of achievements (encouragement of reflection)
- observation of agreed time constraints (development of time management skills).

The emphasis on these and other individual issues will vary with circumstances and some goals may only realistically be achieved in the context of serial sessions.

Stages of group development

All groups go through a series of stages of development before performing in an effective manner. Whilst several models are used to describe this progression, the best known is Tuckman's four stages of group development. For the tutor it may be useful to be aware of these stages.

'Forming'

'Forming' occurs in a collection of individuals who are attempting to establish their personal identities in the group. During this stage group information is exchanged and each member's strengths and weaknesses are determined.

'Storming'

This stage is characterised by conflict, dissatisfaction and competition. Some interpersonal hostility is to be expected but it is during this phase that trust may form within the group. A group member's request to be moved to another group may be an outward display of this stage.

'Norming'

Attempts are made by the group to function effectively as a group through the setting up of rules and norms of behaviour. Clarity regarding roles and responsibilities will be developed and the group starts developing a sense of group identity and ways of behaving.

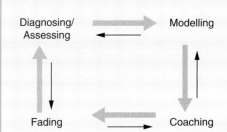

Fig. 7.1 Cyclical leadership roles in small groups (redrawn from Collins et al 1989)

"A fundamental feature of effective facilitation is to make participants feel that they are valued as separate, unique individuals deserving of respect"

Brookfield 1986

Think – cultural diversity
Increasingly, medical schools have a diverse mix of students. The ethnic and cultural upbringing of students must be considered in all learning opportunities. The student-centred approach of small-group work may result in some students, especially those used to a didactic and teacher-centred approach, having difficulty with engagement with the group. The basis of difficulties should be explored.

"Group methods succeed or fail to the extent that work is accomplished"

Walton 1997

Feedback needs to be: linked to actual observation of learners' performance; timely; descriptive of specific behaviours; potentially supportive in nonjudgemental ways and, when possible, tied to the learner's self-assessments.

'Performing'

The final stage requires the successful completion of the three earlier stages. The group is performing at an optimal level. They are focused on their task and are aware of how everyone works. Disagreements and misunderstandings can be effectively accommodated within the group.

Whatever small-group model is envisaged, the importance of according sufficient time to bring the session to an appropriate ending cannot be exaggerated. In a 'stand alone' traditional tutorial this may require only a few minutes but in the kind of session which forms the main focus of this chapter, considerably more time may have to be allocated. Feedback to learners is critically important and is widely regarded as one of the strengths of the small-group process. Reference may be made not only to general points and particular details of the learning content of the session but also to the conduct of the session. The latter may on occasion prompt later counselling of individual students where specific difficulties have been identified that are best dealt with away from the group. In the case of a series of interconnected sessions (e.g. a problem-based model) there will also be a need to agree the topics for discussion at the next session.

What is the role of the student?

While the student is the key figure in any learning event, in small-group learning the positive commitment of the individual learner is absolutely crucial to success. As in the case of the tutor, the learners must accept the principle of this form of learning and realise that what they get out of the process directly reflects what they put into it. This will include undertaking prior reading, actively and constructively contributing to the conduct of the session and effectively reflecting on the issues raised. These types of issues should be discussed when the contracts and ground rules are devised. The student also has an increasingly important role in assessment and evaluation.

It should be remembered that student groups may function entirely satisfactorily in the absence of a tutor.

Assessment

Assessment of learners engaged in small-group activities can be tricky and requires careful consideration. The learners will certainly want to be informed of the nature of the assessment and whether it will be formative or summative or both. They will also want to know who is responsible for the assessment. If the tutor is involved, particularly in summative assessment, this may act as a barrier to the creation of trust within the group and tend to inhibit the spontaneity of discussion. Some learners may be less inclined to 'take the risk' of revealing ignorance if they believe their every utterance is being carefully monitored and scrutinised. Tutors need to be aware of these sensitivities and be prepared to confront the problem – for example, by openly discussing their role in assessment as part of the group process. (It may help to indicate that the tutor's performance will also be assessed and therefore, since they are all 'in the same boat', they may as well 'pull on the oars' together.)

The details of assessment will be discussed in Section 6, Assessment. In general, it is relatively straightforward to construct an instrument for assessing the performance of the group as a whole, particularly if the assessment is formative. The first step is to identify the performance to be assessed. Performance may relate to:

- the attainment of the objectives or task – the 'product'
- the working of the group – (teamworking, collaboration etc.) – the process.

Attainment of the objectives can be assessed in traditional ways, while assessing the group process may be more challenging. This can be achieved in a variety of ways:

- Student self-reporting. Given key guidelines students may report on the success of teamworking and individual contributions.
- Tutor observations. Most small-group assessments occur spontaneously and informally. The dominant or quiet members are easily spotted. These observations, whilst necessary to ensure appropriate facilitation of the group, may also be used to assess the development of the student.
- External or co-tutor observations. A third party may be asked to observe and assess the group process. These observations may involve more in-depth analysis of interaction and frequency of contributions by both students and staff.

Difficulty arises in assessing the abilities of individual learners, especially if the small group sessions are part of a series involving and specifically encouraging teamwork. A recent study (Heathfield 1999) has shown that the learners themselves may assist in this process and, in effect, decide the relative merits of individual performance on the basis of :

- attendance
- contribution of ideas
- research, analysis and preparation of material
- contribution to cooperative process
- support and encouragement of team members
- practical contributions to end-product.

The individual items can be graded and, if accepted as an ongoing part of the small group continuum, can assist individual learners to develop and enhance their abilities, to become aware and reflective of attitudes (both their own and their peers'), and improve their competence as team-players.

Evaluation and development

Course monitoring

Small-group sessions need to be evaluated as much as any other part of the educational programme. The product and the process can be considered:

"We need to continue to develop ways of assessing what we truly value rather than only valuing what we can more easily assess"

Heathfield 1999

Likert type evaluation: the grading of questions or statements using a numerical scale, e.g. between 1 and 5, where 1 = strongly disagree and 5 = strongly agree.

- Evaluation of the product: the achievement of the tasks. This may be best achieved by assessment results related to the objectives of the session. A variety of methods may be used, for example, an objective structured clinical examination (OSCE) might evaluate the success of small-group work in developing communication skills.
- Evaluation of the process: the method (small-group work) used to achieve the objectives. This may be best determined using either a free-text written response or in a Likert-type questionnaire. Questions to ask may include:
  – Did all the group participate?
  – Did you take responsibility for your own learning?
  – Did the group work effectively?
  – Did anyone dominate?

Tutor support

Much has been written recently about the need for undergraduate medical students and young graduates to be supported as they face the increasing pressures of professional life, particularly when responsibilities in their private lives may also weigh heavily upon them. In Section 7, Staff and students the topic of learner support is addressed in detail. It is also worth reflecting on the need for support amongst teachers, particularly when taking on new and unfamiliar tasks.

To quote the approach of Alcoholics Anonymous, the important first step is to realise that help is required and then to take steps to seek help (Walton 1997). There is little merit in soldiering on alone when other more experienced colleagues are around and are willing to assist (Hekelman et al 1994). Both you and those dependent upon you for their learning will benefit from support which is appropriately offered. Most medical schools do in fact offer such assistance but there is still a tendency for teachers to be unwilling or too busy to avail themselves of it. Both medical schools and teachers might with advantage review their approach to this aspect of staff development.

Summary

Small-group work is a powerful educational tool. As with all teaching instruments its benefits are maximised when it is used skilfully in carefully considered situations. The reasons for its deployment have to be clear to both tutor and learner. Advantages include the encouragement of independent self-learning, critical thinking and awareness of the views of others. Successful small groups are based on the creation of trust, fostering of collaboration and achievement of work.

In the context of a medical undergraduate curriculum, the range of small group sessions is limited only by the imagination of the course organisers and tutors. Clinical teaching is invariably small group in character but educational strategies and teaching methods need to be geared to the overall objectives of the curriculum. Staff development is an

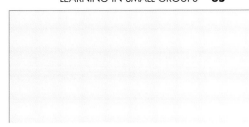

important part of this process. One of the greatest opportunities of small-group work is that of constructive feedback.

As always, assessment and evaluation are critical components of this form of education and should be directed at both the group and its individual members. Increasingly effective methods are being developed to meet this challenge.

References

Bligh J 1995 Problem-based, small group learning. British Medical Journal 311:342–343

Brookfield S 1986 Understanding and facilitating adult learning. Jossey Bass, San Francisco

Christensen C R 1991 Promises and practices of discussion teaching. In: Christensen C R, Garvin D A, Sweet A (eds) Education for judgement: the artistry of discussion leadership. Harvard Business School, Boston, p 15–34

Collins A, Brown J S, Newman S E 1989 Cognitive apprenticeship: teaching the craft of reading, writing and mathematics. In: Reswick L B (ed) Knowing, learning and instruction: essays in honor of Robert Glaser. Lawrence Erlbaum, Hillsdale, N J, p 453–494

Crosby J 1996 AMEE Medical Education Guide no. 8 Learning in small groups. Medical Teacher 18:189–202

Entwistle N, Thompson S 1992 Guidelines for promoting effective learning in higher education. Centre for Research on Learning and Instruction, Edinburgh

Heathfield M 1999 How to assess group work. The Times Higher Educational Supplement, March 26:40–41

Hekelman F P, Flynn S P, Glover P B, Galazka S S 1994 Peer coaching in clinical teaching: formative assessment of a case. Evaluation of Health Professions 17:366–381

Preston-Whyte M E, Clark R, Peterson S, Fraser R C 1999 The views of academic and clinical teachers in Leicester Medical School on criteria to assess teaching competence in the small-group setting. Medical Teacher 21(5):500–505

SNOW (Special Needs Opportunity Windows) http://snow.utoronto.ca/learn2/intoll.html

Walker M 1998 Small group teaching in the medical context. In: Peyton J W R (ed.) Teaching and learning in medical practice. Manticore, Herts, p 139–154

Walton H J 1997 ASME Medical Education Booklet no. 1 Small group methods in medical teaching. Medical Education 31:457–464

Westberg J, Jason H 1996 Generic concepts and issues. In: Westberg J, Jason H (eds) Fostering learning in small groups. Springer, New York, p 9–10

Chapter 8
Teaching in the clinical skills centre

G. Adamo, J. A. Dent

"Medical schools cannot rely on clerkship experience alone to provide adequate basic skills teaching"

Ledingham & Harden 1998

A clinical skills centre:
- is independent of "real" patient availability
- allows clinical teaching to be scheduled
- controls the complexity of the learning situation
- permits mistakes to be made within a safe environment
- encourages direct feedback
- allows repeat consultations and physical examinations
- may directly involve members of the local community in the healthcare learning process
- credibly reproduces the tensions of student interaction with a stranger in an intimate verbal and physical examination.

"Psychological distress is linked to confidence amongst SHOs [senior house officers] in performing clinical tasks"

Williams et al 1997

"Being a successful doctor extends far beyond mere academic ability. Care, compassion and competence are equally important attributes"

General Medical Council 1993

Introduction

The clinical skills centre (CSC) seeks to provide an environment for learning clinical skills in which students can practise without jeopardising patient care or provoking adverse comment. The proliferation of dedicated clinical skills facilities has occurred at a time when hospitals are reserved for shorter stays by the very sickest of patients and when ambulatory care settings for the practice of medicine have eclipsed inpatient hospital care in frequency.

The paradigm of the mentor–apprentice model for bedside teaching and learning has been replaced by the flexible, targeted and explicit learning made possible by a dedicated educational facility and prepared educator faculty. The model is given new life with structured learning that employs discussion and feedback. This may be provided by self assessment, self-reflection, peers, faculty and interactive media and machines, as well as by simulated and standardised patients variously trained to report and feedback on the events of experiential learning from the patient perspective. In general, clinical skills are thought to peak during undergraduate medical education and decline thereafter throughout a physician's career (Chin et al 1997). The role of the CSC is therefore just as relevant in postgraduate education as it is in undergraduate learning.

What do we mean by clinical skills?
In the UK the General Medical Council defined knowledge, skills and attitudes as being of equal importance in the training of a doctor (GMC 1993). Several learning outcomes for clinical skills have been defined and recently adopted by the deans of the Scottish medical schools (Simpson et al 2002):

- Take a history from patients, relatives and others, including the use of good communication skills.
- Undertake physical examination of patients.
- Interpret results of history taking, physical examination and investigation.
- Make a diagnosis.
- Formulate a management plan.
- Record findings – including relevant communication with patients/relatives and colleagues.

Current trends

Since their introduction in the 1990s the role of the CSCs has expanded. Six trends (Dent 2002) illustrate their diversity of activity:

- developing simulated clinical environments
- utilising ancillary technology
- implementing sound educational strategies
- providing self-assessment opportunities
- taking staff development initiatives
- maintaining a supportive learning environment.

Simulated environments

The delivery of a clinical skills programme requires :

- space for the creation of simulated environments
- simulators of varying degrees of sophistication
- simulated and standardised patients and patient-instructors.

Space

Although educational programmes of excellence have flourished without the benefit of a dedicated facility, there is no doubt that the latter makes possible a more comfortable, controllable and predictable programme of curricular activities. In institutions where small-group teaching methods are used regularly, these group sizes and activities should be considered along with the simulation of inpatient and ambulatory settings when designing room dimensions and space requirements. While it may be traditional to crowd a group of learners into a hospital room during rounds it is neither pleasant nor practical for those involved and need not be reproduced when designing a clinical skills centre. Treatment or examination rooms are designed for one-on-one encounters with perhaps one assistant and family member present. A clinical skills centre should simulate a realistic physical approximation of a practice setting (ambulatory clinic, inpatient hospital room or procedures room) but with more open space for student observers than would normally be available. Some medical schools have started with a clinic of six examination rooms while others have anticipated heavy use and built as many as 24 such rooms with additional space for ongoing training of simulated patients to take place.

In CSCs that are supported by a large simulated-patient programme (100–500 different simulated patients are utilised annually in multiple programmes) additional space is needed.

Teaching space should be secure, and inaccessible to casual visitors without explicit permission. It must be designed to maintain separation of learner and simulated patients (SPs) except in the context of the simulated encounter. Other requirements include:

- Separate restroom facilities for SPs.
- A briefing room where they can relax, have snacks, store their personal belongings and be briefed and debriefed as a group by the SP trainer.

"A clinical skills centre reduces the difficulties encountered in medical and nursing colleges in ensuring adequate exposure to clinical problems"

Dacre et al 1996

A clinical skills centre benefits from being:

- accessible to major users
- of adequate size
- designed, furnished and equipped to meet a range of perceived needs
- attractive to students, tutors and 'patients'
- provided with adequate audiovisual and computer facilities.

- Lockers and, less frequently, showers for stage make-up removal.
- Ample dedicated SP training space that simulates the performance environment. This needs to be a separate space which can be used while other programmes are running in the CSC.
- A seminar room for plenary sessions and briefings.
- Office space for the documentation of student pre- and post-encounter activities and for accommodation for the SP trainer and other dedicated staff in the centre.
- A monitoring station to access individual rooms being used in the educational event while allowing privacy in others.
- Room temperatures that are easily adjusted and highly reliable, as gown-clad SPs may be spending hours in a small exam room on a frequent basis. If they are not comfortable their performance may be affected.
- Lighting that must be adequate when it is required, as in treatment/examination rooms. Monitoring rooms function best when lighting is dimmed, as this assists in directing the focus of real-time remote observers to the task at hand on their monitor or computer screen, and reduces the chance of observation rooms becoming social centres.
- Utilities, including air-conditioning, fire alarms, soundproofing and emergency lighting.

Frequently overlooked is space for:

- an additional dedicated server and back-up to store digital recordings and software programs used for educational event administration that involves SPs
- a technicians' workroom
- the photocopier and fax with surrounding space for materials and storage
- an audiovisual presentation room with audio and video teleconferencing capability
- additional rooms for video review and practice
- storage space for current and additional models and simulators
- laundry and janitorial storage.

Simulators

Models and manikins

Simple models are available to simulate intimate or invasive procedures such as bladder catheterisation, or rectal or breast examination. Other more complex simulators allow students to practise intravenous cannulation or intra-articular injections.

The latest generation of simulators (e.g. a pelvic examination simulator) combine a three-dimensional model and a computer-generated performance indicator that records the number of critical areas touched and the maximum pressure used (Pugh & Youngblood 2002). The cardiology simulator, 'Harvey' (Gordon et al 1999), reproduces pulse, blood pressure, chest wall movements and computer-generated heart sounds and

ECGs. The most advanced high-fidelity simulators will reproduce patient reactions to student interventions such as intubation and drug administration (Maran & Glavin 2003; see chapter 23, Simulators and simulation-based medical education).

Once the decision is made to purchase expensive models and manikins, it is essential to determine where they will be stored and by whom and when they will be used. Will they be deployed in treatment/examination rooms and then returned to storage, or will they be better maintained by having a dedicated workbench space in the centre at which they are regularly available?

Practical problems such as the need for the cleaning and sterilisation of real equipment used in simulated encounters require consideration in CSC design and planning.

A new trend combines simulators with the use of SPs who simulate the affective behaviours of the patient, for instance during catheterisation or intravenous cannulation. This approach creates the realistic situation of requiring students to adhere to a procedural algorithm at the same time as they interact and communicate with a person who may present emotional and other communication challenges related to the procedure being performed (Kneebone et al 2002).

Simulated and standardised patients

Simulated environments require simulated patients

Individuals of all ages can be trained to reproduce a clinical history and to respond to physical examination in a consistent manner. SPs may also be trained to accurately report on what was said and done in the encounter. They can be trained to subjectively report on the history-taking, physical examination and communication behaviours of the care provider, and to subjectively assess interpersonal skills and satisfaction with care. Standardisation of performance is particularly important during 'high-stakes' examinations. In other programmes, particularly some formative educational experiences, SPs may be asked to improvise, in response to a medical interview and physical examination, based upon an illness they have experienced in the past or which is currently stable. These are simulated but not standardised and care must be taken to protect confidentiality. The consistency and repeatability of these encounters is not important to the experience. Course and/or centre faculty should specifically address the rights of the simulated patient to confidentiality outside of the class experience.

Depending upon the demands of the specific participation, between 2 and 25 hours of training may be required for simulated patients. Systematic orientation to the setting and goals of the educational event and to their role is key to success. SPs may be trained to portray a clinical condition, document the encounter with a checklist and record and deliver constructive written and/or verbal feedback to the learner. SPs are provided with specific instructions regarding their responses to queries, affective behaviour, level of knowledge and education about their disease. A brief complete patient history should be provided for the SP to call upon if needed to respond to questions. Generalised disease-related education should not be provided to SPs unless the particular patient being portrayed has received the latter. Training materials should provide the SP with information as a specific patient with a specific constellation of symptoms and concerns. It is useful to avoid archetypical improvisation and overly general discussion about what an individual with this disease would be doing and remain specific in training the SP. Even when referring to their actual personal medical history or physical attributes, the SP must be provided with a structured context for their participation in order to avoid the introduction of unintended experiences that may be inappropriate to the level of the learner or foster a negative attitude toward patients. For example, if the task is to provide a simple opportunity for the learner to practise a comprehensive history and physical examination on an adult stranger, they should not encounter a 'difficult physician–patient interaction', such as an overly talkative patient.

Giving feedback

SPs also need specific guidance on how to maintain and define the perspective of themselves as one particular 'patient' in an educational experience which may require them to provide feedback to an individual student or group. Ideally, SPs are trained to structure and limit their feedback to acknowledging specific student behaviours that they felt increased or decreased their comfort with their care and situation as the patient. Training to deliver constructive feedback should prepare SPs to avoid generalisations, global feedback, or references to things that did not occur in the encounter being discussed. The SP can specifically refer to the relationship between discrete student behaviours and their individual feeling in response to that behaviour. At no time is it useful for the SP to become a content expert lecturer or to replace the tutor. Volunteers may be trained to serve as simulated or standardised patients (Collins & Harden 1998), but in many cases this work should be performed by individuals who are compensated and accountable for the quality of the work that they perform.

Patient-instructors

Patients with stable clinical features have always played an important part in teaching clinical skills. They should be asked to participate by a third party and not by their care provider with the understanding that they will not receive personal medical care or advice as a result of participation in this educational event and are participating with informed consent in this capacity.

Patients with appropriate educational backgrounds and extensive training and supervision have been used as 'patient-instructors' (Dacre & Fox 2000, Wykurz 1999). These adjunct educators represent a saving of both costs and faculty and can provide a standardised approach to a specific protocol from a person who is trained to focus on delivery of this particular information. The patient-instructor serves as both demonstrator and model and can do so using only themselves or with a colleague patient-instructor working in a team. This method is thought by some to have made an important contribution to the de-objectification of the patient in the physical examination process. They also offer the advantage of being able to provide direct feedback on accuracy and efficacy of student performance as the student is learning, and to suggest effective methods of communication during stressful and intimate examinations, including, for example, using lay language, interpreting medical jargon and avoiding suggestive language when speaking with a patient

Their role may be substantially extended if they are rehearsed in several modifications of their history as part of the regular teaching sessions.

Ancillary technology

A CSC will require equipment such as semi-permanently and discreetly installed pan-tilt zoom cameras, one-way mirrors, high quality microphones and computer ports inside and outside of rooms. These must be easily accessible for adjustment, repair and replacement as needed. When planning wiring design consider the trends toward wireless operations for computerisation of patient records and the demands of large-scale standardised patient programmes. You may wish to include the capability for overhead announcements and in-room phones and intercoms to facilitate the conduct of timed events. Some CSCs use keycard entry to control camera operation and room utilisation.

It is desirable to build in computers with full sound and video capability for the learner, simulated patient, tutor/remote observer in any formative or summative objective structured clinical examination (OSCE) station. Pre-encounter instructions and patient information is delivered to the learner via computer. Software developed specifically for programmes, event delivery and test data management are now available. The learner can utilize a personal digital assistant (PDA) during the patient encounter just as they would in actual practice to refer to appropriate interview questions for a complaint, record patient responses and conduct information searches. In the CSC, the learner returns to a computer station to record a patient note or to respond to questions about the patient. Post-encounter performance reporting and/or scoring can be carried out by the simulated patient using a checklist or PDA. Tutors or other remote observers can observe in real time and overlay a 'comments' soundtrack on a student encounter. This can also be achieved economically by using a dictaphone to provide students with constructive individualised feedback for a post-encounter tutor activity.

The opportunity for video recording of individual student performance is highly rated by students and tutors. Some schools utilise real-time co-reporting of encounter activities using the same, or an adapted checklist to that which is used by the simulated patients, faculty, or by multiple SPs trained to the same case. SP training extensively uses video review for feedback. A computer routed to the cameras (rather than a traditional video monitor) allows the checklist to be seen on-screen alongside the audio-digital video image. This may be useful to demonstrate interrater reliability in completion of the same checklist or to provide accurate data based on real-time monitoring of each encounter as part of a quality assurance programme.

Planners are well advised to consider recording capability for all rooms including treatment/examination, conference, presentation, training and orientation rooms. It might be helpful for the development of tutor skills to review recordings of their conduct of groups or for the tutor to access this to support feedback to a struggling student. Without remote observation capability, quality assurance of tutor and SP delivery of curricular activities is not possible.

Telecommunications

Telecommunication links are particularly valuable in allowing live clinical sessions (e.g. a patient consultation, physical examination, procedural demonstration or operating theatre activity) to be relayed to larger groups of students, in another room or outside the centre. New applications include such events as video-teleconferenced teaching with participation of SPs and video-teleconferenced training of SPs for the purpose of standardisation across different sites. As video-teleconferenced and streaming video consultations to remote and/or rural patient settings become more frequent, there is a greater need for educators to understand how to best prepare learners for the optimal use of this nontraditional resource to benefit their patients. Streaming video is economical as well as practical and is also useful in sharing educational experiences between distant or multiple learning sites. OSCEs with SPs have been conducted using streaming video to serve distant students (Novack et al 2002). SP encounters featuring phone consultations are becoming frequent as we acknowledge the important triage functions that take place by telephone.

Computers and the internet

The role of the computer to enhance clinical skills learning has yet to be clarified, but its value has been demonstrated in interactive PC-based tutorials and formative assessment programmes.

The strength of this teaching medium lies in its ability to provide instant interactive feedback involving a range of rich media resources, for example high quality medical images, video files, sound clips and access to the internet and its attendant resources (see chapter 22, Virtual learning environments).

Educational strategies

The trend toward increasing demands for practice and research have reduced the dedicated time available for teaching. In many North American programmes this has led to the augmentation of traditional faculty educationalists with personnel such as standardised patient specialists who are sometimes called standardised patient trainers or educators. These educational specialists are faculty/staff who co-design and implement educational programmes in conjunction with educator faculty. At its best, this scheme makes the most of what time educators can devote and uses them to advantage as mentors functioning in a structured and standardised programme of events experienced by the learner. Ideally, this is considered a faculty level role, with the primary responsibilities of this specialist being to collaborate in event design, to develop educational materials and to manage implementation. They have particular responsibility for appropriate recruitment and training of simulated and standardized patients and for quality assurance of all aspects of the educational activities in the centre that utilise SPs. In large, ambitious programmes, that seek to use dedicated facilities during day, evening and weekend educational events, a staff of several educational specialists supported by several administrative and event operations support staff is required to maintain high standards of programme administration and reliable performance of standardised behaviour by simulated patients and faculty.

Curricular activities that build upon the basis of the one-on-one simulated encounter include self-assessment exercises and checklists; traditional post-encounter challenges, such as writing a case history or completing a questionnaire related to the encounter; constructive feedback from different sources; group discussion of a commonly experienced case presentation; group debriefing, and individualised student learning prescriptions developed from formative OSCE participation. A commonly experienced case presentation can take place with simultaneous mounting of multiple iterations of the same case (Hall et al 2004) or by serial rotation through the same group of cases as with an OSCE.

Videotaping or digital recording of one-on-one simulation is a basis for later educational methods that will elaborate learning. Recorded events can be reviewed, rated, discussed and analysed as desired by the tutor, student, SP and/or SP trainer. Quality assurance of standardised behaviour among simulated patients or faculty is essential to development of successful programming at the centre. Without the use of recording, opportunities for faculty-sparing programme development are curtailed. The reliability and validity of reporting and rating methods are called into question.

A collection of prerecorded videos provides a valuable resource for demonstrating aspects of clinical examination.

Traditional faculty, specialist faculty and staff develop instructional materials that can provide specific programmes for targeted learning experiences. Especially useful and faculty-sparing are realistic one-on-one encounters between the learner and a simulated patient, with the additional use of self-assessment instruments and constructive patient, peer and faculty feedback, based on shared simulated experience and remote observation by a tutor.

Examples

Clinical skills teaching may vary from the relatively straightforward didactic demonstration of individual skills to the use of complex, case-based scenarios of which clinical skills learning is an integral component.

Clinical skills teaching embraces the continuum of patient care and can develop in complexity to keep pace with the level of the learner. The usual approach to learning in clinical skills centres involves small-group,

The simulated ward environment . . . gave students their first experience of participating independently in a realistic and safe operational ward setting"

Ker et al 2003

student-centred, interactive sessions (see chapter 7, Learning in small groups) in which tutors act as facilitators rather than information-givers. A typical undergraduate learning session lasts 2 hours and may involve tutors from all the healthcare professions working in an integrated, collaborative manner. Skill acquisition is always in context rather than in isolation. Role playing in loosely structured and relevant scenarios prepare students for subsequent exposure to the 'real thing' in both hospital and community settings (Ker et al 2003).

Example 1   Communication skills

In a plenary session students view two videos illustrating good and bad examples of the doctor–patient interview. In small groups they make notes of the good and bad points in each. They then individually carry out the required history taking and physical examination on a simulated patient. This is videotaped and observed remotely by faculty, peers or other raters. Students then receive written or verbal constructive feedback or formative assessment from these observers. Finally they can review a video of the encounter and reflect on their performance (Dent & Preece 2002).

Example 2   Integrated clinical skills teaching

Each week of the systems-based course is devoted to the study of one core clinical problem. During the 'neck and shoulder pain' week in the musculoskeletal system course, students learn how to take an appropriate history to differentiate between the various possible causes of the presentation. They learn how to examine the neck and shoulder and, during general practice or outpatient attachments, have the opportunity to see a variety of patients with related conditions. In the wards they have opportunities to see pre- and post-operative patients who are having surgery to the shoulder.

Self-assessment opportunities

Peer examination and interview

In communication skills training, for example, structured role playing by students may be a useful experience, particularly prior to exposure to simulated patients. Similarly, in the context of history taking and physical examination, valuable lessons may be learned by allowing the student to assume both the roles of examiner and patient. Cultural competency is one of many curricular themes that can be explored through role play. Experience of peer group activities in one centre (Ledingham & Harden 1998) suggests that once initial reluctance on the part of the students (and some staff) is overcome, the role playing situation is readily accepted and even appreciated.

The attempt should be made to maintain credibility in all assignments. If a role playing task is too absurd, the students will not take the lesson seriously.

One institution uses fourth-year students to portray patient roles and provide feedback to second-year students in a formative OSCE experience

A good clinical skills centre tutor will seek to:
- arrive for the teaching session in good time (preferably 15 minutes before the session starts)
- be suitably prepared (tutor instructions are invariably provided beforehand)
- behave courteously to colleagues, students and support staff.

A meeting with clinical skills centre staff or a visit to the clinical skills centre at least the day before the session generally improves the smooth running of the exercise. Given the involvement of media, machines, SPs and multiple personnel, faculty preparation should go beyond the traditional tutor syllabus and provide extensive hands-on orientation for tutors in the activities that they will facilitate at the centre.

prior to a summative OSCE with SPs. (Sasson et al 1999) Another approach uses self-, peer, faculty and SP remote observation, with checklist recording and rating and verbal feedback, to deliver an accelerated course in health assessment where the number of students outnumber the facilities, SP and budget resources (Gibbons et al 2002).

Staff development

The purchase and use of more sophisticated equipment does not obviate the need for personnel. State-of-the-art facilities require differently qualified and more highly compensated staff than a traditional teaching environment. Among others, CSC staff may include one or more:

- director
- standardised patient specialists
- tutors
- administrative staff
- janitor
- technicians
- computer specialist
- SP recruitment officer.

The effectiveness of simulations in promoting learning can be explained by a variety of learning theories including behaviourism, constructivism, reflective practice, situated learning and activity theory (Bradley & Postlethwaite 2003).

The CSC can nurture a role as a staff development initiator both for its own staff and for clinicians with an interest in teaching.

Clinical skills tutors may be recruited from the various specialties contributing to the course or from individuals with an expressed interest in medical education. They need to be aware of the overall learning outcomes of the course to which they are contributing. Careful consideration must then be given as to how best to address the specific objectives of the clinical teaching session for which they are responsible.

Support mechanisms

The CSC must ensure that it maintains an environment which in every way is supportive of student learning. Students should feel welcome to make use of the CSC for self-directed learning when they can practise procedures either individually or in small groups. If possible one-on-one revision sessions with faculty can sometimes be made available. The CSC is the ideal site for remedial training of students.

Summary

Student training in clinical skills is moving away from exclusive dependence on ad hoc experiences with hospital patients to structured programmes of learning in a CSC. The role of CSCs has continued to expand as they develop the use of a variety of simulated clinical

"The clinician as role model exerts a potent influence – either good or bad"

'Practice makes perfect' is as relevant in the context of clinical skills as with any other group of skills.

environments, a range of simulators being supported by sophisticated ancillary technology.

Simulated and standardised patients are becoming routinely available to facilitate training and in some cases provide constructive feedback. The educational strategies used by CSCs are now being structured to help integrate student learning with other parts of the curriculum, and may be delivered by dedicated skills centre staff and systems-based tutors as well as by simulated or real patients.

The role of the CSC in staff development is still to be fully developed.

Finally, in this supportive environment, students can practise communication and examination skills without embarrassment or negative criticism and without interfering with patient management or wellbeing.

References

Bradley P, Postlethwaite K 2003 Simulation in clinical learning Medical Education 37 (S1): 1–5

Chin D, Morphet J, Coady E, Davidson C 1997 Assessment of cardiopulmonary resuscitation in the membership examination of the Royal College of Physicians. Journal of the Royal College of Physicians 31:198–201

Collins J P, Harden R M 1998 AMEE Medical Education Guide No.13: real patients, simulated patients and simulations in clinical examination. Medical Teacher 20:508–521.

Dacre J E, Fox R A 2000 How should we be teaching our undergraduates? Annals of Rheumatoid Disease 59:662–667

Dacre J, Nicol M, Holroyd D, Ingram D 1996 The development of a clinical skills centre. Journal of the Royal College of Physicians 30:318–324

Dent J 2002 Adding more to the pie: the expanding activities of the clinical skills centre. Journal of the Royal Society of Medicine 95:406–410

Dent J, Preece PE 2002 What is the impact on participating students of real-time video monitoring of their consultation skills? British Journal of Educational Technology 33:349–351

General Medical Council 1993 Tomorrow's doctors. General Medical Council, London

Gibbons S W, Adamo G, Hawkins R et al 2002 Clinical evaluation in advanced practice nursing education: using standardized patients in health assessment. Journal of Nursing Education 41:215–221

Gordon M S, Issenberg S B, Mayer J W, Felner J M 1999 Developments in the use of simulators and multimedia computer systems in medical education. Medical Teacher 21:32–36

Hall M J, Adamo G, McCurry L et al 2004 Use of standardized patients to enhance a psychiatry clerkship. Academic Medicine 79:28–31

Ker J, Mole L, Bradley P 2003 Early introduction to interprofessional learning: a simulated ward environment Medical Education 37:248–255

Kneebone R, Kidd J, Nestel D et al 2002 An innovative model for teaching and learning clinical procedures. Medical Education 36:628–634

Ledingham I M, Harden R M 1998 Twelve tips for setting up a clinical skill teaching facility. Medical Teacher 20:503–507

Maran N J, Glavin RJ 2003 Low– to high-fidelity simulators – a continuum of medical education? Medical Education 37 (S1):22–28

Novack D H, Cohen D, Peitzman S J et al 2002 A pilot test of WebOSCE: a system for assessing trainees' clinical skills via teleconference. Medical Teacher 24:483–487

Pugh C M, Youngblood P 2002 Development and validation of assessment measures for a newly developed physical examination simulator. Journal of the American Medical Information Association 9:554–556

Sasson V A, Blatt B C, Kallenberg G et al 1999 Teach one do one better. Academic Medicine 74:932–937

Simpson JG, Furnace J, Crosby J et al 2002 The Scottish doctor – learning outcomes for the medical undergraduate in Scotland: a foundation for competent and reflective practitioners. Medical Teacher 24:136–143

Williams S, Dale J, Gluckman E, Willesley A 1997 Senior house officers' work related stressors, psychological distress and confidence in performing clinical tasks in accident and emergency: a questionnaire study. BMJ 314:713–718

Wykurz G 1999 Patients in medical education: from passive participants to active partners. Medical Education 33:634–636

Further reading

Wahlstrom O, Sanden I, Hammar M 1997 Multiprofessional education in the medical curriculum. Medical Education 31:425–429

Chapter 9
Bedside teaching

J. A. Dent

Introduction

The clinical application of knowledge and the clinical skills required for practice have traditionally been acquired by apprenticeship in a hospital ward. Fundamental to this experience has been the consultant-teaching ward round, but this has not been without its shortcomings. Students are motivated by the stimulus of clinical contacts but may feel academically unprepared or inexperienced in the learning style required in an unfamiliar environment (Seabrook 2004). Late starts, cancellations and inappropriate comments may discourage and alienate students so that this valuable resource is not used to maximum advantage. In addition, the smaller number of in-patients suitable for teaching purposes and the increased size of the student group attending put further pressure on all resources and on the curriculum timetable for ward-based teaching.

Despite these problems ward-based teaching provides an optimal opportunity for the demonstration and observation of physical examination, communication skills and interpersonal skills and for role modelling an holistic approach to patient care. Not surprisingly bedside teaching and medical clerking were deemed the most valuable methods of teaching by a survey of medical students (Ward et al 1997). Nevertheless, the role of bedside teaching has been declining in medical schools since the early 1960s from 37% to 16% (LaCombe 1997) as interest in clinical acumen declines with the rise in popularity of technology, imaging and laboratory investigations.

The 'learning triad'

Ward-based teaching brings together the 'learning triad' of patient, student and tutor.

Patients

Direct contact with patients is important for the development of clinical reasoning, communication skills, professional attitudes and empathy (Spencer et al 2000). Although it is valuable for junior students initially to have access to simulated patients who will provide valuable experience of normal anatomy and physiology, it is necessary at some stage for students to have teaching with patients in clinical situations.

"To study the phenomena of disease without books is to sail an uncharted sea whilst to study books without patients is not to go to sea at all"

Sir William Osler (1849–1919) quoted by Nair et al 1997

"Most medical students are taught by a system of negative reinforcement in the form of sarcastic remarks and derogatory comments"

Newton 1987

"Bedside teaching is the only site where history taking, physical examination, empathy and a caring attitude can be taught and learnt by example"

Nair et al 1997

"Learners think that BST [bedside teaching] is an effective method for teaching professional skills and that most patients enjoy it"

Nair et al 1997

Seven roles for analysing good clinical teaching:
- medical expert
- communicator
- collaborator
- manager
- advocate
- scholar
- professional.

Prideaux et al 2000

Patients should be invited to participate without coercion and have the opportunity to decline to take part without feeling intimidated. Formal documentation of informed consent to participate in educational events may be required in some centres. Patients should be adequately briefed so that they know what will be expected of them, feel a part of the discussion and even give feedback to students afterwards. The majority then enjoy the experience and feel they have helped the students to learn. Concerns about breach of confidentiality and about provoking increased anxiety have been shown to be unfounded (Nair et al 1997). Depending on the model of ward teaching to be used a variety of patients will be required for varying lengths of time but consideration should be given to patients' needs and the possibility that phlebotomists, radiographers and visitors may also need to see them.

Students

Between two and five students is quoted as the optimal number for bedside teaching. They must be appropriately dressed with white coats and name badges. They should expect to behave professionally on the ward in a manner appropriate for student doctors, introducing themselves to staff and patients and clearly stating the purpose of their visit.

Before beginning, students should be briefed so that they understand the purpose of the session and the goals to be achieved. Any warnings about the patient conditions to be seen should be given and checks made on students' level of initial understanding. When reflecting on their experiences students have found ward-based teaching the most valuable way of developing clinical skills. However, initially, some may feel intimidated by an unfamiliar environment and the proximity of nursing staff and be embarrassed when putting personal questions to a stranger. In addition they may feel anxious if unsure of their knowledge base or clinical abilities and fearful of consultant criticism of their inadequacies (Moss & McManus 1992). As a result some students position themselves towards the back of the group round the bedside to avoid participation while more confident colleagues monopolise conversations with patients and tutors. An observant tutor is required to redress the balance and ensure that all students participate and that anxieties are allayed.

Tutors

Tutors for ward-based teaching may be consultant staff, junior hospital doctors (Busan et al 2003), nurses, trained patients or student peers. Kilminster et al (2001) found that a specialised ward-based teacher helped students in developing history taking and examination skills.

Whether they acknowledge it or not tutors are powerful role models for students, especially for those in the early years of the course. It is therefore important that they demonstrate appropriate knowledge, skills and attitudes. Prideaux and colleagues (2000) describe good clinical teaching as providing role models for good practice, making good practice visible and explaining it to trainees.

Appropriate attitude

Tutors responsible for timetabled ward teaching must arrive punctually, introduce themselves to the students and demonstrate an enthusiastic approach to the session. A negative impression at this stage will have an immediate negative effect on the students' attitude and on the value of the session. Tutors must show a professional approach to the patients and interact appropriately with them and the students.

All those involved in ward teaching bring a different perspective of patient care which is valuable for student learning. Sometimes they will have received no specific preparation for the teaching session and may not know how any particular session fits into the totality of the students' clinical experience at a particular stage of the course. Staff development courses on material are important to help these enthusiastic tutors (Dent & Davis 2004, Ker & Dent 2002). Tutors' individual approaches to clinical examination will also differ as examination technique may not be standardised within the medical school. While it may be of benefit for more confident students to observe a variety of different approaches to clinical skills, weaker ones will find this lack of consistency confusing. Ideally, tutors should be briefed so that they are familiar with the approach to physical examination taught in the clinical skills centre and with the levels of expertise required of students at the various stages of the medical course.

Appropriate knowledge

Experienced clinical teachers are soon able to assess both the patient's diagnosis and requirements as well as the students' level of understanding. This ability to link clinical reasoning with instructional reasoning enables them to quickly adapt the clinical teaching session to the needs of the students (Irby 1992).

Six domains of knowledge have been described that are applied by an effectively functioning clinical tutor (Irby 1994):

- Knowledge of medicine – involving integrated background knowledge of basic sciences, clinical sciences and clinical experience
- Knowledge of patients – a familiarity with disease and illness from experience of previous patients
- Knowledge of the context – an awareness of patients in their social context and at their stage of treatment
- Knowledge of learners – an understanding of the students' present stage in the course and of the curriculum requirements for that stage
- Knowledge of the general principles of teaching, including:
  – getting students involved in the learning process by indicating its relevance
  – asking questions, perhaps using the patient as an example of a problem-solving approach to the condition
  – keeping students' attention by indicating the relevance of the topic to another situation
  – relating the case being presented to broader aspects of the curriculum

"The essential feature is enthusiasm on the part of the teacher"

Rees 1987

If you don't know the answer to a student's question be honest and say so.

You can maintain your relationship with patients while talking to the students by keeping your hand on their shoulder or wrist.

Experienced tutors link
– clinical reasoning with
– instructional reasoning.

"Well, that's something we should both look up this evening"

A senior clinician in answer to a student's question during a teaching ward round

– meeting individual needs by responding to specific questions and providing personal tuition
– being realistic and selective so that relevant cases are chosen
– providing feedback by critiquing case reports, presentations or examination technique
• Knowledge of case-based teaching scripts – the ability to demonstrate the patient as a representative of a certain illness; the specifics of the case are used but added to from other knowledge and experiences in order to make further generalised comments about the condition.

Appropriate skills

If demonstrating clinical tasks to students on the ward tutors must ensure that they are competent in performing them, that they are familiar with any new equipment to be demonstrated and that they do not display inappropriate 'shortcuts'.

The ward

The educational environment of the ward may be affected by many factors (Seabrook 2004) which impact on student behaviour and satisfaction. Often district general hospitals appear more valued than teaching hospitals (Parry et al 2002). However with some thought some simple problems can be avoided.

Ward teaching should not take place when meals, cleaners or visitors are expected. It helps if the staff and patients are expecting the teaching session at a certain time so that X-rays and case notes can be ready and patients do not have to be retrieved from the day room or X-ray department.

The use of a side room for pre- or post-ward round discussion provides a useful alternative venue for discussion once the patients have been seen. Occasionally a member of the nursing staff may be present in the teaching session to add multiprofessional input to the patient care discussion. Stanley (1998) suggests that systematic planning and preparation, especially with increased use of pre- and post-round meetings, would provide more effective and structured training for postgraduate hospital doctors.

A teaching ward round deals with patients not diseases. It develops students' thinking processes and introduces an approach to patients that they will follow for the rest of their working lives as doctors (Rees 1987).

Educational objectives

Many of the educational objectives of the medical curriculum can be experienced to different extents by students at any stage of the course while they are working in the wards:

- Clinical skills. For junior students there are opportunities to become proficient at normal physical examination while more senior students gain practice in eliciting abnormal physical signs.
- Communication skills. Many opportunities exist for students to practise communication skills.
- Clinical reasoning. Students can observe this in practice by junior and senior staff.
- Practical procedures. Venepuncture, bladder catheterisation and cannulation of a peripheral vein are procedures which are readily available on most wards for students to practise.
- Patient investigation and management. There are many opportunities for students to observe and discuss aspects of both of these.
- Data interpretation and retrieval. Interpretation of laboratory reports and accessing scientific papers for reference are examples.
- Professional skills. The observation of both junior and senior doctors in their working relationship with other healthcare professionals should help students develop role models for professional behaviour.
- Transferable skills. Many of the abilities acquired in the ward setting will be of value in other doctor–patient situations.
- Attitude and ethics. It is hoped that appropriate attitudes and ethics can be observed by the students in their ward attachments.

All these aspects can be seen in the context of the patient as an individual rather than in the purely theoretical context presented in lectures. Students should be encouraged to return to the ward in private study time to practise clinical skills further. There is unlikely to be sufficient time for the session to be used formally for formative assessment but opportunities can be used to check on individual students' competencies in small tasks.

Strategies

Planning bedside teaching

A plan of two linked cycles has been described (Cox 1993) to maximise the students' learning from each patient contact. The first, the 'experience cycle', involves student preparation and briefing to ensure that they are aware of what they are going to see and the opportunities available for learning. This is followed by the clinical experience of interacting with their patient which may include discussing the illness, examining physical signs and thinking about management. The 'experience cycle' concludes with debriefing after leaving the patient when the data are seen and interpreted and any misperceptions or misunderstandings are clarified. The 'Experience cycle' maximises the value of time spent with the patients. It is followed by the 'Explanation cycle'. This cycle begins with reflection when students are encouraged to consider their recent clinical interaction in the light of previous experiences. This is done by explication as the clinical experiences are understood at different levels; finally a working

"A good consultant is accessible, approachable and friendly, with the power of a god, the patience of a saint and the sense of humour of an undergraduate"

Lowry 1987

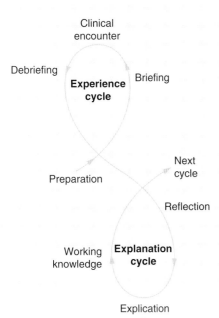

Fig. 9.1 Experience and explanation cycles (redrawn from Cox 1993, with modifications)

knowledge is synthesised which prepares the students for seeing a subsequent patient (see Fig. 9.1).

Logbooks and portfolios

The variety of clinical conditions available for a teaching session at any particular time will inevitably vary so ward-based teaching will of necessity be opportunistic. Some form of documentation is required to ensure that all students see a comparable mix of patients. Logbooks or personal digital assistants (PDAs) can be used to document patients seen and to keep a record of the learning points (Davis & Dent 1994). These can be reviewed periodically and future sessions directed to making good any deficits.

Students' formal documentation of full case presentations can be collated as required and submitted for formative assessment later.

Task-based learning

A list of tasks to be performed or procedures to be observed and carried out is usually a course requirement.

Problem-based learning

The patient's presenting complaint can be used as the focus of a problem-based learning exercise in which basic sciences and clinical sciences can be integrated.

Study guides

A prescribed list of conditions to be seen in the ward may be laid out in the study guide with the learning points to be achieved documented for each.

Models for managing learning in the ward

Shadowing a junior doctor

This model of learning has been formally adopted as part of the final year by some medical schools. Students spend a block of 4 or 6 weeks sharing the work and experiences of a junior doctor. Ideally this takes place in the unit where the students have applied to work once qualified. Opportunities exist to share in carrying out ward tasks, formulating management plans and prescribing.

Patient-centred model

Students attached to a ward for a period of time can be allocated a certain number of patients, each of whom they initially admit and then follow throughout their time in the hospital. They are made responsible for presenting them on ward rounds and should be able to comment on their current investigations, laboratory results and present status. Opportunities exist for practice in examination and communication skills. Patients can be followed for X-ray and to surgery and even visited at home on discharge so the student can assess the impact of illness and convalescence on the patient in the context of their home environment.

Apprenticeship model

The student joins a normal working ward round but does not work as a team member. There are opportunities to observe the input of all those taking part and to practise presentation skills and possibly practical procedures. Students' confidence is increased by interaction with senior doctors and other professionals, by observing the working practice of junior doctors and by seeing patients individually. There may be opportunities to practise decision making. However, if there is no formal teaching the details of the ward round discussion are unlikely to be understood and weaker students may be ignored. Students may find that the only activities available for them are mundane ward chores although others may have opportunities to perform some practical procedures.

Grand rounds

In this traditional model a student group either joins the end of an extensive consultant-led ward round or a side room presentation, which may include other senior clinicians, trainees, junior doctors and other healthcare professionals such as nurses and therapists. There are opportunities to observe multiprofessional interaction and a variety of patients. However, students remain remote from the decision making and are unlikely to understand the issues considered as there may be little opportunity for interaction with clinicians or patients in this model.

Business ward round

This is a challenging environment for both consultant and students. Little time is available for formal teaching, observing student performance or providing feedback (Irby & Bowen 2004). It may be necessary for the clinician to teach at 'different levels' depending on the experience or seniority of others on the ward round.

Teaching ward round

This specially created ward round is aimed at taking students to a small number of selected patients to provide opportunities for them to see physical signs and hear aspects of the case history.

Reserved students may have little opportunity to interact with patients individually compared with more self-confident counterparts, but opportunities to ask and be asked questions exist to a varying degree:

- Demonstrator model (see Fig. 9.2). The clinical tutor demonstrates aspects of the case history and physical examination to the students
- Tutor model (see Fig. 9.3). The clinical tutor stands to the side and critiques each student in turn as they enquire into aspects of the history and carry out aspects of the physical examination.
- Observer model (see Fig. 9.4). The clinical tutor distances him or herself from the student–patient interaction and observes a single student or pair of students in a longer portion of history taking or examination, providing feedback to them all at the end as they discuss their findings and clinical interpretation.

"Excellent clinical teachers model respectful, empathic and professional interactions with their patients"

(Irby & Bowen 2004)

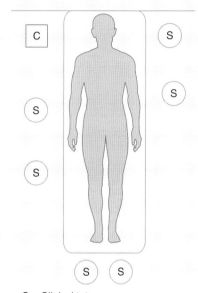

C = Clinical tutor

S = Student

Fig. 9.2 The demonstrator model

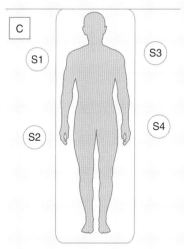

C = Clinical tutor

S = Student

Fig. 9.3 The tutor model

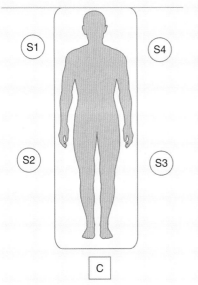

C = Clinical tutor

S = Student

Fig. 9.4 The observer model

⟪ *"a training ward seems to be a very efficient way of improving the ability to work as a team with real patients, and is an inspiring and efficient means of obtaining these skills which . . . are essential in future professional work"*

Wahlstrom et al 1997

Report-back model

Working singly or in pairs, students take a history and examination without supervision and subsequently report back to the tutor in a tutorial room or side room to present the case and receive feedback on content and delivery.

Opportunities are given for students to practise their communication skills in their own time and to demonstrate their presentation skills and knowledge of the case but their bedside technique has been unsupervised so no feedback on this can be given.

Clinical conference

A patient from the ward is presented in a side room at a conference of senior clinicians which students attend. Diagnostic and management problems are discussed by the group once the patient has left. Students have the opportunity to observe the multifaceted management of difficult cases and the spectrum of professional opinion which may be displayed.

Training ward

In Linköping a whole orthopaedic ward has been used as a multiprofessional training ward to provide students with extended opportunities for supervised patient care (Wahlstrom et al 1997).

Summary

Ward-based teaching offers unique opportunities for student learning which, for a variety of reasons, are becoming less efficiently utilised than previously. To attain maximum benefit from ward-based teaching, patients, students and tutors must each be appropriately prepared and the educational objectives must be understood. Various strategies can be used to advantage in both the planning and organisation of ward teaching. A variety of styles of ward-based teaching have been described, illustrating the advantages and disadvantages of each for the students involved.

References

Busan J O, Scherpbier A J J A, van der Vleuten C P M, Essed E G M 2003 The perceptions of attending doctors of the role of residents as teachers of undergraduate clinical students. Medical Education 37:241–247

Cox K 1993 Planning bedside teaching. Medical Journal of Australia 158:493–495

Davis M H, Dent J A 1994 Comparison of student learning in the out-patient clinic and ward round. Medical Education 28:208–212

Dent J A, Davis M H 2004 Getting started . . . a practical guide for clinical tutors. University of Dundee, Centre for Medical Education, Dundee

Irby D M 1992 How attending physicians make instructional decisions when conducting teaching rounds. Academic Medicine 67:630–638

Irby D M 1994 What clinical teachers in medicine need to know. Academic Medicine 69:333–342

Irby D M Bowen J L 2004 Time-efficient strategies for learning and performance. The Clinical Teacher 1:23–28

Ker J S, Dent J A 2002 Information-sharing strategies to support practising clinicians in their clinical teaching roles. Medical Teacher 24:437–446

Kilminster S M, Delmotte A, Frith H et al 2001 Teaching in the new NHS: the specialised ward based teacher. Medical Education 35:437–443

Kroenke K, Omori D M, Landry F J, Ludcey C R 1997 Bedside teaching. Southern Medical Journal 90:1069–1074

LaCombe M A 1997 On bedside teaching. Annals of Internal Medicine 126:217–220

Lowry S 1987 What is a good consultant? As the junior doctor sees it. British Medical Journal 294:1601

Moss F, McManus I C 1992 The anxieties of new clinical students. Medical Education 26:17–20

Nair B R, Coughlan J L, Hensley M J 1997 Student and patient perspectives on bedside teaching. Medical Education 31:341–346

Newton D F 1987 What is a good consultant? 'A worm's eye view'. British Medical Journal 295:106–107

Parry J, Mathers J, Al-Fares A et al 2002 Hostile teaching hospitals and friendly district general hospitals: final-year students' views on clinical attachment locations. Medical Education 36:1131–1141

Prideaux D, Alexander H, Bower A et al 2000 Clinical teaching: maintaining an educational role for doctors in the new health care environment. Medical Education 34:820–826

Rees J 1987 How to do it: take a teaching ward round. British Medical Journal 295:424–425

Seabrook MA 2004 Clinical students' initial reports of the educational climate in a single medical school. Medical Education 38:659–669

Spencer J, Blackmore D, Heard S et al 2000 Patient-orientated learning: a review of the role of the patient in the education of medical students. Medical Education 34:851–857

Stanley P 1998 Structuring ward rounds for learning: can opportunities be created? Medical Education 32:239–243

Wahlstrom O, Sanden I, Hammar M 1997 Multiprofessional education in the medical curriculum. Medical Education 31:425–429

Ward B, Moody G, Mayberry J F 1997 The views of medical students and junior doctors on pre-graduate clinical teaching. Postgraduate Medical Journal 73:723–725

Chapter 10
Ambulatory care teaching

J. A. Dent

Introduction

Well-documented changes in healthcare delivery have focused attention on learning opportunities to be found in ambulatory care settings. There is now a large volume of literature on the development of teaching initiatives in this area for both undergraduates and postgraduates and in both medicine and nursing (Irby 1995, Sullivan et al 2000).

Why teach in ambulatory care?

The ambulatory care setting offers a variety of clinical situations and a range of common clinical conditions not seen in inpatient care. The role of other healthcare professionals and support services can more readily be appreciated here as the patient is seen in an environment more closely resembling their home situation and more closely linked with primary care. However, although large numbers of patients may be present, suitable teaching space and additional teaching staff may not be available.

Where can teaching take place in ambulatory care?

A number of frequently underutilised venues may be available:

- general outpatient clinics
- specialist or tertiary referrals clinics
- multiprofessional clinics where staff from a variety of disciplines see patients together, e.g. hand clinic
- combined clinics where different specialists consult together on a combined management problem, e.g. rheumatology clinic
- 'drop-in' clinics where patients may seek advice from a variety of healthcare workers, e.g. diabetic, foot clinics
- accident and emergency department
- radiology and imaging suites
- clinical investigation unit, e.g. endoscopy suite
- day surgery unit
- physiotherapy and departments of other professions allied to medicine
- self-help group facilities or social services departments.

Finally a dedicated ambulatory care teaching centre (ACTC) can be created where student–patient interaction can take place in a nonthreat-

---

"More medicine is now practiced in the ambulatory setting, making the in-patient arena less representative of the actual practice of medicine and a less desirable place for students to glean the fundamentals of clinical care and problem solving than in the past"

Fincher & Albritton 1993

"Teaching should follow the patient"

Lawson & Moss 1993

Twelve tips for setting up an ambulatory care teaching centre:
Design
1 Allow development time.
2 Integrate curriculum needs and identify organisational constraints.
3 Identify interested parties and their strategic role as a committee.
4 Find suitable accommodation.
5 Secure a budget.
6 Acquire suitable resources and equipment.
Implementation
7 Recruit and train enthusiastic staff.
8 Evolve an implementation function for the steering group.
9 Build up a bank of patients.
10 Implement a teaching plan.
Evaluation
11 Develop a multifaceted evaluation process.
12 Develop a research and development function for the steering group.

(Dent et al 2001b)

ening environment, and where sufficient time and appropriate supervision can be made available to maximise learning opportunities (Dent et al 2001b).

When should ambulatory care teaching be timetabled?

Teaching in the ambulatory care setting may take place throughout the curriculum. In the earlier years, when communication and examination skills are still being developed, visits to the ACTC act as a bridge between practice with simulated patients and manikins in the clinical skills centre and clinical exposure in a routine outpatient clinic. In the later clinical years, when more extensive clinical experience is required, students can either be timetabled for periodic visits or for extended attachments to different venues in ambulatory care.

What educational objectives can be met?

In ward-based teaching, the acquisition of expertise in certain competencies or outcomes is usually emphasised:

- knowledge
- clinical skills
- clinical reasoning
- patient management
- investigations
- information handling.

In the outpatient setting patients are seen nearer the context of their own social circumstances and are therefore considered to be retaining individual responsibility for their own health. Their attendance in the clinic is part of a continuum of the management of their illness. Opportunities are therefore available for students to practise additional competencies or encounter further outcomes (Stearns & Glasser 1993):

- continuity of care
- context of care
- resource allocation
- health education
- responsibility.

There may also be opportunities to practise various practical procedures.

How to facilitate learning in ambulatory care

Logbooks

It is important to organise the content of an ambulatory care session so that the educational objectives required by the curriculum can be met. Strategies are required to regulate the type of medical conditions

Be sure you know the educational objectives which the students should be able to achieve. Identify which of these can be illustrated by the learning opportunities your clinic can provide.

The *EPITOME* logbook is used by students to record:
Enquiry into symptoms
Physical examination
Interpretation of investigations
Technical procedure undertaken
Options of diagnosis
Management
Education of the patient.
Cases recorded in this way come to *epitomise* the clinical condition to be learned by the student.

(Dent & Davis 1995)

Ensure that students recognize opportunities to relate the educational objectives of their course to the experiences provided in the outpatient setting.
Do they have a logbook to complete?

"capture the teachable moment"

Bowling 1993

"The variability and potentially worrisome gaps in the students' experiences in the ambulatory care settings studied are probably representative of students' experiences in such settings"

Gruppen et al 1993

Decide which model you are going to use in your clinic depending on how many rooms are available for you to use and how many members of staff are available to help with the clinic.
Don't be afraid to change models during the clinic to vary the session for the students and yourself.

"It appears that in most cases students have been fitted into existing clinics or patterns of teaching, with insufficient effort given to achieving the maximal educational benefits of the student"

Feltovich et al 1987

to be seen. A structured logbook (Dent & Davis 1995) may be used to list the core clinical problems to be seen during the attachment and to document the student activity and learning achieved with each patient contact.

Task-based learning

A list of prescribed tasks to be carried out in the ambulatory setting are given to the students. These may include:

- participate in consultation with the attending staff
- interview and examine patient
- review a number of new radiographs with the radiologist.

Tasks for future learning can then be built around each task.

Study guides

A two-part study guide described by Mires and colleagues (1998) integrates learning and assessment by asking students to write a structured case report after seeing their patient.

Learning contracts

These have been used to promote adult learning styles in programmes in ambulatory care for postgraduate doctors and degree course nursing students (Chan & Chien 2000, Parsell 1997)

Managing student–patient interactions in a routine outpatient clinic

A variety of management models can be used to ensure students maximise the opportunities to attain educational objectives without disrupting the delivery of the patient service. Students may take part to different extents ranging from full participation to a purely observational role but without satisfactory models their interaction with patients may become either unrestricted and prolong the clinic or inhibited and lead to passivity. Regan-Smith and colleagues (2002) describe restructuring outpatient clinics to allow learners who have already had training to see patients booked in parallel sessions with the tutor's patients. Others report a week's attachment in ambulatory care combining didactic teaching and experiential learning (Frye et al 1998).

The choice of teaching model used depends to some extent on the number of rooms and staff available and on the number of students but in each model the student should be eased away from passive observation towards active learning and participation.

One student, one clinician

'Sitting-in' model
This model works well if there is only one student, if the student is inexperienced in clinical skills or if the clinic is a specialist or multidisciplinary one.

An individual student's requirements are met by one-to-one teaching and students can interact confidently with the clinician and patients. However, student–patient interaction may become limited if the clinician conducts the interview without involving the student while a reserved student may feel vulnerable in this setting and participate minimally (see Fig. 10.1).

Apprenticeship model

A more senior student assumes the role of the clinician and interviews the patient while the tutor acts as observer.

Active student–patient interaction is provided which reinforces the learning experience. Some students may feel intimidated when performing under observation, and aspects of the consultation may have to be repeated by the tutor if relevant points have been overlooked. The duration of the clinic may be prolonged.

Team-member model

If a separate room is available the student can interview and examine a patient alone, before presenting the findings when joined by the clinician or when reporting back to the main consulting room. The student has freedom to interview and examine the patient without constraints and the clinician can proceed with the remainder of the clinic as usual. However, the student will miss other patients attending in the meantime.

Several students, one clinician

It becomes more difficult to organise teaching in a routine outpatient clinic when several students are present.

Grandstand model

Often four or more students are in the consulting room together and crowd around the clinician in an attempt to observe and hear the consultation. Interaction with both patient and clinician is limited as patients feel threatened by the large audience and the clinician's interaction with the patient may also be inhibited.

Supervising model

If several rooms are available, the clinician can select a patient for each student to see individually in a separate room. After a suitable time, during which the clinician can see other patients, it is possible to go to each room in turn to hear each student report on their interview (see Fig. 10.2). The students have time and space to interview and examine their patient at their own pace and benefit from individual feedback on their performance. However, only a limited number of patients are seen by any one student and their time may be wasted while waiting for their turn. The clinician's time is heavily occupied hearing the presentations from each student so inevitably the clinic is prolonged.

Report-back model

Patients are distributed to students as described above, but at an appointed time each student returns to the main consulting room to present their patient in turn. Students have time and space to interview

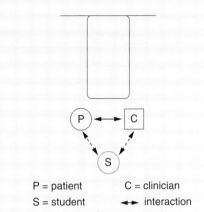

P = patient   C = clinician
S = student   ↔ interaction

Fig. 10.1 'Sitting-in' model: student–clinician and student–patient interaction is variable

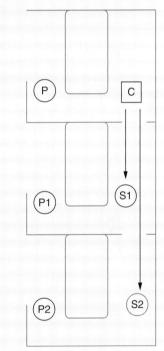

Fig. 10.2 Supervising model: students practise consultations under supervision

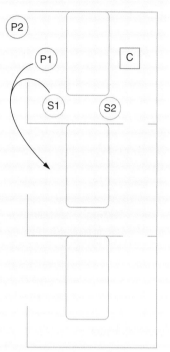

Fig. 10.3 Breakout model: students see patients individually after consultation

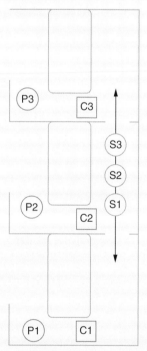

Fig. 10.4 Shuttle model: students see interesting patients but have little opportunity to relate to them

and examine their patient at their own pace and subsequently see something of several other patients. Unfortunately patients may have to wait twice, first to be seen by the student and secondly for the presentation to the clinician.

Breakout model

All the students sit-in with the clinician and observe the whole consultation. This model is particularly appropriate with inexperienced students or in a specialist clinic when particular clinical skills can be demonstrated. Each student then takes a patient in turn to interview or examine at their own pace in another room. Laboratory or radiological request forms may be completed at this time and side-room procedures observed. The clinic can be kept to time as the clinician is saved from completing routine forms. The students have opportunities to interview or examine patients individually and to practise transferable skills. Students see something of most patients attending but miss others while occupied with their own (see Fig. 10.3)

Several students, several clinicians

If two clinicians are available the task of organising students becomes easier.

Division and 'flip/flop' models

The student group can be divided between the clinicians in the clinic who then follow the 'sitting-in' or 'grandstand' models as before and interchange the group at half time. In this model students may see a variety of styles of clinical practice.

Shuttle model

The clinicians see patients simultaneously as usual and call the students in to see selected cases as they present (see Fig. 10.4). This model maintains student involvement in the clinic and interesting cases are not missed. There may be insufficient time for individual student–patient interaction as patients are often only seen as 'demonstrations'.

Tutor model

If several rooms are available the student group may remain with one clinician who may then use any of the previous models as appropriate for the abilities of the students attending. Selected patients are seen for teaching while the remainder attend the other clinicians present. Opportunity now exists for students to see only appropriate, selected patients and the tutor is freed from the time constraints of the routine clinic and can concentrate on teaching.

Managing student–patient interactions in an ambulatory care teaching centre

A specific area in the outpatient department can be developed as an ACTC. This provides appropriate space and serves as a focus for student contact with both patients and the other members of the healthcare team. Appropriate space should be available for small group activities, for individual student–patient interviews (with or without observation by the tutor) and for patient-demonstrations by other healthcare workers. In this protected environment privacy is guaranteed and students feel comfortable to practise and make mistakes free from embarrassment or time constraints.

Supplementary resources which can be made available in the ACTC include abbreviated or constructed case notes for the invited patients attending, laboratory reports, images, videos and equipment for practising practical procedures.

The tutor required to coordinate the session may follow any of the previous models for managing student–patient interactions, and students may be interchanged between different tutors supervising various activities such as practice at history taking, examination or patient demonstration. A store of videotapes to illustrate communication skills and clinical examination provides a useful backup resource.

Managing students in the day surgery unit (DSU)

Although currently underutilised attachments to day surgery units can provide opportunities for students to interact with patients according to the familiar inpatient ward approach or to a skills-based approach (Seabrook et al 1997, 1998). As well as providing experience in general to the students, preoperative assessment and a variety of minor surgical conditions will be seen which are not now managed as inpatient procedures. Experiences in diagnosis, theatre technique, simple operations and postoperative care can be encountered in a multiprofessional environment.

As the numbers of patients attending is usually large, and patients are usually otherwise well, it is relatively easy to structure a teaching session to maximise the educational objectives to be achieved. Various programmes have been described (O'Driscoll et al 1998, Seabrook et al 1998) which may be implemented without compromise to patient care (Rudkin et al 1997). Twelve tips for developing a clinical teaching programme in a DSU have been described (Dent 2003).

Who is available for teaching?

Patients

Referred patients model
Appropriate patients can be invited to visit the ACTC after their outpatient consultation. Clinical histories or signs relevant to the students' stage in the curriculum can then be demonstrated by the tutor in the 'grandstand' format, or students may be given the opportunity to interview patients either independently or under supervision as in the 'report back' or 'supervising' models. Learning opportunities can be developed to focus on particular educational objectives.

The cooperation of clinicians and nurses working in adjacent clinics is required if patients are to be referred for teaching, and patients need to be willing both to be seen by students and to add further unexpected time

"Medical education in general is characterised by the paradox of students' need to learn by trial and error without the luxury and opportunity of making mistakes"

Woolliscroft & Schwenk 1989

Twelve tips for developing a clinical teaching programme in a day surgery unit (DSU):
Preparation
1 Identify the learning objectives that students can achieve in the DSU.
2 Secure institutional support and form an implementation/steering group representing all parties involved
3 Discuss implications, expectations and limitations with DSU staff and tutors.
4 Identify a method for selecting appropriate patients.
5 Identify space for student–patient consultations.
6 Reserve space in a skills training unit.
7 Provide staff development opportunities.
Delivery
8 Provide a study guide/logbook.
9 Employ a DSU-based tutor/supervisor.
10 Provide opportunities for student reflection, tuition and assessment.
Evaluation
11 Evaluate feedback from students, tutors and DSU staff.
12 Discuss research and development opportunities with all parties involved.

(Dent 2003)

"Many patients have actually enjoyed their interactions with students and have been glad to take part in their education"

Krackov et al 1993

"Curriculum-based patient distribution is an administrative intervention at the onset of training that creates patient panels specifically directed towards the educational needs of residents"

Brush & Moore 1994

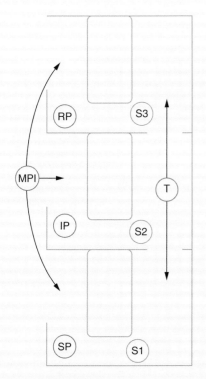

SP = simulated patient
IP = invited patient
RP = referred patient
T = tutor
MPI = multiprofessional input

Fig. 10.5 Ambulatory care teaching centre (ACTC) model

to their outpatient visit. There is little control on the nature of the patients referred and their complaints may be inappropriate for the students' stage of learning so that it may be difficult for the tutor to utilise them efficiently. If no patients are referred the model cannot work and back-up resources are required.

Invited patients model

Patients with good histories or stable clinical signs, or those who have already taken part in teaching sessions, are invited to join a 'bank' of clinical volunteers willing to attend on future occasions. In a systems-based course patients with relevant conditions can be invited at the appropriate time (Brush & Moore 1994).

In this model a patient can be guaranteed to be present at the beginning of the session. The tutor has therefore had time in advance to select a management model for the session and to prepare the content for maximal educational advantage. The same rules of confidentiality of patient data and medical information apply as for a patient seen in other clinical settings.

Selected patients

New patients with appropriate conditions who appear to have uncomplicated histories are chosen from the GP referral letters for outpatient appointments. Patients are advised that they have been appointed to attend a teaching clinic and that although they will be seen and treated by a specialist there will be students present and their appointment may take longer than usual. They can be asked to consent to this arrangement before attending.

Simulated patients

Occasionally simulated patients can be introduced amongst the real patients. Working from a previously arranged script, these volunteers can provide the students with opportunities to practise a particular competence in such fields as attitudes or ethics in a more realistic environment than the clinical skills centre (see Fig. 10.5; see chapter 8, Clinical skills centre teaching)

Staff available

Programme director for ambulatory care teaching

An administrator, preferably with a background in a healthcare discipline, is required to manage the patient bank, timetable tutors and student sessions and ensure the availability of other resource material required.

Tutors

Tutors with a particular aptitude for clinical teaching and who are not required for a concurrent service commitment should be asked to take a teaching session. Effective teaching is facilitated if this person actively involves students in the learning process and sets a good example of patient care skills. If the philosophy is to teach only factual knowledge designated as being of 'core' importance then a 'content expert' (specialist) is not required. The tutor should be able to direct the students to appropriate educational objectives and use additional learning resources to integrate their learning.

Junior staff

A senior tutor can help junior staff unfamiliar with teaching in this venue by demonstrating the approach to teaching required in the ACTC.

Multiprofessional staff

Other healthcare professionals working in the ambulatory care setting can contribute to the teaching programme so students can have the additional opportunity to observe their contribution to patient care. Possible contributors include:

- nurses
- occupational therapist
- physiotherapist
- dietitian
- speech therapist
- chiropodist
- social worker.

Staff development

Formal staff development sessions may be required to help tutors unfamiliar with the delivery of these sessions or with the educational strategy and outcomes being used. Irby and colleagues (1991) list what is required of teaching staff. Simple instructional brochures can be circulated in advance to brief tutors (Dent & Hesketh 2003, Dent & Preece 2001).

Students

Medical students at different stages of the curriculum can be timetabled to a variety of venues in ambulatory care. Tips to help students prepare for their teaching sessions in an ambulatory setting have been described (Lipsky et al 1999). Student nurses may also benefit from learning opportunities in the ACTC and some sessions there may be structured for multiprofessional learning. Dental students learning aspects of general medicine can also be included.

Advantages of teaching in the ambulatory care setting

The ambulatory care setting provides opportunities for undergraduate teaching which are now less readily available in the inpatient setting:

- A wide range of clinical conditions may be seen.
- There are large numbers of new and return patients.
- Students have the opportunity to experience a multiprofessional approach to patient care.
- Unlike ward teaching, increased numbers of students can be accommodated without exhausting the limited number of suitable patients.

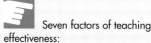 Seven factors of teaching effectiveness:
- knowledge
- organisation and clarity
- enthusiasm
- group instructional skills
- clinical supervision skills
- clinical competence
- modelling professional characteristics.

(Irby et al 1991)

Twelve tips for students to improve their learning in the ambulatory setting:
1 Orientate to the objectives of the session.
2 Share their stage of clinical experience with the tutor.
3 Orientate to the clinical location.
4 Read around the clinical conditions to be seen.
5 Review case notes or summaries provided.
6 Be prepared to propose a diagnosis and management plan.
7 Explain their reasons for these decisions.
8 Seek self-assessment opportunities.
9 Seek feedback time from the tutor.
10 Generalise the learning experience.
11 Reflect on their learning.
12 Identify future learning issues.

(Based on Lipsky et al 1999)

▤ Decide when the teaching session will end!
Announcing this at the beginning will help the students to concentrate and pace themselves. No one can teach or learn indefinitely and the students may have seen as much as they can absorb without staying to the very end of the scheduled session.

◁ *"Ambulatory education is timely and needed, and, to a large degree, ambulatory programmes are being rated highly by the students who participate in them"*

Krackov et al 1993

- Multiprofessional education may be possible in some settings.
- Students' attention can be focused on learning objectives.
- A 'bank' of clinical volunteers can be built up to facilitate the delivery of a systems-sensitive programme.
- Students enjoy this teaching situation and probably prefer it to ward-based teaching (Dent et al 2001a, Lynch et al 1999).
- Medical schools should recognise the role ambulatory care teaching has in relieving pressure on ward-based teaching and provide appropriate resource for its implementation and development.

Summary

The ward setting has become less suitable for clinical teaching as inpatients are now fewer in number and more often acutely ill. Transferring the emphasis of teaching to the ambulatory care setting opens a number of previously underutilised venues for student–patient interaction. In addition a dedicated ACTC may be developed.

The educational objectives to be achieved in ambulatory care are different from those traditionally emphasised in ward-based teaching. Strategies to facilitate learning include a structured logbook and a variety of models to regulate student–patient interaction to maximum advantage.

The educational opportunities available in the ACTC can be developed further by a clinical tutor who can draw not only on the patients attending the clinic, on a bank of invited volunteers and simulated patients but also on colleagues in other healthcare professions who can all contribute to the student's experience of healthcare delivery in the ambulatory care setting.

References

Bowling J R 1993 Clinical teaching in the ambulatory care setting: how to capture the teachable moment. Journal of American Osteopathic Association 93:235–239

Brush A D, Moore T G 1994 Assigning patients according to curriculum: a strategy for improving ambulatory care residency training. Academic Medicine 69:717–719

Chan S W, Chien W T 2000 Implementing contract learning in a clinical context: report on a study. Journal of Advanced Nursing 31:298–305

Dent J A 2003 Twelve tips for developing a clinical teaching programme in a day surgery unit. Medical Teacher 25:364–367

Dent J A, Davis M H 1995 Role of ambulatory care for student–patient interaction: the EPITOME model. Medical Education 29:58–60

Dent J A, Hesketh E A 2003 Developing the teaching instinct: How to teach in an ambulatory care (outpatient) teaching centre. Medical Teacher 25:488–491

Dent J A, Preece P E 2001 'Getting started . . .' in the ambulatory care teaching centre. University of Dundee

Dent J A, Angell-Preece H M, Ball H M-L, Ker J S 2001a Using the ambulatory care teaching centre to develop opportunities for integrated learning. Medical Teacher 23:171–175

Dent J A, Ker J S, Angell-Preece H M, Preece P E 2001b Twelve tips for setting up an ambulatory care (outpatient) teaching centre. Medical Teacher 23:345–350

Feltovich J, Mast T A, Soler N G 1987 A survey of undergraduate internal medicine education in ambulatory care. Proceedings of the Annual Conference of Research into Medical Education 26:137–141

Fincher R M E, Albritton T A. 1993 The ambulatory experience for junior medical students at the Medical College of Georgia. Teaching and Learning in Medicine 5:210–213

Frye E B, Hering P J, Kalina C A et al 1998 Effect of ambulatory care training on third-year medical students' knowledge and skills. Teaching and Learning in Medicine 10:16–20

Gruppen L D, Wisdom K, Anderson D S, Wooliscroft J O 1993 Assessing the consistency and educational benefits of students' clinical experiences during an ambulatory care internal medicine rotation. Academic Medicine 9:674–680

Irby D M 1995 Teaching and learning in ambulatory care settings: a thematic review of the literature. Academic Medicine 70:898–931

Irby D M, Ramsay P G, Gillmore G M, Schaad D 1991 Characteristics of effective clinical teachers of ambulatory care medicine. Academic Medicine 66:54–55

Krackov S K, Packman C H, Regan-Smith M G et al 1993 Perspectives on ambulatory programs: barriers and implementation strategies. Teaching and Learning in Medicine 5:243–250

Lawson M, Moss F 1993 Sharing good practice: innovative learning and assessment. 26 November, 1993, King's Fund Centre

Lipsky M S, Taylor C A, Schnuth R 1999 Microskills for students: twelve tips for learning in the ambulatory care setting. Medical Teacher 21:469–472

Lynch D C, Whitley T W, Basnight L, Patselas T 1999 Comparison of ambulatory and inpatient experiences in five specialties. Medical Teacher 21:594–596

Mires G J, Howie P W, Harden R M 1998 A 'topical' approach to planned teaching and learning using a topic-based study guide. Medical Teacher 20:438–441.

Parsell G 1997 Handbooks, learning contracts and senior house officers: a collaborative enterprise. Postgraduate Medicine 73:395–398

O'Driscoll M C E, Rudkin G E, Carty V M 1998 Day surgery: teaching the next generation. Medical Education 32:390–395

Regan-Smith M, Young W W, Keller A M 2002 An effective and efficient teaching model or ambulatory education. Academic Medicine 77:593–599

Rudkin G E, O'Driscoll M C E, Carty V M 1997 Does a teaching programme in day surgery impact on efficiency and quality care? Australian and New Zealand Journal of Surgery 67:883–887

Seabrook M A, Lawson M, Baskerville P A 1997 Teaching and learning in day surgery units: a UK survey. Medical Education 31:105–108

Seabrook M A, Lawson M, Malster M et al 1998 Teaching medical students in a day surgery unit: adapting medical education to changes in clinical practice. Medical Teacher 20:222–226

Stearns J A, Glasser M 1993 How ambulatory care is different: a paradigm for teaching and practice. Medical Education, 27:35–40

Sullivan M E, Ault G T, Hood D B et al 2000 The standardized vascular clinic: an alternative to the traditional ambulatory setting. American Journal of Surgery 179:243–246

Woolliscroft J O, Schwenk T L 1989 Teaching and learning in the ambulatory setting. Academic Medicine 64:644–648

Chapter 11
In the community
P. Worley

Introduction

Patient care is increasingly moving from hospital wards to community clinics. Recognition of this, and the widening gap between the 'designed' broad-based curriculum advocated by professional bodies and the learning that can be delivered in a tertiary hospital based course, is causing medical schools to search for new sites in which to prepare the next generation of doctors. One solution, for many schools, is community-based medical education (CBME).

What is community-based medical education?

CBME usually refers to medical education that is based outside a tertiary or large secondary level hospital. Community-oriented medical education describes curricula that are based on addressing the health needs of the local community and preparing graduates to work in that community. Community-oriented education is often, quite sensibly, based in the community, but it is possible for large components of such a curriculum to be delivered in a tertiary centre. The medical course at Newcastle University New South Wales, Australia, is a good example of a community-oriented programme largely delivered in tertiary settings.

It may be protested that tertiary hospitals are also 'in the community'. While they are located within the community they are not an integral part of it. Our health system has developed tertiary centres to cater for the high-technology elements of healthcare efficiently and to a high standard. This has resulted in a system that is primarily accountable internally, through processes of audit and peer review; it is not accountable to any one local community as patients are admitted from many different communities, often over significant distances. The centre requires highly developed referral filters to keep people 'out'.

The two principal filters are the primary care system and community-based specialist services. The latter may be consulting medical specialists and the outreach teams from tertiary centres, such as home-based palliative care services. Thus CBME focuses on the care provided to patients both before the decision to refer to a tertiary hospital and after the decision to discharge the patient from such care. In many of these circumstances the traditional doctor–patient relationship will not apply and

Common settings for CBME include:
- general practice
- village/community health centres
- specialist, consulting clinics
- patients' homes
- schools
- factories
- farms
- community fairs
- shopping centres.

"it is possible to cut across the traditional clinical discipline boundaries so entrenched in medical education by teaching in rural general practice but not fundamentally about rural general practice"

(Worley et al 2000a)

patients may be referred to as 'clients' or, even more appropriately, as members of defined local communities.

When discussing CBME in primary care, it is important to understand the difference between the uses of the terms 'primary care' and 'primary healthcare'. The former refers to the first point of contact for members of the community with the health system and will usually not require a referral. Primary healthcare (PHC) concerns a philosophy of healthcare delivery which emphasises health promotion and prevention of illness and advocates strong participation of 'consumers' in healthcare planning. Most CBME curricula are based on a PHC philosophy and are conducted in a primary care setting but it is possible for neither of these two elements to be present, for example, in a rotation based in the private clinic of a psychiatrist with the primary aim of learning advanced psychotherapy.

Uses for CBME

The setting and structure of CBME is principally determined by the aims of the particular component of the curriculum to be delivered. These can usefully be divided into preclinical and clinical aims.

Preclinical aims

CBME is has been used to advantage for learning in such diverse areas as epidemiology, preventative health, public health principles, community development, the social impact of illness and understanding how patients interact with the healthcare system. It is also commonly used for learning basic clinical skills, especially communication skills, and for learning a variety of professional development skills through the mentorship of primary care doctors. These latter aims could also be learned in a tertiary hospital with no particular disadvantage but are often taught in the community because the faculty who have a special interest in these areas, and have been delegated with the responsibility for teaching them, are often general practitioners.

Clinical

The curricular aims of clinical CBME courses usefully fall into three categories.

To learn about general practice

A general practice rotation is the most common clinical CBME attachment and appears in most contemporary medical curricula. It either occurs in a short discrete block of time or in a continuity rotation of perhaps half a day per week for a semester, or even a year or more. There are advantages and disadvantages with both models (Table 11.1).

Whichever structure is chosen, it is essential to have a well planned orientation to the rotation, the practice and the community. This may also involve intensive instruction in relevant clinical skills and in the structure of healthcare delivery in the local community, especially if this is the first such exposure for students. An opportunity to debrief and reflect on their

Table 11.1 Community-based medical education (CBME) general practice attachment

Type of CBME general practice attachment	Advantages	Disadvantages
Discrete block	Immersion experience Allows student to focus entirely on general practice Easy to timetable Intense mentorship relationship Often has a regenerative feeling for the student – 'a change is as good as a holiday' Possibility of using rural and remote practices Easy to conduct evaluation and assessment before and afterwards	Requires accommodation for student Large variation in student experience at different times of the year School and public holidays have significant negative impact Adverse effect on practice income or consulting time Can be tiring for the preceptor
Continuity rotation	Can follow specific patients over time Can see seasonal differences in practice Usually no student accommodation required Can integrate learning with another hospital-based discipline Student can develop a specific role in the practice over time Impact on practice income may be less apparent as only one session per week May appear less tiring to the preceptor as it is spread over a longer period	May be conflicts with activities in the 'feeder' rotation Available sites limited by recurring transport costs and time May be seen by student as less important than the concurrent hospital-based discipline Preceptor may lose interest, leave, get unwell over the extended time period Evaluation often contaminated by variable concurrent learning in hospital rotations

experiences is also helpful to consolidate student learning and conduct course evaluation. These suggestions are relevant to both undergraduate and postgraduate learning about general practice.

To learn about a particular specialty other than general practice
A good example of this type of CBME is the model developed at University College London by Alison Murray (Murray et al 1997). In this internal medicine curriculum students spend 4 weeks in a tertiary hospital and 4 weeks based in a general practice with the specific aim of learning about internal medicine. Evaluation of this model indicates that the student learning at both sites was complementary and students valued the CBME component highly. An interesting randomised cross-over trial,

comparing students who undertook the hospital component first with those who undertook the CBME component first, showed that students learned clinical methods as well in the CBME rotation as they did in the hospital rotation.

In addition to such undergraduate models, postgraduate training programmes in disciplines traditionally taught in hospitals, for example, paediatrics, psychiatry and internal medicine, are creating CBME learning experiences as they seek to appropriately prepare their residents for current and future practice.

To learn multiple disciplines concurrently

This concept takes advantage of the broad patient base in primary care, and, with the exception of the Cambridge model (Oswald 2001), has been situated in rural communities. There are two principal reasons for this that relate to educational opportunities and health policy agendas.

Rural practice, in most countries, has a broader range of patients and involves fewer referrals and the clinicians are more likely to have significant roles in primary care, emergency medicine, obstetrics, and inpatient care. Thus, it is relatively simple for the rural preceptor to give students access to continuity of care through initial diagnosis, investigation, initial management (including as an inpatient) and ongoing care.

Extended rotations of this type have also been shown to be associated with a high number of students choosing a career in rural practice (Verby 1997) and thus have been supported financially by government authorities as a significant strategy with regard to the long-term rural medical workforce. A contemporary example of this CBME model is the Flinders Parallel Rural Community Curriculum (PRCC) (Worley et al 2000a). This programme enables senior medical students to undertake an entire clinical year based in rural general practice learning the disciplines of internal medicine, surgery, paediatrics, women's health, psychiatry, and general practice. Evaluation of this programme has shown that students in the PRCC perform better in examinations than their hospital-based peers (Worley et al 2004).

Based on the Flinders experience, the contrasts between this extended form of CBME and multiple tertiary hospital rotations, combining inpatient and ambulatory outpatient experience, are summarised in Table 11.2.

Practical principles for successful CBME

Although advocates of CBME will talk in passionate terms about its advantages, experienced innovators will rightly point out that success is not guaranteed. It is certainly possible to have poor quality CBME, and even in successful programmes, the issues of sustainability over time and quality control over numerous sites are important challenges that need to be recognised at the outset. Previous analysis of the literature on CBME, combined with authors' experience in CBME development and management, has led to the recognition of four key relationships that are crucial to success (Worley 2000). These factors are

"When they returned to the hospital environment, students did not feel themselves at a disadvantage compared with traditional students"

(Oswald et al 2001)

"rurally based students saw double the number of common medical conditions and assisted in, or performed, six times as many procedures as city-based students, with the result that the majority of the students were sure they had a better educational experience than their city counterparts"

(Worley et al 2000a)

Table 11.2 Comparison of extended CBME and tertiary rotations

Education factors	Extended CBME	Sequential tertiary rotations
Illness spectrum	Greater access to common conditions; many different levels of severity and complexity	Highly filtered case-mix; all of high severity and complexity
Contact with patients	Longitudinal, seeing improvement/relapse/further decision making over time	Cross-sectional snapshot of patients, at similar points in their illness
Role in patient care	Active and valued – extended time in a single setting with the same supervisor enables safe participation to increase over the year	Passive; students feel 'in the way'. As soon as the students have learnt the specific functioning of one team, they move to another ward and discipline with new supervisors and expectations
Student attitude	Regard time in practice as 'work'	Regard time on ward as 'study'
Access to sub-specialist expertise	Either by planned visits, internet resources, or video conferenced tutorials	Face to face, easy to organise
Professional development	See supervising clinicians in clinical and social/family contexts and roles	See supervising clinicians only in clinical context and role
Delegation of teaching	General practitioner supervisors delegate some teaching to resident and visiting specialists	Specialist supervisors delegate significant amount of teaching to junior medical staff
Modelling for future practice	Learning in a low-technology, low-cost environment	Learning in a high-technology, high-cost environment

particularly relevant to clinical CBME, but are also applicable to pre-clinical programmes.

The doctor–patient relationship

Enabling the student to participate, in a meaningful way, in the doctor–patient interaction is a key to medical education in any context. Although the primary care system emphasises the importance of the doctor–patient relationship, successfully integrating the student into this privileged interaction requires explicit attention in CBME. It is not automatic and requires permission, planning and prerequisite skills, knowledge and attitudes.

As clinical CBME often occurs in private consulting rooms in the context of a small business, it is more likely to be successful and sustainable if it can be structured in a way that enhances, rather than detracts from, the doctor's work and the patient's satisfaction with the care provided. Patient consent is a key first step. This is easier to manage if student teaching is seen as a 'norm' within the clinic, rather than an unusual occurrence. That is, the clinic is 'marketed' as a teaching practice where it is expected that students will be part of the healthcare team. Evaluations of patient satisfaction with student participation in such community settings have been extremely positive. In particular, there appears to be a certain 'status' attached by patients to their doctor's being an affiliated university teacher, a recognition of the importance of training the next generation of doctors well, and an appreciation of the extra time and interest a student may give to a patient. In the context of rural CBME, patients may see this as their opportunity to recruit a potential future doctor to their region.

Teaching takes time, and it is important to structure this teaching to have the least negative impact on the number of patients that can be seen. Otherwise the doctor will either decide to discontinue involvement, require significant financial compensation, or encourage purely passive observation by the student. All these are undesirable. Experience with extended CBME programmes indicates that it may even be possible to increase practice capacity by involving the students in useful components of the patient care. It appears that this capacity increases as the student's time in a particular practice increases. This factor alone may eventually lead to the relegation of short-term CBME attachments to medical education history.

Given that there is time to get to know the working of a practice and the trust of the supervisors, how can students become integrated in a meaningful and helpful way? The following practical suggestions have been found to be useful:

- Ensure there is a separate consulting room available for student use.
- Modify the appointment schedule, without reducing the total number of patients, so that patients are booked in simultaneous pairs, one for the student, and one for the doctor. The doctor sees her patient first, then moves to the other room to see the 'student's' patient.
- Encourage patients seen by the student to make their next appointment when the student is consulting.
- Provide a quiet student study area in the practice with internet access.
- Provide a mobile phone or pager for the student to be contacted for after-hours or emergency calls.
- Involve the practice in student selection and matching.
- Employ a regional administrator to timetable and coordinate the multiple learning sites/sessions for each student.
- Encourage academic staff to work clinically in the community selected for teaching.

Shared ownership of curriculum development and student selection enhances commitment from clinicians and the community.

A new set of criteria for modern medical curricula:
- product-focused
- relevant to society
- interprofessional
- shorter
- multiple sites
- symbiotic.

(Bligh et al 2001)

"Symbiotic educational partnerships within a dynamic healthcare system must be diverse and flexible, recognize the extent of different learning styles, modalities and choices that seek to balance student-centred and teacher-centred learning approaches"

(Bligh et al 2001)

The university–health service relationship

In many tertiary centres today there is considerable tension between the research and education agenda of the university and the clinical service targets of the health service. In CBME contexts, the challenge is to enable the presence of medical students to enhance the objectives of both organisations and create a symbiotic relationship between the two. How can this be achieved?

There is much power in perceptions. Bringing medical education to a previously peripheral health service can be seen as recognition of the quality of that service. A university presence may bring with it expectations and expertise in audit, quality control and peer review that improve patient care and further validate this perceived higher status as a teaching centre.

Likewise, in addition to the health service providing access to valuable clinical education opportunities for the university, the community setting can open up new avenues of clinical and health service research and with this the funds to jointly undertake this work. This perspective may be important when innovators seek to encourage tertiary academics to participate in community-based programmes.

University-based clinical research, and the researchers themselves, can improve health service delivery. This principle has been fundamental to tertiary centres for decades; the challenge is to translate this into community settings. One mechanism is to utilise recent advances in information technology. Students and staff in community settings require access to the latest and widest information sources available to supplement their clinical experiences. This may be through internet and university library access, tutorials from visiting academics, specifically developed CD-ROM materials or video-conferenced educational sessions.

These same resources can be put to good use by the health service, and recognition of this, with or without a formal memorandum of understanding, may lead to joint funding of the infrastructure required. For example, visiting academics can include tutorials for health service staff in their itinerary, or combine their teaching with the offer of a new clinical service to the community. Video-conference facilities used for teaching can equally be used for patient care and administrative purposes. High speed internet access can benefit students, staff, and local clinicians.

The principle of redundancy is important in relation to distance education. Students have different learning styles. Some may enjoy searching the web, whilst others may prefer watching a videotape of a lecture. Still others may choose to read a textbook. Electronic resources and power supplies also have a habit of malfunctioning at inconvenient times, especially in remote communities. For high stakes learning, students in the community must be provided with more than one way to learn coursework, to cater both for different learning styles and for unexpected malfunction.

Students quickly perceive whether they are welcome or 'in the way' in a clinical setting, or if they are in a 'second class' academic environment. This perception has a significant effect on their attendance, interest, and subsequent career decisions. The challenge for medical educators is to enable students learning in community settings to see themselves as part of a valued and positive link between the university and the health service.

The government–community relationship

Thus far in this section we have been focusing particularly on clinical learning. However, medical curricula have broader aims than the one-to-one interaction with patients. Gaining an appreciation of the health needs of communities, and methods to address these through local initiative and government policy, are important aspects of most modern medical programmes. CBME can provide excellent opportunities for such learning.

However, there are often tensions between national government policy and local community perceptions of health service priorities. A further key notion that underpins successful CBME is the creation of a university presence in a local community that brings together national policy and local community needs.

The first mechanism for this is through targeted research. Medical students, especially as part of their preclinical learning, can engage in locally driven research that can lead to changes in local understanding and practice. Examples of this may include understanding the occupational health risks of vineyard workers, or factors that improve the local uptake of chemically impregnated mosquito nets. This research may also provide data that enable access to further government funding sources.

Second, students can learn through participation in community development. This may involve local implementation of national priorities such as immunisation, sanitation, food hygiene practices, antenatal care and agricultural safety. This is best undertaken whilst living in the community concerned.

Third, the effectiveness of CBME as a local medical recruitment tool is a powerful synergy of local workforce needs with national workforce policy. This can be both a means to access additional educational funding from national sources and a motivator for continued community participation. This is not, however, inevitable. It will only be effective if the student experience is a positive one. It will be facilitated if both the local community and the potential government funders have a sense of ownership and engagement with the CBME programme. This may be through an advisory committee, student selection, social introductions to community groups, support for student accommodation, or transport subsidies. In light of these potential benefits, it is important for universities to be diligent in collecting appropriate workforce data and maintaining a longitudinal database of their students' career paths.

Thus, if students gain a sense of 'belonging' and appreciation from 'their' community, and an understanding of the relevant government policy agendas, they can become passionate and articulate advocates for the community and see immediate results from their learning at a population level.

Community-based medical education, as an effective long-term workforce redistribution strategy, can provide a point of synergy between a local community's priorities and government policy.

The personal–professional relationship

The final relationship to consider in making the most of CBME is that tension that often exists between the personal values and priorities of the individual physician and the expectations of the profession. Education in primary care settings can result in students spending a relatively large amount of time with one supervisor. This can lead to the development of an effective mentor relationship that can assist the student in analysing their own personal values in the light of professional norms, but it requires vulnerability on behalf of both supervisor and student for this to happen. A well developed mentor relationship may persist after the student leaves and prove influential in future career decisions.

There are practical ways of encouraging this learning to occur. First, it should be explicitly recognised in the curriculum. The best way to do this is to link it with specific assessment. This may involve interviews based on a reflective diary of the student's clinical experiences or written ethical or legal analysis of critical incidents observed by the student. Objective structured clinical examination (OSCE) stations can also be constructed to test this learning.

CMBE courses are an excellent opportunity for students to observe the role of clinicians outside the clinic, both in terms of further professional responsibilities such as community health education, and in terms of how being a doctor impacts on their family and social life in that community. Again, this is best learned if the student is resident in the community. Living with the doctor's family can bring this into very sharp relief but is unsustainable for all but very intermittent short term rotations. Therefore, it is crucial to find comfortable accommodation for students that will support the experience as being a positive one, not an uncomfortable test of sleep deprivation. In this regard, curriculum planners should pay attention to the growing number of students who have partners and children. A community experience may be used by the whole family to determine the benefits and disadvantages of living and working in such a community after graduation.

One factor that is important to be aware of is student safety. This may entail carefully managing physical risks to students in communities where violence is a significant issue, managing the risk to the student of exposure to communicable diseases and assisting students to deal with relative isolation, cultural change and, for some, living away from home for the first time. Students also, from time to time, become unwell, or have family or social crises and need to have access to assistance independent of their teacher/assessor. Such resources should be arranged before any need arises and students should have written and verbal explanation of the arrangements. These pastoral care issues can make the difference between a student recommending a CBME experience to future students or not, even if they do not wish to mention this explicitly in their reference.

CBME academic and administrative staff who support the personal and professional development of their students will find that the students not only gain cognitive and psychomotor knowledge and skills during their attachment, but also have the opportunity to gain affective skills and find themselves changed by the experience.

Pay as much attention to the students' learning of 'heart' knowledge as you do to their 'head' knowledge.

Summary

Community-based medical education is an increasingly popular tool in the medical educator's toolbox. Its use reflects the growing importance of community-based practice in the 21st century health system. There are many forms of CBME allied to the various curricular aims it is intended to deliver and many curricula are developed through necessity or opportunity rather than being based on clear medical education research. Whilst it is clear that further research is urgently required, it is hoped that the principles outlined in this chapter can help innovators to avoid major pitfalls and increase the likelihood of positive feedback from all the stakeholders involved. Moving medical education from tertiary centres into the community involves institutional change and requires proactive leadership and significant resources. Successful change involves rethinking problems as opportunities and having the creativity to find practical solutions. Organisations such as the Network: Towards Unity for Health can provide a forum for exchange of ideas and support for change agents. Become aware of the CBME initiatives worldwide through the Network's regular international conferences – you will be inspired and invigorated.

"The field of shared education between community and hospital settings remains open for research"

(Oswald et al 2001)

References

Bligh J, Prideaux D, Parsell G 2001 PRISMS: new educational strategies for medical education. Medical Education 35:520–521

Murray E, Jolly B, Modell M 1997 Can students learn clinical method in general practice? A randomised crossover trial based on objective structured clinical examinations. BMJ 315:920–923

Oswald N, Alderson T, Jones S 2001 Evaluating primary care as a base for medical education: the report of the Cambridge Community-based Clinical Course. Medical Education 35:782–788

Verby JE 1997 The Minnesota rural physician distribution plan, 1971 to 1976. JAMA 238:960–964

Worley P, Silagy C, Prideaux D et al 2000 The Parallel Rural Community Curriculum: an integrated clinical curriculum based in rural general practice. Medical Education 34:558–565

Worley P 2002 Relationships: a new way to analyse community-based medical education? (Part one). Education for Health 15:117–128

Worley P, Esterman A, Prideaux D 2004 Cohort study of examination performance of undergraduate medical students learning in community settings. BMJ 328: 207–209

Further reading

Boaden N, Bligh J 1999 Community-based medical education. 1st edn. Arnold, London

Hays R 1999 Practice-based teaching. A guide for General Practitioners. Eruditions Publishing, Emerald, Victoria, Australia

Schmidt H, Magzoub M, Feletti G et al 2000 Handbook of community-based education: theory and practice. Network Publications

Worley P S, Prideaux D J, Strasser R P et al 2000 Why we should teach undergraduate medical students in rural communities. Medical Journal of Australia 172:615–617

http://www.the networktufh.org (The Network: Towards Unity for Health)

Chapter 12
Distance education

J. M. Laidlaw, E. A. Hesketh

Introduction

Distance education as an approach to learning is not a new concept but it has rapidly developed since its pioneering days as simple correspondence courses.

This decentralised, flexible method of learning is expanding in tandem with the new technologies such as the internet and multimedia initiatives. The increasing emphasis being placed on the concept of lifelong learning is also giving distance education a higher profile.

Defining distance education

There are several definitions of distance education in the literature. Here are just two of them:

Distance education consists of all arrangements for providing instruction through print or electronic communications media to persons engaged in planned learning in a place and time different from that of the instructor or instructors.

Moore 1990

The term 'distance education' covers the various forms of study at all levels which are not under the continuous, immediate supervision of tutors present with their students in lecture rooms, or in the same premises, but which nevertheless, benefit from the planning, guidance and tuition of tutorial organisation.

Holmberg 1977

Two key factors, of time and place, distinguish distance education from other types of learning. Distance education allows the learners to study in their own place and at a time of their choice. This can be seen more clearly from Figure 12.1. For example a self-study module in a learning resource area would lie in the window of 'same place' (i.e., to be studied at a fixed place) and 'different time' (i.e., study at any time), whereas distance learning lies in the 'different time and different place' window.

What then distinguishes distance learning from, say, studying a textbook? As alluded to in the definitions, in distance education there is an ongoing responsibility to build a teacher–learner interaction into the learning experience.

"Throughout the world, confidence is growing that open and distance learning will be an important element of future education and training systems and may offer some responses to the world's educational challenges"

[Williams et al 1999]

The actual distance between learner and tutor is irrelevant.

	Same	Different
Different	Learning resource area	Distance learning
Same	Lectures	Video conference

Place

Time

Fig. 12.1 Time–place windows

Why distance education?

The popularity of distance education lies in its ability to overcome many of the barriers that face traditional education. It has been stated that access to continuing medical education (CME) activities depends on factors such as geography, funding, time constraints, service pressures and specialty-specific problems (Scottish Office 1998). Distance education can certainly address some of these constraints, if not all! For example learners may have work patterns that prohibit them from attending a specific course at a particular time; learners may simply be too busy to attend, or the location of the course may not be convenient and result in considerable travel time and travel expenses for the learner. Other barriers may also concern finance: for example from the employer's perspective it can be costly to release someone from work during the day to attend a course.

In addition there may be educational barriers inherent in traditional learning. Distance education can allow learners to study a topic to the depth they desire and at a pace that suits them. After all not everyone has the same learning needs or the same preferred learning style. Distance Education therefore can cater for individual needs both with regard to content of the topic and method of study.

In the medical profession distance education has been used extensively in the field of continuing education, particularly to keep healthcare professionals up to date with new techniques and therapies.

The educational approach

Distance education is an applied field and, as such, borrows from a variety of theoretical frameworks

Dillon & Walsh 1992

As far as main educational principles are concerned, there really is very little difference between designing a course for face to face participants and for those learning at a distance. Indeed Shale (1990) makes a plea for theoreticians and practitioners to 'stop emphasising points of difference between distance and traditional education but instead to identify common educational problems'.

The components of distance education

In designing a distance education programme the following key areas need to be addressed:

- the educational needs of the learners
- the design of the materials
- the support mechanisms for students.

The educational needs of the learners

Preparing distance education programmes for the medical profession or indeed the healthcare professions is a challenging task. Rowntree (1994) suggests a variety of facts which should be known about distance learners

Doctors would like to know their strengths and weaknesses in order to address their deficiencies.

Knowing some of these facts, if not all of them from the outset, may help in understanding distance learners better, and perhaps prevent 'drop out' if things get too tough.

"Distance education can only be designed and delivered with the highest quality by teams of specialists"

Moore 1997

'CRISIS' criteria:
- **C**onvenience
- **R**elevance
- **I**ndividualisation
- **S**elf-assessment
- **I**nterest
- **S**peculation and systematic approach.

before you start to design a course. These include a range of educational, social and economic characteristics such as:

- Age, sex, place of study, occupation – you need to know and 'understand' the type of person for whom you are writing.
- Motivation – reason for enrolling on the course. For example, do learners wish to gain a higher qualification or are they simply studying for interest? This will have implications for the content of the programme. Someone studying for a qualification is likely to do only what is required for the assessment/assignment, whereas an individual studying purely for interest may engage with the optional activities.
- Learning factors – preferred learning styles, learning skills, experience of distance learning. Ideally programmes should offer learners a choice of study methods. For example some learners prefer a problem based approach while others like a more traditional information approach.
- Subject knowledge – attitude to the subject, prior knowledge/skills, misconceptions, relevant interests. Designers of a programme on fissure caries found that dentists fell into three categories: those who were not up-to-date with the recommended sealant techniques; those who were aware of the techniques but needed to change their attitude to using them, and those who were familiar with the techniques. The design and content of the programme had to cater for all three groups.
- Resources – available time for study, access to media/facilities, access to human support, funding. These factors have implications for a distance-learning programme. For example if learners do not have access to library facilities or specific journals, they should be able to access the basic information from the core text(s) provided in the programme. Further references would be for optional reading only.

The design of distance-learning materials

The main players in any distance education development are the content expert, the education expert, the instructional designer and an editor. Team members vary depending on the method of delivery which is chosen. If it is intended to make use of CD-ROMs or the internet then it would make sense to have a computer expert on the team. It is also common practice to have a member of the target audience in the team. This helps to ensure that the programme is relevant and appropriate for that audience and not written by a subject expert remote from the 'real world'.

The CRISIS model (Harden & Laidlaw, 1992) is of value to those developing distance education programmes. CRISIS is an acronym for the following criteria, all of which can contribute to the effectiveness of continuing medical education:

Convenience

Voluntary participation must be easy. It has long been recognised that doctors educate themselves at home through reading books and journals. The role of the self-directed learner is therefore not really new to them. A distance education approach offers busy doctors the opportunity to study in their own home or workplace and at a time best suited to them.

Relevance

The user's day-to-day role in medical practice must be reflected.

The presentation of facts alone is of little use. It is how these facts are applied to the learner's everyday practice that is important. It is important therefore to identify precisely the target audience's educational needs and present the material in a context with which the learner can identify. Patient management problems and everyday scenarios are often used to make the link between theory and practice.

Individualisation

Learners must have a say in what is learnt and be able to adapt the programme to their own needs. After all they are likely to have different starting points on the topic as well as wanting different endpoints. It is also about offering a choice of learning style. How distance learning can cater for the needs of individuals and provide them with different learning pathways is best illustrated by the following example.

A distance learning programme on management, aimed at doctors and nurses working in hospitals and in the community, was designed to encourage multidisciplinary learning and could be used as a teaching resource for individuals or groups. The programme consisted of three booklets all interlinked. The distance learners could start learning about the topic using any of the booklets depending on their preferred method of study. There was a booklet for those seeking a quick practical insight to the subject, a booklet for those wishing to study the topic in greater depth and a booklet which adopted a problem-based approach.

Self-assessment

Self-assessment encourages doctors to evaluate their understanding of a subject, to identify their strengths and weaknesses and to remedy any gaps. As far as distance education is concerned, it is a key component of programmes as it motivates the learners and enables them to plot their progress. To a large extent the interaction of receiving feedback alleviates the isolation that some distance learners experience.

With regard to feedback there should be an element of choice as to the method by which distance learners can assess themselves. Feedback can be contained within the programme, it can be mailed, given by telephone or email, or given via audio- or video-conferencing. This list is by no means complete.

It is of help to learners to receive feedback not only from the 'experts' but, as shown in the feedback sheet in Figure 12.2, from their own peers who have responded.

Computers can be used successfully to generate tailored responses to individual distance learners, but this necessitates some advance computer programming. One of the most effective forms of feedback and perhaps the most educational is to offer explanations regarding all the options that might have been selected by the learner.

Option	You	Your colleagues (%)	The authors
(a)		05	
(b)	*	40	
(c)		42	*
(d)		08	
(e)		05	

Fig. 12.2 A sample feedback sheet

Individualisation refers to building into the programme the ability to cope with the different levels of detail/study required by the target audience.

We all learn in different ways and bring our own experiences to what we do.

Self-assessment is a three-stage process. The question is asked; there is a response; and there is feedback.

More attention should be paid to the feedback to the learner, especially if the prime purpose of self-assessment is diagnostic. Consider including peer comparisons and directions to learning material if a deficiency has been identified.

"for the distance educators the Internet is a land of infinite possibility"

Colyer 1997

Think

In what circumstances might the surgical patient face an increased risk of hypercapnia, and what methods are available to reduce this risk?

Make a point of familiarising yourself with relevant monitoring systems in the operating theatre and intensive care unit

Fig. 12.3 Use of icons

A 'trigger' leaflet, usually the smallest component of any distance-learning package, is often the key to its success.

If a learner is not able to allocate enough time to a distance education programme, it is better to advise the learner to postpone participation to a more appropriate period.

Interest

Attention should be aroused, encouraging learners to participate in the programme and sustaining the learner's motivation to complete the course.

There is now a wide choice of media other than print to deliver distance learning. These include audio and video cassettes; interactive video; computer-assisted learning (CAL), CD-ROMs and the internet; audio, video and computer teleconferencing, and television and radio. All can add interest to a programme and encourage interaction, providing they have been designed on sound educational principles.

Despite this technological revolution distance education in the printed format is still popular, but the trend is to augment and enhance it with electronic support materials. Desktop publishing materials can look very professional providing the principles of good layout and design have been applied. Text can also be made more stimulating by applying various educational strategies such as using advance organisers, headings, illustrations and summaries. Also, by introducing colour and various print styles, you can create a programme with impact. Even the style of writing is vitally important. The most effective materials have been written in a conversational style.

Icons too are being used more often in printed materials, to enable learners to select various types of activities that are flagged up, and in a distance education programme, activities are a main feature. An example from the 'SELECT' distance education programme of the Royal College of Surgeons of Edinburgh shows how effective the use of icons can be (Fig. 12.3).

An ever-increasing number of distance-learning courses are available today, covering a wide range of topics. Competition is healthy but calls for the use of marketing strategies. Leaflets help raise awareness of distance-learning programmes. Spending time and money on the design of the 'triggers' is well worth the effort.

Speculation and systematic approach

Speculation is about recognising controversial and grey areas in medicine and making it clear that sometimes not everything is known about a subject. It is important that such areas of uncertainty are addressed and not glossed over. The systematic element is about offering a planned programme with coverage of a whole subject or an identified part of it. The distance learning teacher needs to consider the topic areas to be studied, identify these for the learner and show him or her how their studies will cover these areas.

Support mechanisms

There are a variety of mechanisms which can be used to provide the distance learner with support. Even although Knowles (1984) describes the adult learner as relatively independent and internally motivated in distance education, support for learners is crucial and can often determine whether a learner will continue with a programme of study or drop out. The support you can provide depends greatly on your funding and the technologies available to you and your learner. Here are just some support mechanisms worth considering:

- Offer support when needed by the learner. This is usually in a one-to-one situation where the learner seeks tutor support.
- Offer a planned session between tutor and an individual or a group of learners, or simply between a learner and their peers. If a group of learners are conveniently situated near each other, a face-to-face peer group meeting may be organised, in which learners are encouraged to support each other. More recently the electronic chatroom is being used as an additional support mechanism.
- Offer a planned summer school or series of face-to-face workshops which are part of the distance-learning course.

Remember you can also build in support through 'embedded support devices' within the distance-learning materials.

There is also a trend today to incorporate study guides into distance-learning packages. These are basically tools to help self-directed learners manage their learning more effectively and efficiently. Study guides are dealt with in more depth in chapter 21, Study guides.

Study of 'embedded support devices' such as margin texts, summaries, examples, questions with feedback, text in italics, etc, has shown that they assist learning.

Guard against making your study guide too voluminous or it will become a less effective tool for the distance learner.

Summary

Distance education continues to grow in popularity amongst adult learners and will expand further as technologies develop. In the medical profession a large percentage of doctors have used this approach to learning to keep up to date with new techniques and therapies. It differs from other approaches to learning in that the learner is separated from the tutor, and there is no fixed time or place for study.

There are three key areas to address when developing a distance-learning programme. First the educational needs of the learners must be determined. If a distance-learning course does not meet the learners' needs in terms of many aspects, of which relevance, content, depth of study, preferred learning style, cost and accreditation are just a few, then it will either fail to attract enrolments or result in drop outs.

The second key area involves the design. Although there is no recognised theory underpinning distance education, designers have leaned heavily on Gagne's principles of learning (Gagne 1970), as well as on the CRISIS model, to create innovative educational programmes.

The third issue is that of learner support. Even if the programmes are educationally sound, distance learners need additional support to help them in their self-directed role. These support mechanisms can vary from simply incorporating embedded support devices into the programmes, through to planning scheduled tutorial sessions using electronic media, organising kick-start or face-to-face courses, making use of study guides or providing tutor support on demand.

As the demand for lifelong learning increases, the number of distance learners is likely to increase and, more importantly, be valued by institutions worldwide.

References

Colyer A 1997 Copyright law, the internet and distance education. American Journal of Distance Education 11(3):41–57

Dillon C L and Walsh S M 1992 Faculty: the neglected resource in distance education. American Journal of Distance Education 6(3):5–21

Gagne R M 1970 The conditions of learning, 2nd edn. Holt, Rinehart and Winston, New York

Harden R M and Laidlaw J M 1992 Effective continuing education: the CRISIS criteria. Medical Education 26:408–422

Holmberg B 1977 Distance education: a survey and bibliography, Kogan Page, London

Knowles M S 1984 Andragogy in action. Jossey Bass, New York

Moore M G 1990 Contemporary issues in American distance education. Pergamon Press, New York

Moore M G 1997 The study guide: foundation of the course [editorial]. American Journal of Distance Education 11(2):1–2

Rowntree D 1994 Preparing material for open, distance and flexible learning. London, Kogan Page

Scottish Office 1998 Scottish Joint Consultants' Committee and representatives of NHS trust chief executives. Continuing medical education for career grade hospital doctors an dentists. Health Bulletin 56(3):624–630

Shale D 1990 Toward a reconceptualization of distance education In: Moore M G (ed) Contemporary issues in American distance education. Pergamon, Oxford, p 333–343

Williams M L, Paprock K, Covington B 1999 Distance learning – the essential guide, Sage, California

Chapter 13
Peer-assisted learning

M. T. Ross, A. D. Cumming

Introduction

There has been a considerable increase in the number of medical schools incorporating student-led teaching into their curricula in recent years. This chapter looks at the background to this development, issues to consider when planning such a programme and some practical examples from the medical undergraduate literature.

What is peer-assisted learning?

Peer-assisted learning in its broadest sense would include any situation where people learn from, or with, others of a similar level of training, background or other shared characteristic. In the undergraduate curriculum this could include virtually any small-group work (Learning in small groups, chapter 7, Problem-based learning, chapter 16) and feedback from peer review or peer assessment. In postgraduate medicine there are also many examples such as peer review of journal articles, critical incident review, clinical team meetings and appraisal.

The specific term peer-assisted learning (PAL) has been accepted in the UK medical undergraduate literature to mean organised educational programmes where students tutor or teach their peers. In this sense a 'peer' is someone doing the same course of study and may be either in the same year or somewhat more advanced. This more specific learning situation will be the focus of this chapter which will refer to those assisting the learning of their peers as 'tutors' and those being assisted as 'tutees', although in some reciprocal forms of PAL these roles are exchanged.

Historical and educational background to PAL

The concepts of teaching by students and of groups of peers learning by sharing experiences are not in any way new. In her book on the history of peer teaching, Lilya Wagner (Wagner 1982) presents the evidence of Aristotle's 'archons' (c. 340 BC), Quintilian's view that 'one who has just acquired a subject is best fitted to teach it' (c. 80 AD), Johann Sturn's 'decurions' in German gymnasia (1507), Andrew Bell's 'mutual instruction system' developed in Madras (c. 1800) and Joseph Lancaster's 'monitorial system' in Great Britain (1803). Essentially, at various points in history, the great potential of students to assist in the learning of their

"To teach is to learn twice"

Possibly Isocrates, but attributed to Joseph Joubert.

"Acquire new knowledge whilst thinking over the old, and you may become a teacher of others"

Confucius

peers has been recognised and encouraged in formally organised teaching and mentoring programmes.

Because the PAL concept has been developed in different ways across a wide spectrum of educational fields, from primary school through secondary to business education, catering, law, sciences and medicine the terminology is very diverse. Current designations include: peer teaching or tutoring, peer-supported learning, peer-assisted study, cooperative or collaborative learning, students helping students, student tutoring or facilitation, student mentoring, study advisory schemes, teaching assistant schemes, supplemental instruction and proctoring. Not all are entirely synonymous, but all have common features.

Various educational and sociological theories have been suggested to explain the success and appeal of PAL programmes. Most students involved in these programmes agree that the experience is enjoyable, that there are benefits for both tutor and tutee, and that there seems to be a level of understanding and rapport between peer tutor and tutee which is different from that between students and members of staff. In his review of peer tutoring in further and higher education, Keith Topping discusses the theoretical cognitive, pedagogical, attitudinal, social, economic and political processes involved in PAL (Topping 1996). Contributing factors discussed in the review include the cognitive aspects of verbalisation and questioning, scaffolded learning in the tutee's 'zone of proximal development' and modelling, as well as the processes involved in preparing to be a tutor, tutees' increased access to support and teaching, empowerment of students generally and the social aspects of the peer relationship. Topping also gives an overview of findings from PAL programmes in schools, showing that students who have had supplemental peer tutoring outperform control groups, that same-age tutors seem as effective as cross-age ones, and that offering specific training to tutors improves tutee outcomes and the attitudes and self-concept of both tutor and tutee.

Training-grade doctors and medical students have a very long history of supporting and assisting the learning of their peers. This has, however, tended to be informal, opportunistic, and largely undocumented. The origins of the phrase 'see one, do one, teach one' are obscure but the legacy lives on, although most doctors would now justly be wary of this approach.

A more regulated form of PAL called 'supplemental instruction' (SI) has been developed from the University of Missouri–Kansas City (UMKC), where it was originally conceived as a way of reducing the dropout rate of students in medicine, pharmacy and dentistry. The basic idea was to train successful senior students to tutor more junior students of the same discipline, as a supplement to their usual coursework. Since 1973 the SI model has been researched, developed and applied across the USA and abroad in numerous disciplines, but is still supported and coordinated by the UMKC-SI centre. There is also a group in the United Kingdom, the UK SI Network, which has identified and attempted to unite the diverse approaches to PAL being developed in this country in various disciplines; only some of these approaches follow the UMKC-SI model (see References for website address).

"The authority of those who teach is often an obstacle to those who want to learn"

Cicero

In February 2003 the UK medical governing body, the General Medical Council, issued the second edition of *Tomorrow's doctors* detailing the standards by which the quality of UK medical schools is judged (GMC 2003). Section 8 states that students should 'Be able to demonstrate appropriate teaching skills' and 'Be willing to teach colleagues and develop their own teaching skills'. Section 24 states 'Graduates must understand the principles of education as they are applied to medicine. They will be familiar with a range of teaching and learning techniques and must recognise their obligation to teach colleagues.' PAL approaches are a practical way to allow medical students to participate in training and gain experience in teaching.

What are the advantages of PAL?

There are many advantages to peer assisted learning over professional teaching or self-directed learning. Findings from the references at the end of this chapter can be categorised into advantages for tutor, tutee and medical school.

Advantages for tutors
- Provides opportunities to reinforce and revise their learning.
- Encourages responsibility and increased self-confidence.
- Develops teaching and verbalisation skills.
- Enhances communication skills, empathy and observation.
- Encourages reflection and self-direction in their own learning.
- Develops appraisal skills (of self and others) including the ability to give and receive appropriate feedback.
- Enhances organisational skills.
- Enhances teamworking skills.

Advantages for tutees
- Relaxed and informal approach means that they feel less threatened and more supported.
- Provides a good opportunity to formulate and ask questions, even 'silly' ones.
- Provides opportunity to obtain detailed feedback on their knowledge or skills.
- Peer tutors may be more aware of problem areas than staff.
- Associated with social benefits, role-modelling and increased motivation to learn.
- It is efficacious: peer tutors seem to be as good as staff in certain areas.
- Can discuss learning strategies and study skills.

Advantages for the medical school
- Cost and resource-effective (but should not be the primary aim).
- Students feel more involvement in the course and ownership.
- Some evidence to suggest it is easier to standardise tutoring from peers than from professional teachers.

"I found myself not just listening to the conversation but assessing the dynamics of the group at the same time. This was very new and difficult at first and is something I probably should have been doing as a group member all along"

Student tutor (Solomon & Crowe 2001)

"The peer tutors were great teachers. They are students as well, so they know what and how we think, the mistakes we tend to make"

Tutee (Howman et al 2003)

- Meets obligation to train medical students in teaching skills.
- Encourages a culture of collaborative learning instead of competitiveness.

Are there concerns about PAL?

Concerns have been raised about the PAL approach, and some studies report opposition from teaching staff to the implementation of PAL schemes, because of perceived problems. Potential concerns include:

- Student tutors may have inadequate depth of knowledge.
- Student tutors may teach 'the wrong thing' or give incorrect information.
- There may be overload of information and reduced tutee confidence.
- Tutors lack experience and may transfer knowledge and skills poorly.
- Tutor ego and personality issues may cause groups to be dysfunctional.
- Tutors lack experience in group facilitation and may have difficulty retaining focus and discipline.
- Students may be encouraged to examine each other, with potential peer pressure, embarrassment and inappropriate behaviour.
- Time and effort are required to organise PAL programmes, train tutors and monitor outcomes.
- Student tutors may be used as 'cheap labour', teaching on established courses, where there is no real benefit for the tutor, because there are insufficient faculty staff.

These are very real and important issues that have been reported from various centres (medical and nonmedical) involved in PAL. When developing a PAL programme it is worth considering these problems and how they can be minimised.

Having well-defined and structured subject areas will increase tutor familiarity with material and can also provide a structure and focus to sessions. Involving more than one peer tutor per session increases the breadth of tutor knowledge, reduces the effect of an individual tutor's personality and may minimise idiosyncratic teaching. Providing additional tutor training in the subject matter and in educational approaches may increase the standardisation of the material covered and increase the functionality of the sessions. Specific training could also be used to encourage a facilitative tutee-centred approach rather than a more didactic tutor-centred one, to draw on the pre-existing knowledge of the tutees rather than the tutor. These suggestions are largely speculative, however, as there has not yet been enough research into PAL tutor training to allow programme developers to use an evidence-based approach.

What is involved in a PAL programme?

Different centres have developed peer-assisted learning in different ways, with variations in how tutors and tutees are selected, the training tutors

Beware thinking of student tutors as trained faculty or cheap teaching staff. If there are no apparent benefits for tutors, or the tutees would be better served by faculty tutors, or both, then it would be hard to justify continuing the programme.

receive, the scheduling of sessions and what actually takes place in terms of format and content. The administration of such programmes varies considerably depending upon the material tutored, the amount of training and support given to tutors and whether the sessions are timetabled and organised by members of staff or by the students themselves. The financial costs of such a programme also vary depending upon the staff involvement in terms of numbers and frequency, the resources required and whether or not student tutors are paid. The following characteristics have been described in the literature.

Recruitment of tutors

Tutors can be recruited comprehensively or compulsorily or both as part of a course, on a voluntary basis, or because of high achievement. They can either be from the same year as the tutees or from a more advanced year. Tutors may or may not have the same level of ability as tutees. Some reciprocal PAL programmes involve tutors swapping their roles to become tutees and vice versa.

Recruitment of tutees

The majority of programmes seem to be open to all who are interested, although some tutees are comprehensively recruited as part of their timetabled course. Other programmes offer PAL to particular subgroups of students such as those with poor academic achievement.

Training of tutors

Some PAL programmes do not specifically train tutors beyond what they would be learning anyway, for example, in reciprocal peer teaching. Some provide supplementary training in the subject to be tutored and others combine this with basic educational training in pedagogical approaches, facilitation, groupwork, communication skills and giving feedback. Depending upon the programme, resources or special facilities may be required to train tutors.

It is important that the tutors feel confident enough to undertake the task well and understand what is expected of them.

Try to ensure tutors know what is expected of them, ideally giving them an opportunity to practise in a simulated setting.

Scheduling of sessions

PAL sessions can either be incorporated into the timetabled curriculum, be formally organised outwith normal working hours or be held on an ad hoc basis depending upon the availability or needs of tutees. There is wide variation on how often sessions run, how long they last and how many tutors are present. There may be the same number of tutors as tutees in reciprocal teaching and 'dyads'. Alternatively, individual or groups of tutors can work with differently sized groups of tutees. Sessions may be organised by staff or by students themselves at a variety of locations.

If tutees are to select from a list of tutorials to attend, the use of a 'group selection tool' or 'online sign-up sheet' greatly reduces the amount of administrative time required.

Format and content of sessions

The majority of published programmes are modelled on facilitative small-group tutorials, with varying content which may include anatomical dissection, simulated or real patients for examination, or other special facilities. They are most commonly supplementary to the formal taught curriculum, and may be revision (exam practice, past papers, discussion), remedial (help with content or study skills) or practice of clinical skills (observed practice, review of videos, reflection). Some peer-led sessions are more didactic lectures or formal tutorials, where new information may be presented to tutees. Some forms of PAL do not involve face-to-face contact at all, but rather the production of resources such as written summaries, revision aids and computer-assisted learning (CAL) programmes.

The content and approach used in different PAL programmes is usually clearly defined to the students, and will vary depending upon the desired learning outcomes. Thus the structure will be different if the intention is to supplement exam revision or study skills, compared with developing practical skills or critical thinking (although there are likely to be multiple supplementary outcomes in addition to those planned).

How can PAL be used in medical education?

All teaching modalities and strategies are available for use in peer-assisted learning. The most common methods used in the literature are revision tutorials which reinforce material already familiar to tutees. Below is a brief summary of selected examples from the medical and related education literature which illustrate different approaches to PAL, with some indication of feedback and response where available.

Course organisation, delivery and assessment: Bibb & Lefever (2002) Los Angeles

Year-4 dental students participated in a student-selected elective course in which they created a 'microcourse' for incoming year-1 students during their orientation week, under the guidance of an anatomy lecturer and an educationalist. They were introduced to learning theory, selecting and sequencing content, presentation skills, writing of test questions and assessment of outcomes. Staff tried to remain nondirective in the actual creation of the microcourse. The year-4 participants then presented a didactic 20-minute lecture each, administered a brief test and collected feedback from the year-1 class. The microcourse delivered to year-1 students was entitled 'Welcome to dental anatomy' and lasted only 2 to 3 hours.

Feedback from year-1 students revealed that they felt their knowledge had significantly increased as a result of the microcourse and were also more confident and enthusiastic about studying the material. They also felt the course had been useful preparation, when asked after an anatomy exam 5 weeks later (following the usual dental anatomy teaching by staff). Student tutor feedback suggested the experience was positive and rewarding, increasing their confidence, understanding of the educational process and presentation skills. Interestingly all but one of the tutors wanted to be involved in teaching again in the future, the other realising that he did not enjoy teaching.

You may want to explore a variety of approaches to PAL to provide diverse teaching experiences for tutors (such as large-group, small-group and individual teaching, facilitation, giving feedback, creating resources, course organisation and student support).

PAL may be particularly useful to new students joining a course or in a situation where the context of learning changes acutely (e.g. moving from a pre-clinical to a clinical environment).

Revision and study skills tutoring: Walker-Bartnick et al (1984) Maryland

Supplementary tutoring may be offered to students who have difficulty in various subjects. This paper discusses a programme in which senior students provide extracurricular tutoring to more junior students who experience difficulty in basic medical sciences. Tutors are carefully screened for academic ability and study habits, but the programme is open to all junior students who perceive themselves to be having difficulty. As with many similar programmes, there is recognition that tutees may have multiple factors contributing to their poor academic performance. The tutorials are not solely aimed at reinforcing and explaining course content; they also aim to provide support to students trying to cope with very wide subject areas, and specifically focus on the need to help tutees with generic study skills and study schedules.

There was no control group; however, the programme received positive feedback from both tutors and tutees and the authors felt the grades tutees subsequently received indicated the effectiveness of this intervention.

Reciprocal teaching of basic sciences: Nnodim (1997) Benin

Some studies from the 1980s looked at reciprocal peer teaching in anatomy, where students would research a topic and then present it to their peers. An interesting variation is to split the class into two groups and have the first group complete a dissection unit while the second group engages in private study. At the next session the first group demonstrates the findings of their dissection to the second group before retiring to the library, whereupon the second group does the next dissection unit, and subsequently demonstrates this to the first group at the next session, and so on. Thus each group does only half of the dissection units themselves and has the alternate ones taught to them by the other group.

In the study cited, students learning by this method performed significantly better in a theoretical exam on the subject than those who had been present in the dissection room throughout the dissection of all units (although the authors felt this could have been due in part to increased time for independent study).

Preparing resources and computer-assisted learning (CAL): Shanks et al (2000) Minnesota

In this study, year-2 medical and dental students organised a 'knowledge co-op' which provided academic support to year-1 students in the form of group reviews and peer-led tutorials as well as electronic resources. A website was created where year-1 students could obtain information on the support available, e-mail addresses to contact year-2 students, handouts for the review sessions and also online practicals created and collected by the year-2 students which they felt would be useful practice for year-1 students.

There are many other examples in the literature of students creating resources for the use of their peers, including CAL packages, poster presentations and the reciprocal sharing of work in study groups and during exam revision.

"The requirement to educate others has sharpened my attention during dissection and challenged me to work harder"

Reciprocal tutor (Nnodim 1997)

Peer feedback on video recordings of patient encounters or simulations can be useful. This does not interfere with the orginal encounter, can be carried out at a time convenient for the students and is very amenable to quality assurance.

"At times I felt like giving my opinion on certain issues but I felt like if I spoke my word was 'it'. I felt I had to clarify, 'This is my opinion only, I don't know if it is right' "

Student tutor (Solomon & Crowe 2001)

Communication skills training: Escovitz (1990) Pennsylvania

After suitable training, senior student tutors have been used to view, assess and provide constructive feedback on junior students' video interviews with simulated patients. In the cited example, tutors spent 10 hours being trained in interview techniques, video assessment and feedback. They then spent an average of 2 hours viewing the taped interview of each student before meeting with them individually for about an hour to discuss the interview and provide feedback to the tutees. The programme was quality-controlled, revealing an 80% concurrence between video assessments made by student tutors and those made by the author.

The sessions were very well received by the tutees who felt their self-confidence and skills had increased and that the tutors were knowledgeable and nonthreatening. Tutors also reported feeling that they were better observers and more comfortable giving and responding to feedback.

Problem-based learning facilitation: Sobral (1994) Brazil

Early studies which looked at problem-based learning (PBL) groups with student tutors suggested that the tutees had poorer educational outcomes than those tutored by faculty. A 7-year study at the University of Brasilia compared the educational outcomes and overall satisfaction with a PBL course before and after substituting a teacher with a trained student for the second (problem-solving) session, while continuing to use teachers to tutor the first (problem-definition and question-generation) session. The results suggested no disadvantage in educational outcome compared with teacher-tutored sessions, and significant improvement in tutees' ratings of the usefulness and meaningfulness of course experience. It should be noted, however, that these tutors attended a detailed tutor training course with orientation before the PBL sessions.

Some other very helpful insights into the experiences and challenges of PBL student-facilitators can be found in Solomon & Crowe, 2001.

Examination skills teaching and assessment by objective structured clinical examination (OSCE): Howman et al (2003) London

This article describes a student-selected project of 5 weeks' duration in which senior clinical students attended a 2-day training course on teaching, received revision of clinical skills from consultants, taught clinical examination skills to groups of junior students (for whom this was their first real clinical experience) and subsequently set and ran an OSCE for the junior students. A control group of junior students taught basic clinical skills by general practitioners also sat the OSCE and performed similarly.

The project seems to have been well received by both parties and the peer-tutored group do not seem to have been disadvantaged in terms of OSCE result compared with those trained by GPs. Unfortunately, however, there was no longer term follow up.

Rehearsal of examination skills: Culver et al (2003) Edinburgh

Proficiency in clinical examination, as with all skills, requires a considerable amount of practice – preferably in a supportive environment with constructive feedback. Edinburgh medical students are taught and tested on systematic clinical examination in year 2, but report a need to revise and practise this when starting clinical placements in year 3. Volunteer year-4 tutors are recruited and trained to facilitate sessions in which year-3 students can rehearse their clinical examination skills on one another or on simulated patients (depending upon the nature of the examination). They then receive detailed feedback from the year-4 tutor and other year-3 tutees. A similar approach has been employed for sessions using the 'Harvey' cardiology simulator manikin. These sessions are open to all year-3 students who feel they would benefit from this extracurricular activity. Because the year-3 tutees already have a grasp of the subject area, tutors are not required to teach the subject, but are rather encouraged to draw on the knowledge that the tutees already have and encourage them in the practical rehearsal of their examination skills.

Feedback suggests that the programme is well received by tutors and tutees, and most tutees subsequently feel more confident in their clinical examination skills.

Critical-incident review

A very good example of peer-assisted learning which is widely used in postgraduate medicine, and is also starting to appear in undergraduate study, is the practice of critical-incident review, also known as 'significant event analysis'. In postgraduate medicine there are often patient safety issues such as drug errors, complaints and missed diagnoses. Undergraduates may also consider these areas or other more personal ones, such as a failed exam or an unexpected response from a patient. This component of continuous professional development uses such incidents as stimuli for discussion and nonjudgmental feedback, to review practices and policies, to identify how any mistakes could have been avoided and to try to identify individual learning needs in the context of a peer group or clinical team. As yet there is very little in the literature discussing the use of critical incident review amongst peer groups in undergraduate education, but the situation is likely to change.

Where to start when considering a PAL programme

Most of the examples discussed above could easily be extended to cover other subject areas and desired learning outcomes. The educational basis for peer-assisted learning is sound. However it is not appropriate for all aspects of medical teaching and is unlikely ever to become the main teaching method of any course. The PAL approach is particularly useful for well-defined subject areas such as basic sciences or practical clinical skills, but has also been successfully applied to the more complex areas of training in communication skills, facilitation of self-directed learning and course organisation. PAL is probably not an appropriate method for subjects where teachers need a broad general knowledge or grasp of diverse concepts, such as those required for the teaching of ethics, some of the more advanced consultation skills, differential diagnosis and in constructing management options.

Think carefully about your learning objectives for both student tutors and tutees before designing a PAL programme.

"I learn more and better when I discuss the topic. I am able to learn from others by exchanging ideas with them."

Reciprocal tutor (Nnodim 1997)

In developing a PAL programme it is important to consider what are the relevant learning outcomes, which educational approach is most suited to achieving these, and the detailed practicalities of organising such a programme. This information should be readily accessible and open to comment at an early stage to all parties involved.

Summary

Peer-assisted learning (PAL) can be defined as an organised educational programme in which students tutor or teach their peers. The concept dates back to ancient times, but has come to the fore recently in medical education with the desire to provide new graduates with some teaching skills and experience. There is a growing medical undergraduate literature on PAL which includes applications in teaching and assessing knowledge-based subjects, training and reinforcement of clinical examination and communication skills, revision and help with study skills, course organisation, resource preparation, and the facilitation of self-directed learning in areas such as problem-based learning. Many of these programmes report considerable benefits for both student tutors and tutees. There are some potential pitfalls and drawbacks; however, with careful planning these can be minimised.

References

Bibb C A, Lefever K H 2002 Mentoring future dental educators through an apprentice teaching experience. Journal of Dental Education 66(6):703–709

Culver E L, Green E J, Glassford N J, Evans P 2003 Peer-led clinical skills facilitation programme: student and tutor perspectives. Poster presentation at ASME annual scientific meeting 2003. Online. Available: http://www.mvm.ed.ac.uk/clinskill_poster.htm

Escovitz E S 1990 Using senior students as clinical skills teaching assistants. Academic Medicine 65(12):733–734

GMC 2003 Tomorrow's doctors: recommendations on undergraduate medical education. General Medical Council, London. Online. Available: http://www.gmc-uk.org/med_ed/ tomdoc.htm

Howman M, Bertfield D, Needleman S 2003 The PAL project – peer assisted learning in medicine. Online. Available: http://www.ucl.ac.uk/acme/dev/PAL.htm

Nnodim J O 1997 A controlled trial of peer-teaching in practical gross anatomy. Clinical Anatomy 10:112–117

Shanks J C, Silver R D, Harris IB 2000 Use of web-based technology in a peer-teaching program. Academic Medicine 75:538–539

Sobral D T 1994 Peer tutoring and student outcomes in a problem-based course. Medical Education 28:284–289

Solomon P, Crowe J 2001 Perceptions of student peer tutors in a problem-based learning programme. Medical Teacher 23:181–186

Topping K J 1996 The effectiveness of peer tutoring in further and higher education: a typology and review of the literature. Higher Education 32:321–345

UK SI Network. Online. Available: http://www.peerlearning.ac.uk/national_network.html

UMKC University of Missouri–Kansas City Supplemental Instruction. Online. Available: www.umkc.edu/cad/si

Wagner L 1982 Peer teaching: historical perspectives. Greenwood Press, Westport, CT

Walker-Bartnick L A, Berger J H, Kappelman M M 1984 A model for peer tutoring in the medical school setting. Journal of Medical Education 59:309–315

SECTION 3
EDUCATIONAL STRATEGIES

Chapter 14
Outcome-based curriculum

S. R. Smith

"The only way to get somewhere, you know, is to figure out where you're going before you go there"

[Updike 1960]

Introduction

A story frequently told by educators concerns a young lad and his dog, Fido. 'I taught Fido how to whistle,' the boy proudly tells his father. When asked to demonstrate this remarkable achievement, the boy commands, 'Fido, whistle!' Fido wags his tail vigorously but does not whistle. 'I thought you said you taught Fido how to whistle. I didn't hear him whistle,' the father says to his son who replies, 'I taught him how to whistle, but he didn't learn!'

All too often, we, as teachers, focus too much on what we teach rather than on what our students learn. Outcome-based education emphasises what we expect students will have achieved when they complete their course. These learning achievements go beyond just knowing; rather, they describe what learners can actually do with what they know.

Outcome-based education defines what we expect of our graduates and holds us accountable to provide an education that achieves those endpoints. It is not only good education, it is good public policy.

Medical schools around the world are increasingly embracing the concepts of outcome-based education (Simpson et al 2002, Smith et al 2003). National and international bodies in medical education have espoused these principles, urging and even requiring their constituents to comply (ACGME 2003, Schwartz & Wojtczak 2002).

Planning backwards

The traditional model of medical education ('planning forwards') begins with the delineation of the knowledge fundamental to medicine, teaching that knowledge, then testing whether students have learned that information, typically by some form of closed-book examination (Fig. 14.1). The hope is that acquisition of this knowledge base will lead to students becoming good doctors.

The outcome-based model ('planning backwards') goes in the opposite direction, starting with the good doctor and working backwards (Fig. 14.2). The faculty designing the curriculum begin by defining the attributes of the successful graduate, then they figure out how they would know whether students had attained those outcomes, then they create learning opportunities that would enable the students to achieve them.

Choosing outcomes

The easiest way for a medical school to create an outcome-based curriculum is to adopt outcomes that others have defined. Abilities in nine areas were described at Brown Medical School (Smith et al 2003):

1. effective communication
2. basic clinical skills
3. using basic science in the practice of science
4. diagnosis, management, and prevention
5. lifelong learning
6. professional development and personal growth
7. the social and community contexts of healthcare
8. moral reasoning and clinical ethics
9. problem solving.

The 'Scottish doctor' model has 12 outcomes, categorised into three elements (Simpson et al 2002):

- *What the doctor is able to do*
  – clinical skills
  – practical procedures
  – patient investigations
  – patient management
  – health promotion and disease prevention
  – communication
  – medical informatics.
- *How the doctor approaches his or her practice*
  – basic, social and clinical sciences
  – attitudes, ethical understanding and legal responsibilities
  – decision-making skills and clinical reasoning.
- *The doctor as a professional*
  – the role of the doctor within the health service
  – personal development.

The US Accreditation Council on Graduate Medical Education (ACGME 2003) lumps the outcomes into a smaller set of six general competencies:

- patient care
- medical knowledge
- practice-based learning and improvement
- interpersonal and communication skills
- professionalism
- systems-based practice.

Using an already established list of outcomes has the advantages of ease, simplicity, comparability and established credibility. However, simply adopting someone else's list has its own drawbacks. The faculty and students may not feel the same sense of ownership, unique characteristics of the school may not be represented or sufficiently emphasised, and the outcomes may be interpreted differently from what was originally intended.

Flexnerian Model

Define "Fundamental knowledge"

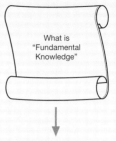

Teach the fundamentals

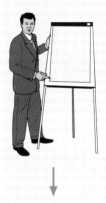

Test for knowledge of fundamentals

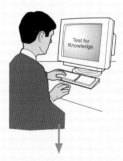

Hope for the best

?

Fig. 14.1 The Flexnerian model

Competency-based model

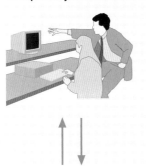

↑↓

Develop learning experiences

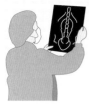

↑

Design measures and standards of performance

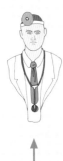

↑

Define the successful graduate

Fig. 14.2 Competency-based model

 Outcomes should be few in number, self-evident, and easily understood.

If a school chooses to create its own list of outcomes, it ought to maximise the amount of participation in the process to increase the buy-in from students and staff. Since the only requirement of participants is that they have an opinion on what qualities they appreciate in their own doctors, everyone can be part of the process, from PhD basic scientists to students to clinical professors.

A nominal group process technique can be used to maximise participation and minimise the impact of overbearing personalities. Each person in the group is allowed to add a desirable attribute of a good doctor. This continues in a 'round-robin' fashion until no new attributes are suggested. Attributes may be grouped together, with the permission of the persons who proposed them. Participants then vote by placing a star next to the attribute they believe is most important and ticks alongside to the three attributes they feel are next most important. The stars are counted as two points and ticks as one point. The votes are tallied and the attributes with the highest votes are selected as the outcomes.

Defining outcomes

Having chosen the outcomes, the curriculum planners must define each more fully. This is best accomplished by small writing committees comprised of individuals with a particular interest in that outcome.

The definition should be relatively short, but detailed enough to be clear (Harden 2002). The following is an example from the nine abilities described at Brown Medical School:

Ability 7: The social and community contexts of healthcare The competent graduate provides healing guidance by responding to the many factors that influence health, disease and disability, besides those of a biological nature. These factors include sociocultural, familial, psychological, economic, environmental, legal, political and spiritual aspects of healthcare seekers and of healthcare delivery. Through sensitivity to the interrelationships of individuals and their communities, the graduate responds to the broader context of medical practice.

Another example is drawn from the 'Scottish doctor' learning outcomes:

Outcome 6: Communication Good communication underpins all aspects of the practice of medicine. All new graduates must be able to demonstrate effective communication skills in all areas and in all media, e.g. orally, in writing, electronically, by telephone, etc.

Developing criteria

Once the definition of the outcome is agreed upon, the next step is to delineate criteria. The criteria describe specific tasks that students will be expected to undertake to demonstrate mastery. For example, procedures such as taking a blood pressure, performing a urinalysis and interpreting a chest X-ray could be delineated as criteria under the medical procedures outcome.

The group charged with delineating the criteria should also provide examples of ways in which the criteria could be demonstrated. An example for the lifelong-learning outcome might be: 'presents findings of research to other students in problem-based learning group'. These illustrations help other teachers think of ways to incorporate the outcomes in their own teaching activities.

Levelling

The competence of students grows as they progress through their education. Teachers' expectations should also increase in parallel fashion. Tasks assigned to students at the beginning of their course of study should be simpler than those assigned at the end of their training.

Faculty should classify learning expectations into a minimum of two levels: one appropriate for the novice or beginning student and another that specifies the expectations necessary for graduation. A third level of achievement higher than the minimum required for graduation should also be specified. Students should be allowed to differentiate themselves at this advanced level, based on their individual interests and talents.

The complexity of the challenge should increase at the intermediate and advanced levels. For example, novice students should be expected to demonstrate good communication skills with patients who are relatively free of significant communication impairments, whereas more advanced students could be challenged with patients who are not native language speakers or who have hearing or speech impairments.

Evaluating outcomes

Performance-based assessment (see chapter 35, Performance assessment) goes hand in hand with outcome-based education. Satisfactory performance requires students to skilfully apply the knowledge they possess to a specific task.

Performance-based assessment is not a radical departure for clinical medicine. Clinical teachers are accustomed to asking students to demonstrate physical examination skills or to interpret a diagnostic image. In outcome-based education, the same approach is applied systematically across all outcomes.

Much of this can and should be accomplished using real patients in real clinical situations. Certain practical limitations, however, preclude the use of real patients in all teaching situations. Basic science courses, for example, do not usually involve real patients. Even in real clinical situations, the variability of clinical practice means that there can be no guarantee that every student will have the opportunity to work with patients with specific medical problems. Also, not every patient with the same problem presents in the same way.

Simulations can be substituted when the use of real patients is impractical. Readers should refer to section 6 to learn about the various forms of assessment that can be employed, with chapter 35 on objective clinical examinations being particularly relevant. The objective structured clinical examination (OSCE) enables the faculty to design an assessment that can measure particular outcomes very precisely.

Faculty should specify which outcomes they wish to assess with an OSCE, then build the OSCE around that blueprint. For example, at Brown Medical School, the OSCE given in the last year of medical school

"It is a highly questionable practice to label someone as having achieved a goal when you don't even know what you would take as evidence of achievement"

[Mager 1962]

Tasks for beginner, intermediate, and advanced students should present greater challenges to their skills at each level.

Assessment should reflect as authentically as possible the real tasks that doctors do.

measures four of the nine abilities required for graduation: effective communication; basic clinical skills; diagnosis, management, and prevention; and moral reasoning and clinical ethics. The OSCE consists of eight standardised patient stations with an interstation exercise following each of the cases.

The following are examples of performance-based assessments that could be used to measure attainment of each outcome in the curriculum at Brown Medical School. The purpose is simply to stimulate readers' imaginations regarding how outcomes might be evaluated at their own institutions.

Effective communication

Oral communication (see chapter 26, Communication skills) can be assessed even in basic science courses by incorporating speaking assignments in the course. Students in our anatomy course, at Brown Medical School, must give a 10-minute presentation that relates the anatomy to a clinical situation. The students demonstrate the anatomy on a prosection as they present their clinical correlation. Faculty rate the students' oral communication skills on the basis of clarity, organisation, fluency of speech, volume, tone and pace.

Students can also be evaluated on their oral communication skills in problem-based learning groups or in case presentations on clinical clerkships. Faculty must concentrate on the communication skills apart from the content in order to properly evaluate students and give them adequate feedback. Focusing on the communication for the first 30 seconds of an oral presentation enables the observer to make fairly reliable characterisations. Selecting another 30-second segment later in the presentation enhances the reliability of the observations after students' initial nervousness has subsided.

More advanced oral communication skills can be assessed using real or standardised patients who represent a greater communication challenge to students. Examples include telling a woman with previously treated breast cancer that metastases have been detected, obtaining a history through an interpreter or communicating with a reticent adolescent. Faculty should directly observe students, either through live direct observation or through an audio or preferably video recording. Recorded interactions have the advantage of enabling faculty to review the students' performances in short segments, stopping, and providing feedback. If the observation was direct and not recorded, faculty should focus on a short segment of the interaction, then provide feedback based on specific behaviours observed during that segment rather than broad generalizations based on the entire interaction.

Written communication skills are easily assessed through formal writing assignments such as having students write a short opinion piece on a controversy in healthcare policy. The writing sample can be evaluated based on its ease of readability, clarity, organisation, tone and the degree to which it is free of errors in spelling, grammar and usage.

Writing skills can also be assessed in clinical settings. Legibility can be assessed in students' entries in patient records. Students can be asked

Assess communication skills by focusing on how the student is speaking rather than on what is being said.

to draft consultation letters to assess their ability to write clearly, concisely and correctly.

Basic clinical skills

Bedside teaching
Bedside teaching (see chapter 9) represents the way in which clinical skills have traditionally been assessed. Clinical tutors observe students obtaining a history or examining the patient or performing a clinical procedure. Procedure logs can help ensure that this actually happens. Students are required to obtain faculty members' signatures attesting to the adequacy of specific clinical skills that have been directly observed. Assigning responsibility to students to obtain the signatures increases the likelihood that the observations will actually be done.

Videotaping
Given the hectic schedules of students and faculty, videotape recordings of encounters between students and patients offer the advantage that they can be jointly viewed at more convenient times. Videotapes are particularly useful to assess the history-taking skills of students. Videotapes are less ideal when used to assess physical examination skills or clinical procedure skills because of limitations of fields of vision.

Standardised patients
Standardised patients (see chapter 8, Teaching in the clinical skills centre) can be used very effectively to assess physical examination skills. Standardised patients have proved particularly useful in teaching and assessing female breast and pelvic examination skills and male genitourinary and rectal examination skills.

Simulations
Nonhuman simulations can be used safely and efficiently to assess skills in clinical procedures. Plastic manikins can be used to teach students how to perform lumbar punctures, catheterise the bladder, insert nasogastric tubes, obtain arterial blood samples and many other common procedures.

Using basic science in the practice of medicine
Students can become excited about the relevance of basic science when they are asked to demonstrate their knowledge of the underlying scientific facts and principles through clinical correlations (see chapter 25, Basic and clinical sciences). At the Memorial University of Newfoundland, the physiology faculty designed a three-stage paper-based 'triple-jump' examination in which students were presented in class with a clinical situation, then asked to list the topics in biomedical science necessary for understanding the physiological responses in such a person. Students pursued their own learning objectives outside of class, followed by an in-class examination derived from the students' own work (Hansen & Roberts, abstract presentation, 1993).

During the clinical years, students can be assigned to present an update on the latest scientific explanations of the mechanisms of disease related to the patients they are caring for. This can be done either as an oral presentation to their faculty supervisor and fellow students or as a written report as part of the patient record.

Diagnosis, management and prevention

Medical teachers are comfortable with assessing students' skills in diagnosis, management and prevention. Student ability is most often assessed through oral presentations to faculty preceptors and by written lists of differential diagnoses and management plans as part of the medical record.

OSCEs also can be used to assess these outcomes, both during the interactions with standardised patients and in exercises following the encounters with them. Examples of standardised patient cases that assess these outcomes are: offering the standardised patient an opinion about the nature of a headache after obtaining a history, diagnosing depression in a patient presenting with somatic complaints, offering the patient a management plan for the treatment of low back pain and providing the patient with contraceptive options. Examples of exercises without standardised patient present include: interpreting a chest X-ray, electrocardiogram or Gram stain, and writing a prescription for an antihypertensive drug in a patient newly diagnosed with hypertension.

Diagnosis, management and prevention can be applied to populations as well as to individuals and families. Students can be told to undertake a community diagnosis in which they ascertain the health status of the population, then propose plans for better management of the health problems, including public health measures designed to prevent or minimise illness and injury.

Lifelong learning

Lifelong learning comprises both skills and attitudes. The skills involve being able to identify one's own learning needs, to undertake the appropriate learning activities, and to apply what one has learned. Attitudes of curiosity, a drive for excellence, a willingness to honestly appraise one's own weaknesses and a motivation for learning fuel the quest for lifelong learning.

Problem-based learning groups (see chapter 16, Problem-based learning) are an excellent venue in which to assess this ability in students. The faculty facilitator can observe the degree to which students contribute to the delineation of learning issues, adequately investigate the learning issues and apply what they have learned to the case under discussion.

The attitudes of lifelong learning can be observed in the clinical setting when students take the initiative themselves to learn more about their patients. This can be observed when students cite sources they have explored in learning more about their patients' problems.

Structuring the curriculum to allow students to pursue independent interests provides another excellent opportunity to assess lifelong learning. In designing their projects, students should be asked to explicitly state what incident or event made them think about what they needed to learn. Students should also be asked to explicitly describe their proposed learning strategies and resources. Students should suggest ways in which faculty could determine whether the student had successfully achieved the learning goals. This model of assessing lifelong learning in students closely parallels the model for continuing professional education for practising clinicians.

Professional development and personal growth

Portfolios (see chapter 37, Portfolios, projects and dissertations) may be the best way to assess professional development and personal growth, since self-reflection and self-awareness are such an important component to this outcome. Students select the material that they wish to put into their portfolios that is important and meaningful to them. For example, some students may wish to write a short reflection essay about their feelings after having first encountered a cadaver or after their first interview with a patient. Ideally, students should discuss these reflections with a trusted faculty advisor.

Faculty advisors assess students' achievement of this outcome not so much on the specific content of the discussions as much as on the degree to which students have thoughtfully reflected on the incidents, honestly confronted their own feelings and values and drawn lessons that help them grow both personally and professionally.

Professional development and personal growth are best assessed over a long period of time by the same faculty advisor. Specific time for these activities must be built into the curriculum because they are unlikely to happen on their own, given the other pressures on students.

The social and community contexts of healthcare

Service learning enables students to make connections between what they have learned in class about the healthcare system and the reality that their patients actually encounter (see chapter 11, In the community). By reflecting on their experiences, students can bring their own values into their analysis of what they have seen. Journals are a particularly good way to capture these reflections. Faculty can assess the journal entries on the degree to which they demonstrate evidence of careful observation, curiosity, connections, self-awareness, empathy and social consciousness.

Students' ability to understand the nonbiological factors that influence health can be assessed by involving students in discharge planning for patients with complex health and social service problems. Students can make home visits to assess the home situation and the patient's progress, accompany patients to community health resources and work with other health professionals involved in the patient's care.

Community health projects initiated by students reflect an advanced level of competency, demonstrating a commitment to public health and social justice. Formal assessment of such initiatives can be undertaken in a seminar format in which the student leaders present an overview of their efforts to a panel of faculty, perhaps augmented by community representatives.

Moral reasoning and clinical ethics

Students can be asked to present ethically challenging cases to faculty supervisors. The ensuing discussion enables the faculty to assess the

The staff in community practices are in an excellent position to assess professionalism in students.

"The intended output of a competency-based programme is a health professional who can practise medicine at a defined level of proficiency, in accord with local conditions, to meet local needs"

[McGaghie et al 1978]

student's ability to identify ethical issues in a clinical context and to analyse them appropriately (see chapter 27, Ethics and attitudes). OSCE stations can be designed with the same goals in mind. The OSCE format has the advantage of being able to demonstrate whether students can detect an ethical component and allows direct observation of the students' clinical ethics skills during interactions with patients (Smith et al 1994).

Students can also write formal papers on ethical controversies. This approach is particularly useful to assess students' ability to explore the moral dimensions of issues of health policy. The evaluation focuses on how well students can argue their positions on the basis of moral principles rather than the particular position they take.

Problem solving

Problem solving means more than calculating the correct answer to a computational question in physiology. Problem solving as an educational outcome means being able to get the job done in messy situations. In a very real sense, problem solving is a meta-outcome, requiring students to utilise all the other previously enumerated skills to assess a situation, frame the problem, devise an action plan, negotiate with multiple players, mobilise resources, execute the plan, respond flexibly and creatively to unanticipated obstacles and constantly monitor progress. Being a good problem solver is the essence of being a professional.

The best way to assess problem solving is to put learners into real clinical situations in which they have primary (but closely supervised) responsibility for patient care. Clinical supervisors must restrain themselves from giving too much direction, instead observing how students set priorities, juggle multiple tasks simultaneously, filter and interpret large amounts of data and respond agilely to changing circumstances. Of course, clinical supervisors must be ready to intervene to safeguard patient safety and assure appropriate care, but should do so only when necessary and with the least amount of intervention needed to get things back on track. Ideally, this could be done by suggesting to students that a new approach is needed and asking the students to come up with alternative plans.

Summary

An outcome-based curriculum rests on sound, practical, time-tested principles of good education:

- Define what you want students to come away with from your course. We must go beyond simply knowing, to being able to implement what one knows.
- Design assessment methods to ascertain whether students have achieved the learning you expected.

The goal of teaching is to help students learn. Therefore, we make our expectations of learning clear, precise and public. Since assessment drives student learning, we create assessments with the primary purpose of helping students learn. The assessment should reflect, as authentically as possible, the actual tasks that students will be expected to perform in actual situations.

The course of study should present students with repeated opportunities to experience, practise, and gauge their progress in the assessment tasks in varied contexts and situations, at increasing levels of challenge and complexity. Faculty should repeatedly assess student performance and ask themselves how the learning experience might be improved to enhance student performance.

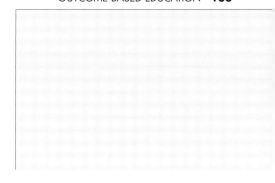

References

ACGME (Accreditation Council on Graduate Medical Education) ACGME Outcome Project 2001 Online. Available: http://www.acgme.org/outcome/comp/compFull.asp 19 Dec 2003

Harden R M 2002 Learning outcomes and instructional objectives: is there a difference? Medical Teacher 24:151–155

Mager R F 1962 Preparing instructional objectives. Fearon, Palo Alto

McGaghie W C, Miller G E, Sajid A W, Telder T V 1978 Curriculum models. In: Competency-based curriculum development in medical education. World Health Organization, Geneva, p 18

Schwartz M R, Wojtczak A J 2002 Global minimum essential requirements: a road towards competence-oriented medical education. Medical Teacher 24:125–129

Simpson J G, Furnace J, Crosby J et al 2002 The Scottish doctor – learning outcomes for the medical undergraduate in Scotland: a foundation for competent and reflective practitioners. Medical Teacher 24:136–143

Smith S R, Balint J A, Krause K C et al 1994 Performance-based assessment of moral reasoning and ethical judgment among medical students. Academic Medicine 69:381–386

Smith S R, Dollase R H, Boss J A 2003 Assessing students' performance in a competency-based curriculum. Academic Medicine 78:97–107

Updike J 1960 Rabbit, run. Knopf, New York

Chapter 15

Independent learning

R. M. Harden

"Self instruction may be an alternative to other forms of teaching, but it can also be combined with them"

Rowntree 1990

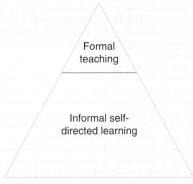

Fig. 15.1 The formal learning 'iceberg'

"a strategy that promotes self-directed learning is likely to be the most effective"

Spencer & Jordan 1999

Introduction

Other chapters in this book look at how students learn in large-group settings such as lectures, in small groups and 'on the job' working with their colleagues. What matters, irrespective of the approach adopted to teaching and learning, is the learning achieved by the individual. In postgraduate and continuing education, and in traditional and innovative undergraduate education programmes, learners spend a significant proportion of their time learning on their own. Indeed, the formal learning in the taught part of an educational programme may represent only the tip of the iceberg (see Fig. 15.1).

After a lecture, students master the topic by reading their notes or the relevant sections in a textbook. Students prepare for small-group work and follow up such sessions by studying on their own. In the clinical setting, too, students need to find out more about the underlying problems of the patients they have seen, from further reading or the use of electronic information sources. The intensity of independent learning in the traditional undergraduate curriculum usually increases before a formal examination, with students attempting to revise or master the contents of a course over a relatively short period of time, sometimes at the expense of attendance at other scheduled sessions. In distance learning, independent learning is the major or sole activity.

The importance of independent learning may not be fully recognised – time for it is not formally scheduled in the curriculum and appropriate learning resource material and support for students are often not provided. The increasing emphasis on independent learning acknowledges that learning is not something that someone else can do for students but that it must be done by students for themselves.

In this chapter we will consider:

- what we mean by 'independent learning' and related terms such as 'self-learning'
- why independent learning makes a key contribution to the curriculum

- some current trends in independent learning and the rapid advances in e-learning.

What is independent learning?

Six key principles

The concept of independent learning means different things to different people. It incorporates six key principles:

- Students learn on their own.
- Students have a measure of control over their own learning. They may choose:
  - where to learn
  - what to learn
  - how to learn
  - when to learn.
  Learners take responsibility for:
  - deciding the context for learning
  - diagnosing personal learning needs
  - identifying resources
  - deciding time for learning and the pacing of learning.
- Students may be encouraged to develop their own personal learning plans (Challis 2000).
- The different needs of individual students are recognised and appropriate response is made to the specific needs of the individual learner – 'just-for-you' education.
- Student learning is supported, to a greater or lesser extent, by learning resources and study guides prepared for this purpose.
- The role of the teacher changes from a lecturer or transmitter of information to a manager of the learning process – a more demanding but a more rewarding role (Harden & Crosby 2000).

Terms used

A number of terms have been used to describe this approach to learning. These terms are often used interchangeably although different meanings may be implied.

- Independent learning – emphasises that students work on their own to meet their own learning needs.
- Self-managed learning, self-directed learning or self-regulated learning – emphasises that students have an element of control over their own learning, with responsibility for diagnosis of learning needs and identifying resources. Implicit in this approach is that students have a clear understanding of the intended learning outcomes.
- Resource-based learning – emphasises the use of resource material in print or multimedia format as a basis for students' learning, and the freedom this gives to the student.
- 'Just-for-you' or flexible learning – emphasises the wide range of learning opportunities offered to students and a flexibility in responding to individual student needs and aspirations.

Independent learning is based on discovery-guided mentoring rather than on the transmission of information.

"Flexible learning is a generic term that covers all these situations where learners have some say in how, where or when learning takes place"

Ellington, in Bell et al 1997

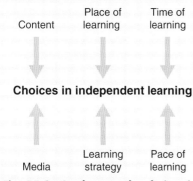

Fig. 15.2 **Students make choices in independent learning**

- Open learning – often used interchangeably with flexible learning. It emphasises the provision of greater access for students to their choice of education.
- E-learning – learning is facilitated by information and communication technology.
- Distance learning – emphasises that students work on their own at a distance from their teacher. Implicit in the approach is that the teachers interact with students at a distance and facilitate the students' learning.
- 'Just-in-time' learning – resources are made available to learners when required. This facilitates 'on-the-job' learning and the integration of theory and practice.

The two ideas underpinning the above concepts are:

- learners study individually on their own
- learners have charge of the learning process.

Both features are absent in the lecture and present in independent learning where students direct their own studies to achieve the prescribed learning outcomes (see Fig. 15.2). In many education programmes, students work on their own, e.g. reading prescribed texts, but have little control of their learning. In other situations, students may control their learning, as in problem-based learning, but greater emphasis is placed on group rather than on individual work.

The importance of independent learning

There are many reasons why independent learning has become more fashionable as a paradigm of learning in medical education.

Developments in the new learning technologies and e-learning are occurring at an astonishingly rapid pace, and the implications for traditional approaches to education, and indeed for medical schools as we know them today, are profound. The dramatic developments taking place in e-learning cannot be questioned, bringing a whole new dimension to what is possible in independent learning (Harden 2002). This is discussed further in chapters 22, 23 and 24.

The modular and flexible curriculum
There has been a trend to modularity and flexibility in curriculum planning. Students, individually or in small groups, may rotate through a series of attachments. In electives or special study modules, they can choose to study areas in more depth. Independent learning has a useful role to play in these situations and can help to avoid unnecessary repetitive teaching by staff. Different groups of students may use the same resource pack and study guide, leaving the teacher free for one-to-one contact with students.

Different contexts for learning
With the development of e-learning, distance learning has increased in popularity in undergraduate, postgraduate and continuing education.

"Web and Internet technologies are transforming our world, presenting opportunities we could only imagine a few years ago"

Horton 2001

"Self directed learning enables progressive educators to give greater expression to their philosophies"

Collins & Hammond 1987

Technophobes may choose to minimise contact with the computer. Encourage them to try e-learning.

Students are remote from the teacher and have to rely more on working on their own. Distance learning is particularly appropriate in postgraduate and continuing medical education (see chapter 12). The CRISIS criteria for effective continuing education, developed in the context of distance learning, recognise the potential advantages implicit in independent learning (Harden & Laidlaw 1992):

- **C**onvenience for the student in terms of pace, place and time ('just-in-time' learning)
- **R**elevance to the needs of the practising doctor
- **I**ndividualisation to the needs of each learner ('just-for-you' learning)
- **S**elf-assessment by the learner of his or her own competence
- **I**nterest in the programme and motivation of the learner
- **S**ystematic coverage of the topic or theme for the programme
- **S**peculation – the grey areas where there may be uncertainty.

Active learning

Independent learning, if planned appropriately, encourages a more active approach to learning. Students adopt a deep rather than a superficial approach to learning and search for an understanding of the subject rather than just reproducing what they have learned. Students are encouraged to think and not just recall facts they have learned.

The needs of individual learners

Learners are not a homogeneous group – they have different needs and different aspirations and learn in different ways. The adoption of an independent learning approach encourages these needs to be recognised and allows for learner choice in terms of content, learning strategy and rates of learning (see Fig. 15.3). In 'just-for-you' learning, the learning programme is customised to the needs of the individual student or doctor.

Students can choose the learning method or approach which suits them best. They can skim learning material rapidly if they already understand it and spend more time with what is new or challenging to them. In mastery learning, students work with appropriate resource material until they reach the level of mastery required.

Student motivation

Independent learning gives students more responsibility for their learning and greater participation in the learning process. It allows them to choose the appropriate level for their studies. This in turn gives them a sense of ownership of their learning which has a positive effect on student motivation.

The role of the teacher

The teacher's role as a manager of the students' learning is well accepted and consistent with an independent learning approach (Harden & Crosby 2000). This facilitative role leaves teachers to develop new relationships with students and may result in greater trust between teacher and student.

"Their aims have been to promote greater active learning, more experiential learning and to encourage reflective learning"

Hudson et al 1997

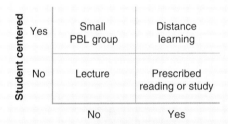

Fig. 15.3 **Control of learning by student**

Do not settle only for learning experiences with which the students are comfortable. Stretch the students both individually and personally.

"There is no right way to develop self-instructional materials. But there are lots of wrong ways"

Rowntree 1990

While many teachers feel most comfortable in the traditional role of information provider, others have discovered talents in developing resource material, a role which is also being recognised and rewarded.

Cost-effectiveness

There are pressures on academic staff to provide coherent and effective teaching and learning programmes despite increasing student numbers and decreasing units of resource. There is strong opposition to these pressures and there are concerns that quality may suffer.

The justification for the introduction of independent learning lay previously with improved quality of learning rather than with cost savings. Independent learning can now, if used appropriately, contribute to cost savings. This is likely to require the sharing of resources between institutions as in the International Virtual Medical School (IVIMEDS). Careful timetabling is also required. If all students are scheduled to use a learning resource at the same time, then many copies may be required. If the period of time when students are 'ripe' for a resource is extended, fewer copies are required and the exercise is more likely to be cost-effective. In an integrated endocrinology course made up of four modules and based on the use of resource material, for example, the timetable was so arranged that only a quarter of the students studied a module at any one time. This greatly reduced the need to duplicate resources. However, this is less of a problem with computer- or internet-based resources.

Areas of controversy

The traditional curriculum emphasises the views on a topic of the teacher or lecturer with whom the student is in contact. The student may be seduced into the notion that there is one right answer or one approach to a problem. Independent learning allows him or her to be exposed to the rich environment of many visions and interpretations.

Outcome-based education

There is a move away from a process model of curriculum planning to a product one where the learning outcomes are made more explicit and where outcomes influence decisions about teaching and learning and about assessment.

With the destination to be reached clearly charted, students may wish to plan their own route. Independent learning thrives in such an environment.

The development of self-learning skills

The acquisition of the skills of self-learning and the ability to keep up to date with developments in medicine are learning outcomes about which there is general agreement.

Traditional teaching methods do not emphasise the development of these skills. In contrast, independent learning encourages not only mastery of the content area being studied but also the development of generic skills of self-learning.

A greater emphasis on independent learning can be seen as a response to many of the challenges facing medical education.

"Uncertainty should not be hidden away as an embarrassment"

Alderson & Roberts 2000

"The only man who is educated is the man who has learned how to learn"

Rogers 1983

Trends in independent learning

Independent learning is not new. To a greater or lesser extent, students have always worked independently. One can identify, however, a number of changes in current approaches to independent learning, many triggered by developments in e-learning.

An increasingly important role

It was demonstrated almost four decades ago in a randomised controlled trial (Harden et al 1969) that medical students learn as or more effectively when they work independently, using learning resources prepared for the purpose, compared with students who attend lectures. Until recently, however, teachers have been slow to move away from a curricular emphasis on lectures. There has been a significant change and independent learning is now playing an increasingly important role in the curriculum:

- Time previously scheduled for lectures or small-group work is often rescheduled for independent learning.
- Independent learning is now an explicit planned part of the learning activities, and protected time is allocated for it in the timetable.
- The role of the lecture is changing. Lectures are used to support independent learning rather than independent learning being used as an adjunct to support the lecture.
- Students make increasing use of the internet as a learning resource.

A planned and supported programme

Independent learning, it is now appreciated, has to be carefully planned and not left to chance. The choice is not between a planned programme of lectures and other activities on the one hand, and on the other, students being left to fend for themselves.

Planning by the teacher for independent learning includes:

- Recognising the role of independent learning in the curriculum, making this explicit to students and scheduling it in the timetable.
- Ensuring students have the necessary study skills with which to engage in independent learning in the first instance. Study skills training needed may include:
  — how to assess needs
  — how to plan learning
  — how to manage time
  — how to locate and use appropriate resources including electronic resources
  — how to evaluate outcomes of learning.
- Identifying the tools to be used by students in their studies, including library facilities, personal textbooks, computer-based simulations and the internet.

A wide range of tools available

An increasingly wide range of tools to support independent learning has become available. Regrettably, however, the technical sophistication of

"The curriculum must motivate students and help them develop the skills for self-directed learning"

GMC 2002

"Medical faculties should examine critically the number of lecture hours they now schedule and consider major reductions in this passive form of learning"

Association of American Medical Colleges 1984

"If students are to learn effectively in resource-based learning courses, then they need more and better learning skills than those currently exhibited by students on conventional courses"

Brown & Smith 1996

Technology should enrich teaching not substitute for it.

To develop learning resources, expertise is needed in the content area, in the delivery medium and in instructional design.

"A study guide can be seen as a management tool which allows teachers to exercise their responsibilities while at the same time giving students an important part to play in managing their own learning"

Harden et al 1999

"A peer support website can broaden student interest in learning independently and is especially pertinent to the needs of less confident students seeking to improve their academic performance"

Baker & Dillon 1999

the resources available is often not paralleled by their educational sophistication. Many lack the basic principles of educational design such as the incorporation of meaningful interactivity and feedback.

Too often computers have been used merely as mechanical page-turners and the internet has been abused, encouraging passive learning rather than a deeper understanding and reflection. The need is now recognised to incorporate proven effective educational strategies into the instructional design for self-learning.

E-learning, as adopted for example, in the International Virtual Medical School (IVIMEDS), is supporting a self-directed, an integrated and a problem-based curriculum. It is of value in bringing together and integrating in various ways a range of resources and experts from a number of fields.

The provision of support for students

The adoption of independent learning does not imply that the teacher abandons the student to work on his or her own. The role of the teacher as a facilitator in independent learning is an important one. This is achieved through interactions between student and teacher, face-to-face, by telephone or on the internet. The teacher can also prepare study guides to support the student's learning as described in chapter 21.

Study guides can:

- provide information not readily available to students in the information sources to which they have access
- provide guidance for students on the management of their learning, with advice on what they should learn, how they should learn it and how can they assess whether they have learned it
- suggest activities for students which reinforce their learning and relate it to clinical practice.

Study guides vary in the extent to which they emphasise each of these facilities, and the relative importance of each in a guide can be indicated by placing the guide in a triangle (the study guide triangle), with each function identified at one of the three points of the triangle (Harden et al 1999). A guide placed equidistant from each of the points has all three functions equally represented.

Study guides may be in print or electronic format.

Students may also get support from their colleagues. This concept of peer-to-peer collaborative learning has gained increased recognition. Students may be helped by:

- their peers
- students in the later years of a course who are assigned to help more junior students
- working in pairs as a basis for their studies.

The range of contexts

The wide range of contexts in which independent learning can occur is now recognised. These include:

- at home
- in areas in a learning centre or teaching institution developed for this purpose
- on the job or in the workplace.

A focus for assessment

Portfolios prepared by students as part of their independent work serve not only as an aid to learning but as a powerful tool for assessment alongside more traditional tests based on written examinations and/or objective structured clinical examinations (OSCEs) (Friedman Ben-David et al 2001). This emphasises the importance of independent learning. What the students are intended to achieve and how they will record this should be documented.

Summary

Independent learning should occupy a key role in the curriculum with e-learning making a major contribution. The twin aims are mastery of the topic under consideration and the development of the skills of self-learning. Teachers and curriculum planners should decide:

- How much time should be scheduled in the curriculum for independent learning? It is unlikely to be less than 25% or more than 75%.
- How to recognise and institutionalise the position adopted with regard to independent learning through:
  — protected time in the curriculum identified in the timetable
  — provision of appropriate learning resources
  — recognition in the assessment procedures
  — a staff development programme to orientate staff.
- The range of methods or tools to be offered to the learner, e.g. printed material, videodiscs, curriculum-based simulations, virtual patients and the internet.
- How students will be supported as they work through the programme. Study guides can be seen as a tutor to which they have constant access.

"Traditional exams cannot test many of the skills and abilities developed by resource-based learning"

Brown & Smith 1996

"Having students acquire skills as active learners will require considerable effort and increased dedication to this goal of faculty members"

Anderson & Swanson 1993

References

Alderson P, Roberts I 2000 Should journals publish reviews that find no evidence to guide practice? British Medical Journal 320:376–377

Association of American Medical Colleges 1984 Physicians for the 21st Century: report of the project panel on the general professional education of the physicians and college preparation for medicine. Journal of Medical Education 59, Part 2:1–208

Anderson M B, Swanson A G 1993 Educating medical students – the ACME-TRI report with supplements. Academic Medicine 68 (Suppl):S1–46

Baker J, Dillon G 1999 Peer support on the web. IETI 36(1):65–70

Brown S, Smith B 1996 Resource-based learning. Kogan Page, London

Challis M 2000 AMEE Medical Education Guide no.18. Personal learning plans. Medical Teacher 22(3):225–236

Collins R, Hammond M 1987 Self-directed learning to educate medical educators: why do we use self-directed learning? Medical Teacher 9(4):425–432

Ellington H 1997 Flexible learning – your flexible friend! Keynote address. In: Bell C, Bowden M, Trott A (eds) Implementing flexible learning. Aspects of educational and training technology vol XXIX. Kogan Page, London, p 3–13

Friedman Ben-David M, Davis M H, Harden R M et al 2001 AMEE Medical Education Guide no. 24. Portfolios as a method of student assessment. Medical Teacher 23(6):535–551

GMC 2002 Tomorrow's doctors: recommendations on undergraduate medical education. General Medical Council, London

Harden R M 2002 Myths and e-learning. Medical Teacher 24(5):469–472

Harden R M, Crosby J R 2000 AMEE Education Guide no. 20. The good teacher is more than a lecturer – the twelve roles of the teacher. Medical Teacher 22(4):334–347

Harden R M, Laidlaw J M 1992 Effective continuing education: the CRISIS criteria. AMEE Medical Education Guide no. 4. Medical Education 26:408–422

Harden R M et al 1969 An experiment involving substitution of tape/slide programmes for lectures. Lancet 1:993–935

Harden R M, Laidlaw J M, Hesketh E A 1999 AMEE Medical Education Guide no. 16. Study guides – their use and preparation. Medical Teacher 21(3):248–265

Horton W 2001 Leading e-learning. American Society for Training and Development (ASTD), Alexandria VA, p 130–131

Hudson R, Maslin-Prothero S, Oates L 1997 Flexible learning in action: case studies in higher education. Staff and Educational Development Series. Kogan Page, London

Rogers C R 1983 Freedom to learn for the 80s. Charles E. Merrill, Columbus, Ohio

Rowntree D 1990 Teaching through self-instruction: how to develop open learning materials. Kogan Page, London

Spencer J A, Jordan R K 1999 Learner-centred approaches in medical education. British Medical Journal 318(7193):1280–1283

Chapter 16
Problem-based learning

A. Sefton

Introduction

What is problem-based learning?

Problem-based learning (PBL) in small groups is an effective student-centred approach to learning (Norman & Schmidt 2000). It differs substantially from programmes based on didactic teaching supplemented with case-based activities (Boud & Feletti 1998, Maudsley 1999). The tutor is a facilitator rather than a content expert. PBL in medical programmes is usually implemented early, although it may extend into later years. For over 30 years evidence has accumulated to demonstrate that the method successfully encourages effective and self-directed learning, critical thinking, teamwork, understanding rather than memorisation, and facility with professional language. Both students and staff enjoy the process. Different, well-established medical examples are provided by Tosteson and colleagues (1994), Henry and colleagues (1997) and Des Marchais (2001). PBL is enriched if aligned with computer-based resources (Carlile et al. 1998).

A problem initiates the activity. The group (of 10 or fewer) is stimulated to explore basic scientific and clinical mechanisms together with social, psychological, ethical or professional issues. Knowledge is integrated and applied. Because the process is potentially open-ended, teachers have an obligation to design well-structured problems that meet explicit goals.

The problem stimulates students to reason, think critically and weigh evidence; they seek out and share relevant information. Groups do not need prior knowledge to generate lively ideas as they identify areas for further collective and personal learning. Each student brings individual experience and makes a distinctive contribution (Woods 1994). The tutor's role is to manage the interactions (Fig. 16.1) rather than supply information (Fig. 16.2).

An effective group provides a safe environment for sharing and testing new knowledge. Students practise the language of science and medicine, evaluate ideas and receive feedback from peers and tutor.

When clinical exposure is introduced concurrently, intellectual and practical skills develop in parallel. Clinical experiences enrich tutorial discussions.

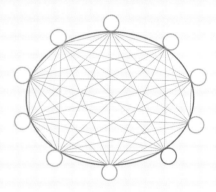

Possible interpersonal communication links for nine students and a tutor. These complex interactions must be facilitated and managed.

Fig. 16.1 A problem-based group

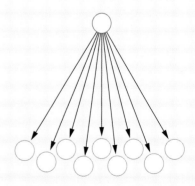

A typical didactic session with one-way communication.

Fig. 16.2 A didactic session

"A particular goal of this student-centred, problem-based approach is to develop physicians who practice 'science in action' rather than attempting to apply learned formulas to clinical situations"

Tosteson et al 1994

"the key for problem-based learning is...to use a problem to drive the learning activities on a need-to-know basis"

Woods 1994

Trust the collective curiosity and motivation of the group to identify the issues arising from the problem and determine their learning goals.

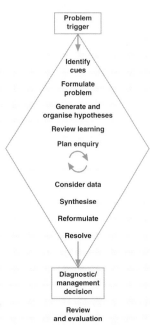

Fig. 16.3 Model of problem-based learning. A trigger (text or image) stimulates wide brainstorming to encourage the generation of hypotheses and ideas that are tested in discussion. The group breaks (once or twice) to explore relevant information to bring back to the discussion. An agreed resolution is reached.

In preparing students for professional practice, PBL:

- Encourages independence as students identify and meet individual learning needs.
- Stimulates reflection and self-direction for lifelong learning.
- Supports ongoing self-assessment.
- Introduces clinical reasoning, later refined with clinical experience.
- Enhances critical thinking and evidence-based decision making.
- Ensures that knowledge is transferred, applied and retained by providing a relevant, integrated context.
- Offers practice and experience in introducing professional concepts and medical language.
- Supports effective teamwork and peer communication.

Developing and mapping a sequence of learning problems structures a modern, relevant, integrated curriculum, minimising redundancy, overload and gaps. It supports evaluation and continuing evolutionary change (Field & Sefton 1998).

Experiencing a problem-based tutorial

Observing an effective tutorial group in action provides an opportunity to experience the basic characteristics. The initial impression is usually of an open, lively and free-flowing discussion in which all participate. The atmosphere is friendly and informal.

In different schools, the number, structure and sequence of tutorials may vary. As students and tutors gain experience, groups become more targeted and efficient.

Effective tutors do not dominate or instruct. Indeed, it may not be immediately apparent which individual is the tutor. She or he quietly observes and monitors the process, ensuring that all are included and that interactions focus on relevant issues.

Frameworks and sequences for problem-based learning

Well-designed problems are underpinned by a structure for reasoning, equally explicit to tutors and students (Fig.16.3). Typically:

- A trigger initiates the problem (on paper, computer, video).
- Groups brainstorm to identify cues and key issues for discussion.
- Broad thinking produces a rich array of mechanisms and ideas.
- Hypotheses are critically explored through reasoning and organised by priority or likelihood.
- The need for additional information is identified.
- Hypotheses are tested and refuted or supported by information that is progressively revealed.
- A conclusion is reached on diagnosis and/or management.
- The group reviews the process.

In breaks between tutorials, students identify learning issues to be pursued. They are encouraged to adopt an evidence-based approach. When they reconvene, they share and review the learning.

Characteristics of an effective PBL group

An effective group is cohesive, motivated, mutually supportive and actively engaged in learning. The group understands the process and energetically pursues its task.

Members respect each other's contributions but examine them critically. Discussion flows as students cooperate rather than compete. Quieter members are encouraged while the more confident restrain their tendencies to dominate. Individuals are supported during times of personal stress.

The atmosphere is friendly and good-humoured. Discussion is open but tactful and constructive. Difficulties that arise are not ignored, but dealt with sensitively in a climate of mutual tolerance.

Members are proud of their successful group. They look forward to tutorials and may spend time together outside sessions. Successful groups induct new tutors and restrain excessive interference from overly directive teachers.

Roles are shared; all take turns in scribing, leading discussion or accepting responsibility for acquiring information. If the tutor is delayed, well-established groups confidently start the tutorial and proceed effectively.

Groups often share food and drink, inside the rooms if permitted or by taking 'time out'.

Staff development

The importance of tutor training to equip teachers for their new roles cannot be overemphasised (Farmer 2003). Indeed, basic training is usually mandatory and further development may be a requirement. Some teachers find it hard to relinquish more didactic roles that allow them to display content expertise, but most enjoy the new experience.

Before starting as a tutor, it is usual (and may be required) to observe a group in the same school. In new programmes, tutors who initially observed groups elsewhere must be aware of differences in goals, expectations or organisation.

The nature of staff development and ongoing support varies. Initial training may involve observation and practice with a group from the programme or recruited for the purpose. Alternatively the PBL process may be modelled amongst the trainees themselves.

Effective training ensures that the necessary background, goals and local strategies are considered, together with information on assessment and evaluation. Specific issues of institutional emphasis (e.g. evidence-based medicine or information technology) require explanation and practice. Tutors need skills in monitoring the process and giving feedback.

In addition to materials supplied to students, tutors are usually issued with handbooks or guides, highlighting issues for each problem. They may also contain essential information to be revealed progressively.

Making explicit the underlying framework, as well as the sequence and structure of the tutorials, encourages groups to work efficiently.

Relax! Students in problem-based groups will certainly:
- Learn and understand content.
- Think critically.
- Use scientific and medical language.
- Correct errors.
- Learn how to learn.

"I learn so much science and medicine from being a PBL tutor!"

Senior clinical academic

"...PBL is very different from traditional teaching methods and requires that administrators, teachers and students adapt."

Schwartz et al 2001

To become a confident tutor:
- Sit in on a class.
- Seek staff development.
- Review the sequence of problems.
- Study tutor guides and websites.
- Understand assessment requirements.

Seek information about the characteristics of your group from previous tutors and get to know the individuals as quickly as possible.

Make sure that you can communicate directly with your group for messages (e-mail, phone call, bulletin board, mailbox). Plan ahead and be prepared:
- Understand the model used.
- Know the students' level.
- Review the goals.
- Read tutor information.
- Identify key discussion points.

"I thought the group I sat in with was doing really well for second year students – their collective knowledge and understanding was impressive. Then I found out that they were actually only a few months into first year!"

Visitor from UK to Graduate Medical Program, University of Sydney

One important source of continuing support is engagement with other tutors. Frequently a meeting is scheduled to discuss current and upcoming problems, ideally with case writers or subject experts present. Issues of content and process are discussed, and difficulties or confusions resolved; experiences are shared and strategies reviewed. Such meetings encourage tutors to contribute to the quality control of the programme. To summarise, participants in a tutor training session will:

- Review the goals.
- Understand the tutor's role.
- Clarify local practices and requirements.
- Acknowledge and share concerns.
- Identify resources and support.
- Practise new strategies.
- Share experiences.
- Meet fellow tutors.
- Participate enthusiastically!

Starting as a PBL tutor

Would-be tutors need some crucial information before embarking on teaching:

- Are the students beginners or 'old hands'? What have they learned already? What are their expectations?
- What model of PBL is used? How many tutorials? What are the reasoning steps?
- Are guides or handbooks supplied to tutors?
- What is the tutor's role in guiding the breadth and depth of learning?
- What additional learning activities are provided? Are other resources available? What support is offered to students in difficulties?
- How are students assessed? Do tutors assess?

At your first tutorial, introduce yourself and allow time for each student to introduce himself or herself as an individual. Nervous new tutors generally find it easiest to start with an established group. Helping students to form a new group requires particular skills but some tutors prefer that role.

Who makes a good PBL tutor?

Good tutors encourage appropriate interaction by maintaining an open and trusting environment. They reflect on their own performance.

PBL teachers enjoy facilitating learning and enhancing reasoning skills. With training, senior undergraduates, research students and staff at all levels of appointment have become effective tutors.

Does subject expertise matter? Successful tutors may be drawn from diverse disciplines but the majority are most comfortable tutoring in areas related to their own expertise. Some prior knowledge or experience may allow tutors to enhance a group's effectiveness provided that they facilitate and do not dictate. Relevant experience leading to a sense of comfort may come from prior research, teaching or clinical practice or from previous tutoring on the same problems (Wilkerson 1994).

Any trained tutor who facilitates group learning is appropriate. Thus individuals with educational, scientific, health professional or humanities backgrounds have been effective medical PBL tutors. By contrast, subject experts who direct, deliver mini-lectures or interrupt the free flow of a group's discussion are inappropriate since they circumvent the essential exploration and interaction that underpin the success of PBL.

Some teachers who are expert in an area find it difficult to adopt the facilitative practices needed. That shift in role requires an understanding of the goals of PBL flexibility and an awareness of students' needs.

Good tutors encourage behaviours that enhance the sessions, ensuring that all participate appropriately. They help set expectations and provide thoughtful insights to the group.

At the end of the session a tutor should reflect on the following questions to formulate an impression of his or her performance:

- Are we achieving our goals?
- Could I have done better?
- Were there high or low points?
- Did I intervene appropriately?
- Should I have a word with student...?
- Is the time well balanced?
- Did everyone participate?

Group dynamics

Encourage the group to articulate concerns, make suggestions and own the solutions. *Problem-based learning* by Schwartz, Mennin & Webb (2001) is a useful resource.

Examples of difficulties and solutions are:

- *Dominant students, confident and perhaps wrong*
  Encourage the group to examine all statements critically, and maybe have a quiet word with the student outside the tutorial.
- *Silent students – personality or failure to keep up?*
  Sensitise the group to the needs of the shyer or less confident; make 'space' for contributions, suggest particular roles so that they are included.
- *Uncooperative, disruptive students*
  Encourage group discussion and solutions; interview the student privately; in extreme cases consult the course director.
- *Students who persistently seek information from the tutor*
  Respond with open questions; encourage others to contribute.
- *A group that fails to 'gel', or in which personality clashes develop*
  Raise the issues; elicit suggestions for diagnosing the problem(s) and developing practical solutions.

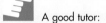

A good tutor:
- is clear on the aims and goals
- maintains a friendly and open atmosphere
- recognises the characteristics of the individual students
- knows when to intervene
- handles difficulties with tact and sensitivity.

Once a group is firmly established, members can cope with a session in the absence of a tutor.

When difficulties arise it is better to deal with them rather than let them fester:
- Tactful directness is appropriate.
- Seek support/solutions from the group.
- Offer practical assistance where possible.
- Deal with personal issues in private.
- Know local resources for student assistance.
- Do not be tempted to undertake a counselling role.

- *A group that bogs down, reporting on detailed information retrieved rather than advancing discussion of the problem (common)*
  Suggest that the group exchanges information beforehand by e-mail, paper summaries or in a prior meeting, or help the group to structure its reporting back.

What is the tutor's role in assessment?

Tutors must be familiar with local assessment policies. Individual students and/or groups may be assessed summatively (determining progression) or formatively (for feedback).

The group

At the end of each problem, groups review their processes, to encourage self-reflection and enhance their collective performance. Some students, however, are uncomfortable with self-assessment and personal discussion; differences reflect national characteristics, cultural backgrounds, fluency in the local language, confidence and personality. Overall, the comfort of students with PBL, as well as trust in the tutor and fellow members, affects their willingness to engage in meaningful reflection and revelation.

The skills of a tutor are tested when their group is unwilling to take responsibility for the process or to participate effectively. Trust is essential and must be established early; students who fear a penalty or negative outcome are unlikely to commit themselves honestly and openly. Useful questions to discuss include:

- How did we go as a group? What went well?
- What could I have done better as a tutor?
- Were there difficult situations? What could we have done better?
- What have you found to be particularly helpful?

Facilitative strategies include posing open-ended questions or inviting comments on particular situations.

Formative group assessment can occur when tutors change groups for one problem in order to provide independent feedback to the group and the regular tutor. More formal reviews require expert observation or the use of group assessment instruments.

Individual students

Tutors are usually expected to provide formative feedback to each member. One useful device is to ask students to complete a simple self-assessment questionnaire reviewing appropriate behaviours; the tutor returns them with comments and may interview each individual privately.

Students will be assessed using a variety of written, oral and/or clinical tests that will determine their progression and ultimate graduation. Students who are competitively graded in examinations may be less willing to share knowledge and contribute to the group process. In that circumstance, tutors need particular skills to encourage cooperation.

Tutors are usually expected to note absences and to assist and perhaps report on students who experience difficulties. They may be required to judge each student's performance summatively, but it can be difficult to do that objectively, even when criteria are established and training is provided.

Evaluating PBL tutorials

Students value the opportunity to comment on the effectiveness of teaching and learning, providing that the demand is not excessive, their views are taken seriously and consequent action is evident. At the end of each problem, and particularly in the final tutorial of a term, time is usefully allocated for evaluation.

Both the process and the learning in PBL tutorials can be evaluated against explicit goals. The tutor's review of the effectiveness of group processes offers insights for the members. In addition, specific questions of content can be resolved and common confusions noted. Tutors can pass on their group's views to curriculum managers who should then notify students of any changes that result.

Students normally evaluate their tutor. The explicit skills considered most important for effective facilitation should be identified so that constructive feedback is provided to teachers and managers.

Sample issues for tutor evaluation include:

- tutor characteristics: helpfulness, interest, enthusiasm
- support of clinical reasoning
- encouragement of independent learning
- enhancement of group process
- appropriate intervention
- provision of effective feedback.

Summary

The characteristics of teaching in PBL tutorials have been outlined. The tutor is a facilitator rather than a source of information, a role that requires training. Broad goals of PBL include the encouragement of self-directed learning, clinical reasoning and teamwork. Implementation varies so tutors must clarify local expectations and practical details. They need to know what parallel educational activities are offered, the students' previous learning experiences and resources available for students and staff. The roles of tutors differ, so local expectations in terms of tutorial process, assessment and evaluation must be understood.

Acknowledgement

I am grateful to Jill Gordon who made helpful comments on a draft of this chapter.

Understand the overall assessment process

Support anxious students and encourage self-assessment

If you are to assess summatively:
- Be clear about the criteria.
- Maintain objectivity.

Compared with didactic methods, PBL:
- is active and self-directed
- is enjoyed more by staff and students
- offers 'safe', cooperative learning
- introduces early clinical reasoning
- incorporates relevant scientific, social, ethical issues
- knowledge is integrated, readily applied
- encourages use of medical language

but:
- students are more anxious about the boundaries of knowledge expected.

References

Boud D, Feletti G 1998 The challenge of problem-based learning. Kogan Page, London

Carlile S, Barnet S, Sefton A J, Uther J 1998 Medical problem-based learning supported by intranet technology: a natural student-centred approach. International Journal of Medical Informatics 50:225–233.

Des Marchais J 2001 Learning to become a physician at Sherbrooke. Network Publications, Maastricht

Farmer E A 2004 Faculty development in problem-based learning. European Journal of Dental Education 8:59–66

Field M J, Sefton A J 1998 Computer-based management of content in planning a problem-based medical curriculum. Medical Education 32:163–171.

Henry R, Byrne K, Engel C 1997 Imperatives in medical education, University of Newcastle Faculty of Health Sciences, Newcastle, New South Wales, Australia

Maudsley G 1999 Do we all mean the same thing by 'problem-based learning'? A review of the concepts and a formulation of the ground rules. Academic Medicine 74:178–185

Norman G, Schmidt H 2000 Effectiveness of problem-based learning curricula: theory, practice and paper darts. Medical Education 34:721–728.

Schwartz P, Mennin S, Webb G 2001. Problem-based learning: case studies, experience and practice. Kogan Page, London.

Tosteson D C, Adelstein S J, Carver S T 1994 New pathways to medical education. Harvard University Press, Cambridge, MA, USA.

Wilkerson L 1994 The next best thing to an answer about tutor's content expertise in PBL. Academic Medicine 69:646–648.

Woods D 1994 Problem-based learning: how to gain the most from PBL. Donald R Woods, Hamilton, Ontario.

Chapter 17
Integrated learning

D. Prideaux

Introduction

Medical education courses draw on disciplines from the physical, human and biological sciences, humanities and the social and behavioural sciences and clinical sciences. Traditionally the disciplines were taught separately with an emphasis on the basic sciences in the early years and clinical experiences in the later years. Students, however, were expected to combine all the knowledge and skills from the disciplines and apply them to their clinical work.

In the later part of the twentieth century medical education reformers advocated the combination of the disciplines and the organisation of integrated learning experiences for students where they called upon knowledge and skills from across the disciplines in addressing patient cases, problems and issues. Integration was promoted in teaching and learning approaches rather than assuming that students would somehow integrate their disciplinary knowledge on their own. For example, integration was one of the key criteria for assessing the degree of innovation in a medical education programme in the SPICES curriculum model first published in 1984 (Harden et al 1984). Courses could be ranked on a continuum from discipline-based to integrated. This was further refined in 2000 through the concept of an 'integration ladder' which described 11 steps from treating the disciplines in isolation from each other to transdisciplinary models of integration (Fig. 17.1) (Harden 2000).

Types of integration in medical education

Grundy (1994) has distinguished between approaches and contexts for integration. In the first of these the programme is deliberately structured to organise or facilitate learning across the disciplines around key concepts, themes or problems. There are two common approaches in medical education. These are:

- horizontal integration
- vertical integration.

In horizontal integration there is integration between the various disciplines within any one or each year of the course such as in courses organised on a body systems basis. In vertical integration there is integration

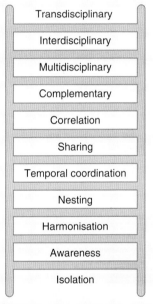

Fig. 17.1 The integration ladder

Transdisciplinary
Interdisciplinary
Multidisciplinary
Complementary
Correlation
Sharing
Temporal coordination
Nesting
Harmonisation
Awareness
Isolation

Approaches (how to) to integration
- horizontal
- vertical.
Contexts (places) for integration
- integrated clinical environments.

of disciplines taught in the different phases or years of the course. The early introduction of clinical skills and their development alongside basic and clinical sciences is a good example of vertical integration.

Integrated learning contexts are more common in the clinical components of medical courses. As clinical services become more integrated so too do the learning experiences available for students. The increased emphasis on clinical experience in primary care and general practice settings has brought additional opportunities for integrated learning in current medical school curricula.

The rationale for integrated learning

The rationale for integrated learning is frequently unstated or not argued strongly. It is assumed that integrated learning will result in a more relevant, meaningful and student-centred curriculum but the assumption often remains untested.

A rationale for integrated learning can be found, however, in some of the writings in cognitive psychology. Regehr & Norman (1996) refer to the concept of 'context specificity'. The ability to retrieve an item from memory depends on the similarity between the condition or context in which it was originally learned and the context in which it is retrieved. There are at least three ways to address context specificity. One is to promote the elaboration of knowledge in 'richer' and 'wider' contexts. Horizontally integrated system or case-based curricula can provide such elaboration. Repeated opportunities to use information in different contexts can also reduce the effects of context specificity. Such opportunities can be found in vertically integrated courses where there is revisiting of knowledge in different situations and in different combinations of disciplines.

An additional way of reducing the effect of context is to make the learning contexts as close as possible to the context in which the information is to be retrieved. This provides an argument for integrated learning within integrated clinical contexts such as in primary care, family medicine or general practice.

Context specificity – what is learned in one context is more readily retrieved in a similar context.

Approaches to integration

Horizontal integration

In horizontally integrated courses the disciplines are combined together around concepts or ideas in each year or level of the course. Commonly this is done using a body system approach. For example in the medical course at Flinders University in South Australia the first two years are organised into blocks or units corresponding to body systems such as:

- cardiovascular
- respiratory
- renal
- gastrointestinal
- endocrine/reproductive
- musculoskeletal.

Within these blocks students learn the basic sciences of anatomy, physiology and biochemistry together with social and behavioural sciences and clinical sciences as applied to normal and abnormal structures and functions within the systems (Fig. 17.2).

Horizontally integrated courses are becoming more popular as increasing numbers of medical schools around the world adopt problem-based or case-based learning approaches. In these approaches, specifically constructed cases become the focus for a week or two weeks of study. The cases may be organised by system blocks but each case in itself is also integrated. They are designed so that students must draw on knowledge, ideas and concepts from across the disciplines in order to generate and pursue learning goals. Problem-based learning, in particular, emphasises elaboration of learning as students generate learning goals and discuss them in small groups calling on all relevant knowledge across the disciplines.

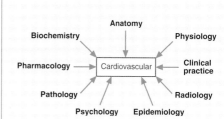

Fig. 17.2 Horizontal integration

Vertical integration

In vertically integrated courses the disciplines are organised into themes or domains which run throughout all years of the course. Many medical courses are now organised around four main themes which, while given different names, generally deal with the following:

- clinical and communication skills
- basic and clinical sciences
- social, community and population health
- personal and professional development.

Within each of the themes there may be sub-themes or blocks which provide the basis for integration across the years of the medical course. The programme at St George's Hospital Medical School in London uses a life cycle approach where sub-themes such as life support, life maintenance and life cycle, which integrate across the disciplines, are present in each year of the course. The studies in each year revisit those from the previous year or years, build upon the sub-theme and extend the learning to higher levels and greater complexity. This is known as a spiral approach to curriculum design. Each turn of the spiral represents an extension of the studies from the previous turn (Fig. 17.3).

There are few medical courses which now rigidly maintain a preclinical/clinical divide with the former presented in the earlier years of the course and the latter towards the end. Students now have early clinical learning experiences which increase in emphasis as they proceed through the course. There is a corresponding decrease in emphasis on the basic sciences but they still have an important part to play in the clinical years in providing an explanation of the mechanisms of disease and disease processes. This increases the potential for integration of clinical and science disciplines (Fig. 17.4).

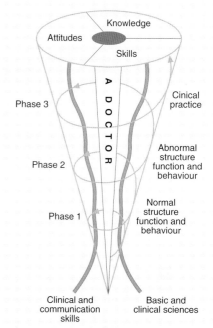

Fig. 17.3 Vertical integration – a spiral curriculum (redrawn from Harden et al 1997)

Contexts for integrated learning

In the rationale for integrated learning set out here it is argued that one way to achieve such learning is to ensure that the learning context is itself

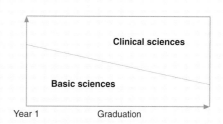

Fig. 17.4 Emphasis on basic and clinical sciences

"information in isolation is inert and unhelpful"

Regehr & Norman 1996

In a symbiotic curriculum, education and clinical service are mutually enhanced.

"organisational practices can be seen as a lever that can support cross-curricular practices"

Grundy 1994

integrated. With medical practice becoming more specialised, particularly in large teaching hospitals, this is becoming increasingly difficult to achieve. This is one of the reasons underlying the calls for more clinical experiences for students in general practice, family medicine or primary care. It is claimed that these contexts will provide opportunities for students to experience a patient-centred approach rather than a disease-oriented one and will enable them to experience a broad spectrum of illness to which they can apply the integrated knowledge from the studies in their medical courses.

The Parallel Rural Community Curriculum (PRCC) in the School of Medicine at Flinders University enables students to take a whole year of clinical studies in rural general practices and associated small rural hospitals. They learn the same content from the major clinical disciplines as those students in the Flinders course who take the year in a teaching hospital, but do it in an integrated patient-based approach. Students in this integrated approach perform better in end-of-year examinations than their teaching hospital-based peers, thus providing evidence for the importance of matching integrated learning programmes with integrated learning contexts (Worley et al 2004) (see chapter 11, In the community).

One of the additional features of the PRCC programme is that students make a contribution to the clinical and other services of the general practices and hospitals in which they work. This idea is encapsulated in the PRISMS model of medical education which emphasises that medical schools should enter a 'symbiotic' relationship with their health services (Bligh et al 2001). In such a relationship, student learning should be enhanced by the health services and, in turn, the students and their programme should make a contribution to the enhancement of the clinical services in which they are placed. This can be achieved by enabling students to have longer placements in clinical services and by providing guidelines and support for students to direct their own learning from patients rather than expecting them to be constantly directly 'taught' by busy clinical staff. In this way students can have extended placements across clinical services with opportunities for integrated learning facilitated by study guides or learning logs. The Peninsula Medical School in the south west of England has organised its clinical studies around such arrangements. A model of 'pathways of care' is used where students follow a patient-oriented programme across the different services accessed by patients for various conditions.

Achieving integration in medical education programmes

It is regarded as paradoxical by some medical educators that integrated curricula require a greater degree of structuring than those based around traditional disciplines. In a course based on separate disciplines, concepts and key ideas can be defined by the well-structured approaches existing in the disciplines. In an integrated curriculum, concepts and key ideas from several disciplines must be combined together in some logical way. Hence there has been increasing interest in medical education on approaches to the organisation and articulation of curriculum and curriculum content.

There is much contemporary interest in medical education in outcomes-based approaches to curriculum design and development (Harden et al 1999). In an outcomes approach those responsible for the course define broad and significant outcomes that students must attain on graduation. There is then a process of 'designing down' so that learning and assessment systems match the outcomes. In the medical curriculum at the University of Dundee the course is guided by 12 outcomes across all areas of the course. These then become the central organising statements for the curriculum and a focus for drawing on ideas from across the disciplines. It is the integrated outcomes that are designed to drive student learning not necessarily the bodies of knowledge found in the disciplines.

In a similar manner, integrated curricula can be defined by key concepts or ideas that transcend disciplines. For example, 'homeostasis' can be used as a key concept to integrate content from biochemistry and physiology. Clinical studies can be integrated by examining the effects and outcomes of disordered homeostasis. The key is to define a set of concepts that will effectively integrate all the content required in the course (Fig. 17.5).

Curriculum maps can be employed effectively in this process. One way of designing maps is to place the key concept or idea in the middle of a diagram and then to draw the content from across the disciplines that will contribute to the understanding of the concept. There then can be a selection of the linked content to provide the material for study in the medical course. Maps can also be used as a double-check on the curriculum. Those responsible for the disciplines can draw up their own maps of essential concepts and content to be covered. This can be matched against the material covered in the integrated approach to identify omissions or overlapping content.

Searchable computer databases provide an effective way of determining the coverage of content in integrated courses and are increasingly employed in medical schools across the world. Course content can be logged onto the computer and can be subject to searches according to a number of criteria, including discipline, key concepts, common presentations or illnesses and system complexes. Students can have access to the data bases as a guide for their own learning and preparation for assessment. They can match what they learn in their integrated programmes to what is expected in the course as a whole, by careful examination and searching of the database. This gives them responsibility for their own learning.

All these approaches require a greater degree of central rather than departmental control of the curriculum. Indeed, they require the breaking down of so-called departmental 'silos'. In most medical schools the responsibility for curriculum content and organisation now lies in a central committee or decision-making body representative of the disciplines and groups in the course. It is this body which oversees curriculum content and the contribution of the disciplines.

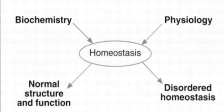

Fig. 17.5 Homeostasis is an example of a key learning concept

"The curriculum is not the intention or prescription but what happens in real situations."

Stenhouse 1976

"the point of education is to improve the quality of the meanings we construct"

Newman et al 1996

Problem- or case-based learning provides a strong foundation for integrated learning.

Learner integration

Lawrence Stenhouse (1976), one of the seminal writers on curriculum design and development, has distinguished between curriculum as 'intention' and curriculum as 'reality'. There may well be a difference between the curriculum as it is intended by its designers and how it is received by the students who experience it. Thus the real measure of the degree of integration of a curriculum is not what is written down in plans, statements and booklets but rather how much integration takes place in student learning.

Contemporary medical education curricula emphasise self-direction in learning and there is much interest in the concept of 'constructivism'. In constructivist approaches students actively construct or develop their own learning from the range of experiences available to them. Again this makes the question of achieving integration more problematic. In a didactic approach the integration can be presented to students in a prepackaged way although, of course, the question still remains as to whether it will necessarily be received in that way. In more self-directed and constructivist approaches, learning plans and goals, study guides and learning pathways should be designed to facilitate integrated learning, but in the final analysis it will be up to the students to construct their learning in an integrated or nonintegrated way.

Newman and colleagues (1996) have provided a critique of constructivist approaches where student engagement has become an 'end in itself' rather than the pursuit of quality learning and 'intellectual' outcomes for students. They use the term 'authentic learning' which they argue has three central components. These are:

- the construction of knowledge
- disciplined inquiry
- 'value beyond' the school or educational context in which the learning takes place.

These three components bring together some of the earlier discussions presented here. As indicated above, a major task for curriculum designers will be to design learning tasks that enable students to construct their learning in integrated ways. This can be facilitated through the use of:

- study guides
- learning logs and portfolios
- online materials
- independent projects.

This construction of knowledge should be underpinned by a process of rigorous inquiry. The central elements of the process of inquiry as set out by Newman and colleagues are:

- building on a prior knowledge base
- providing for in-depth learning
- providing for elaborated learning.

These match the central elements of problem-based learning. Thus problem or case-based approaches will provide a strong foundation for authentic integrated learning.

Finally, providing integrated clinical contexts for learning will demonstrate the value of what is being learned beyond the medical school environment and indicate its relevance to clinical practice. This potentially is the most important area of all. If student learning is to be meaningfully integrated it must be anchored in the realities of clinical practice. There must be a high degree of involvement of students in the actual tasks and activities of integrated clinical services so that they can clearly see that integrated learning is not just something important for success in medical school, but will be an important part of their continued development as medical professionals. The interprofessional learning experiences offered at Linköping University in Sweden are an example of this. Students from different health disciplines work together in the authentic tasks of actually running an interprofessional patient care service.

The frequently quoted adage in medical education that 'assessment drives learning' must not be ignored. If integrated learning is to be achieved it must be driven by integrated assessment. As in the process of structuring the curriculum, integration must be deliberately incorporated into the assessment process. The most important step is to ensure that integrated learning is represented in assessment blueprints. This requires a central process of test and examination construction, with responsibility for assessment residing with the medical school overall rather than with individual departments, similarly to the design of the curriculum as indicated earlier.

There are now established methods for assessing integrated clinical learning once it has been represented in the blueprints. The objective structured clinical examination (OSCE) format is ideal for assessing integrated clinical learning. Similarly, portfolio-based evaluation lends itself to integrated assessment. Written assessments too can be focused on integrated learning. Many medical schools using problem-based formats have adopted case-based assessment methods which attempt to evaluate the processes of problem-based learning as well as the integration of student knowledge. Multiple-choice and short-answer questions which are directed towards the lower levels of recall and comprehension in Bloom's taxonomy (1956) are less readily applied to the assessment of integrated learning. However, when such tools are focused on the assessment of processes of application, analysis, synthesis and evaluation they do provide opportunities for students to demonstrate that they can integrate and apply their learning and knowledge base.

Conclusion

Building an evidence base about integrated learning

Despite the advocacy of integrated learning, many of the claims made for it remain largely untested. As yet there is not clear evidence about the impact of integrated learning nor about the best ways to achieve it. Certainly Newman and colleagues found some support for their concept of authentic pedagogy and the interrelationship between pedagogy, assessment and performance in the school population. However, there have been few studies of integrated learning in the medical education context.

Assessment items that assess higher-order cognitive skills allow students to demonstrate integrated learning.

There will be a need to pay careful attention to questions of research design. Simple comparison of student performance in integrated and nonintegrated programmes raises a number of design questions about the interrelationships of variables, the ability to maintain blindedness about the intervention and the very real difficulty in classifying programmes as wholly integrated or nonintegrated. Difficulty in addressing issues of this kind has restricted findings for example, about the effects of problem-based learning in medical education (Norman & Schmidt 2000).

Some of the approaches to research and research methodologies advocated by Norman & Schmidt in their critique of research on problem-based learning may be usefully employed in researching the claims about integrated learning. It is important to ask and to seek responses to questions such as those below.

- What factors promote integrated learning?
- What factors limit it?
- What curriculum designs promote integrated learning?
- What is the perceived relevance of integrated learning for students?
- What is the effect of integrated assessment on integrated learning?
- Does integrated learning provide value beyond medical school?
- Is integrated learning promoted by student participation in authentic integrated clinical contexts?

Answers to these questions will assist in establishing both the nature and place of integrated learning in medical education and, ultimately, in assessing the effect of student engagement in integrated learning on subsequent practice as a medical professional.

Summary

Contemporary medical educators have increasingly called for the integration of student learning across the disciplines contributing to medical courses. A rationale for this kind of learning can be drawn from cognitive psychology through the concept of 'context specificity'. Retrieval of learning is enhanced where there is similarity between the context of initial learning and the context of retrieval. Horizontal integration addresses context specificity by enabling elaboration of learning in richer and wider contexts such as those provided in case-based or systems-based curriculum designs. Vertical integration provides repeated opportunities for use of information in different contexts in theme-based or spiral curricula. Integrated learning is also promoted where the learning context itself is integrated, as in general practice or family medicine clinical services.

Integrated curriculum designs require structure around outcomes, concepts or maps. Nevertheless, irrespective of what is intended, it is the reality of integration for the learner that is important. Constructivism and authentic learning can promote integration and integrated assessment will drive integrated learning.

However, despite widespread advocacy of this approach, there is little evidence about integrated learning. There is a need for research evidence about its nature and place in medical education so that its contribution to the ongoing medical practice of medical graduates can be assessed.

References

Bligh J, Prideaux D, Parsell G 2001 PRISMS: new educational strategies for medical education. Medical Education 35:520–521

Bloom BS 1956 Taxonomy of educational objectives: the classification of educational goods. Handbook 1 Cognitive domains. McKay, New York.

Grundy S 1994 Reconstructing the curriculum of Australian schools: cross-curricular issues and practices. Occasional paper 4. Australian Curriculum Studies Association, Canberra

Harden R M, Sowden S, Dunn W R 1984 Some educational strategies in curriculum development: the SPICES model. Medical Education 18:284–297

Harden R M, Davis M H, Crosby J R 1997 The new Dundee medical curriculum: a whole that is greater than the sum of the parts. Medical Education 21:141–143

Harden R M, Crosby J R, Davis M H 1999 An introduction to outcome-based education. Part 1 AMEE no. 14 Outcome-based education, pp 7–16

Harden R M 2000 The integration ladder: a tool for curriculum planning and evaluation. Medical Education 34:551–557

Newman F M, Marks H M, Gamorgan A 1996 Authentic pedagogy and student performance. American Journal of Education 104:280–312

Norman G R, Schmidt HG 2000 Effectiveness of problem-based learning curricula: theory, practice and paper darts. Medical Education 34:721–728

Regehr G, Norman G R 1996 Issues in cognitive psychology; implications for professional education. Academic Medicine 71(9):988–1001

Stenhouse L 1976 An introduction to curriculum research and development. Heinemann, London

Worley P, Esterman A, Prideaux D 2004 Cohort analysis of examination performance of undergraduate medical learning in community settings. BMJ 328:207–209

Chapter 18
Interprofessional education

H. Barr

Introduction

Much that you are learning as you dip into this book is as relevant to interprofessional education as it is to professional education. If and when you apply that learning to interprofessional education may be a matter of inclination, although you may find that it is expected of you as such education becomes more widespread. Becoming an effective interprofessional educator, however, entails more than the transfer of knowledge and skills from medical education as you will soon discover.

You will need:

- to find your bearings in an unfamiliar field
- to distinguish between interprofessional and multiprofessional education
- to capture the distinctive qualities of interprofessional education
- to exploit its potential in college and workplace before and after qualification
- to work as an equal with teachers from other professions
- to embrace the distinctive approaches to learning that they bring.

Learning together

Opportunities are increasing in many countries for medicine, allied health, nursing, social work and other professions to learn together:

- to gain economies of scale by sharing common curricula
- to sustain the viability of specialist studies across professions
- to optimise the use of specialist teaching expertise
- to enable professions to substitute for each other
- to accelerate progression from one profession to another
- to cultivate collaborative practice between professions.

This chapter focuses on the last of these. It explores ways to promote, develop and deliver interprofessional education to help students and workers from different professions to understand each other better, surmount barriers to collaboration and work together to improve services and patient care (Barr et al 2005, Freeth et al 2005 Meads et al 2005).

"The days when courses are designed exclusively for doctors, or exclusively for nurses, should be behind us"

Sir Ian Kennedy in the Bristol inquiry (cited in Meads et al 2005)

"Improve reciprocal attitudes Understand each other's roles Establish common foundations Reinforce collaborative competencies Prepare for teamwork"

Barr 2003a

Sorting out semantics

The World Health Organization (WHO 1988) called this 'multiprofessional education' which it defined as:

> The process by which a group of students or workers from health related occupations with different educational backgrounds learn together during certain periods of their education, with interaction as an important goal, to collaborate in providing promotive, preventive, curative, rehabilitative and other health related services.

The term multiprofessional education has, however, come to be used more widely to cover learning together to address many or all of the objectives listed earlier. A more precise term is therefore needed to recapture the original intention. The one which has gained most currency is 'interprofessional education', although others coexist confusingly, ranging from the grandiose such as 'transdisciplinary education' to the prosaic such as 'shared learning' or 'joint training'.

The UK Centre for the Advancement of Interprofessional Education (CAIPE) distinguishes between multiprofessional and interprofessional education. Multiprofessional education is defined as 'occasions when two or more professions learn side by side', while interprofessional education is described as 'occasions when two or more professions learn from and about each other to improve collaboration and the quality of care' (Barr 2003a).

Defined thus interprofessional education is a subset of multiprofessional education (Fig. 18.1) with value added. It includes common learning, but also comparative learning. It is interactive and collaborative. It explores differences in culture and custom. It equips each profession with essential knowledge about relevant others to inform intelligent referral, co-working and teamworking. In so doing it exposes prejudice and negative stereotypes to challenge by those to whom they are directed, and exerts peer group pressure to modify attitudes and change behaviour.

Interprofessional education includes learning which is:
- common
- comparative
- collaborative
- interactive
- challenging.

Remedying the problem

Interprofessional education starts from the assumption that all is not well in working relations among the health and social care professions, that ignorance and prejudice impede collaboration exacerbated by rivalry and miscommunication. But to blame practitioners would be unfair. Many work effectively together across professional and organisational boundaries despite differences in perception, policy, practice and priorities, although findings from inquiries into the abuse of children, tragedies when support networks fail in psychiatric aftercare and unacceptably high mortality rates resulting from medical error tell another story. They point to failures in communication, collaboration and trust between professions that occur with such regularity that they can no longer be ignored.

The nub of the problem may lie less with professions than with professionalism which, notwithstanding its virtues, can be divisive, erecting barriers between professions, making invidious comparisons, exaggerating

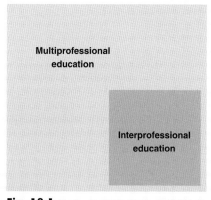

Fig. 18.1

*"Modify reciprocal attitudes
Establish common values, knowledge and skills
Build teams
Solve problems together
Respond together to community needs
Change practice
Change the professions"*

World Health Organization 1988

	Before qualification	After qualification
At work		
At college		

Fig. 18.2

"Learning for work; learning at work; learning from work"

Seagrave, cited in Burton & Jackson 2003

	Before qualification	After qualification
At work		
At college		

Fig. 18.3

differences and justifying claims to exclusive knowledge and skill. Professional education must carry some of the responsibility for this problem, being the means by which students are socialised into the culture and mores of their chosen profession, while prejudices towards other professions become more pronounced. If education is part of the problem, it must also be part of the solution, as the WHO (1988) argued.

Taking account of dimensions

Interprofessional education has many dimensions with different implications for structure, content, methods and outcomes.
It may be:

- before or after qualification
- college-based, work-based or independent of both
- short or long
- for two or more professions
- generic or focused on a particular role, field or patient group
- discrete or integral to multiprofessional education
- discrete or integral to two or more professional programmes.

This chapter uses the first two of these dimensions to form an interprofessional education matrix, focusing on each of four 'domains' in turn and relationships between them. (Fig. 18.2).

The same domains can also be adopted to classify uni-professional and multiprofessional education, which makes it easier to relate interprofessional education to them in a structured and an ordered fashion.

Work-based post-qualification interprofessional education

Interprofessional learning occurs in everyday practice, for example, when a worker provides background information to a colleague from another profession, or an interprofessional team meeting breaks off from its business agenda to reflect from different perspectives on an interesting, puzzling or troublesome question (Figs 18.3 and 18.4).

Such exchanges typically pass unrecognised as learning, still less as interprofessional learning, under the pressure of a working day, but learning is more likely to be remembered, reinforced and transferred when it is made explicit. Making time for reflection and explanation is less likely to seem indulgent when benefits are tangible and lasting.

Much lip service is paid in health care to the notion of the learning organisation, although good examples may be hard to find. A learning organisation fosters a culture of questioning and enquiry. It reframes information as learning, adopting a cyclical process of change. It respects differing roles, experience and expertise, and values them as learning assets. It mobilises its own capacity to respond to learning needs from its internal teaching resources, bringing in college and freelance teachers when needed. It responds as a good employer to the needs and expectations of the individual, within and beyond his or her present post, as well as those of the organisation. It recognises the limits of its inner learning capacity, valuing the distinctive qualities of extramural learning by making provision to release staff to attend courses.

The notion of the learning team is similar. It synthesises theories from adult learning and group dynamics. It sees individual learning as necessary, but collective learning as essential for an organisation to survive and flourish. It moves beyond teambuilding as a linear process towards a predetermined goal, making realistic allowance for chronic instability in many teams as members come and go.

Modern management mechanisms can help to set the learning agenda. At best, performance appraisal is a positive opportunity to identify the learning needs of both individuals and groups. So too is clinical governance when it exposes shortfalls in services which call for more skilled workers to effect improvement. Individual and team learning needs are perhaps met most effectively in practice professional development planning (PPDP), as pioneered in primary care in the UK (Wilcock et al 2003).

Continuous quality improvement (CQI) has been widely introduced in the United States and other countries, including the UK, as a means to empower teams, many of them interprofessional, to effect change for the better. Each team selects the particular improvement which it is intent on effecting and embarks on a four-stage 'plan', 'do', 'study' and 'act' (PDSA) cycle for learning and change, often assisted by an external facilitator. Numerous evaluations demonstrate not only that the chosen objective was achieved, but also that participants learned from each other and team cohesion was strengthened (Wilcock & Headrick 2000).

PPDP and CQI are the mechanisms which have been employed most effectively so far to realise the latent potential in the workplace for interprofessional learning. Of the four domains, however, this is the one where most remains to be done to convince management that professionally and interprofessionally driven learning will further organisationally driven strategies.

College-based post-qualification interprofessional education

Arguably, the need for externally provided post-qualification interprofessional education (Fig. 18.5) will diminish as the interprofessional dimension is built into work-based learning. Workers released to attend college programmes can, however, take a broader view as they learn from teachers from diverse practice professions and academic disciplines, and from fellow students drawn from other agencies, other work settings and other professions. They can stand back from immediate preoccupations at work to see the wood from the trees. They can question conventional wisdom. They can think the unthinkable. They can raise emotive issues. They can look beyond their present posts with their sights set on career progression. They can even indulge intellectual appetites whose application to work may not be immediately obvious, but enrich the organisation nonetheless.

Many post-qualification programmes are convened by colleges, voluntary organisations, specialist institutions or pressure groups. Most fall

---

The learning organisation

The learning team

Action learning sets

Practice professional development planning

Continuous quality improvement

Fig. 18.4 Examples of work-based, post-qualifying interprofessional education

"A powerful way of ensuring change and improvement"

Sir Kenneth Calman on practice professional development planning, in Wilcock et al 2003

"Understand community health issues
Connect the institution and the community
Understand the people whom you wish to serve
Identify appropriate short term projects
Practice interdisciplinary teamwork"

Keys to continuous quality improvement, Gelmon et al, in Wilcock & Headrick, 2000

	Before qualification	After qualification
At work		
At college		

Fig. 18.5

Reinforcing academic foundations

Introducing academic disciplines

Promoting new models of care

Learning additional roles

Fig. 18.6 Examples of college-based, post-qualifying interprofessional education

within the wider bounds of multiprofessional education, for example (Fig. 18.6).

- reinforcing academic and scientific foundations, e.g. in research methods
- introducing perspectives from academic disciplines, e.g. gerontology
- promoting new models of care, e.g. in mental health or learning difficulties
- learning additional roles, e.g. counselling, education or management.

Once underway, many such programmes, especially for students studying and working concurrently, build in interprofessional dimensions or emphases in response to the demands of practice, and to students' needs and expectations. This may be the most effective way to ensure that interprofessional education finds a lasting home in college-based post-qualification studies, replacing freestanding interprofessional programmes which are often marginal to the mainstream of such studies, vulnerable to budgetary cuts and, as a result, short-lived. Discrete interprofessional programmes make uneasy bedfellows for college-based multiprofessional education. Many find a warmer welcome in the independent educational sector where freelance trainers can respond more flexibly to the vicissitudes of the education market place.

Experience gained from those programmes can, however, inform interprofessional perspectives introduced into multiprofessional education.

The following are just some of countless examples of interprofessional workshops:

- for general practitioners and health visitors to understand each other's roles
- for general practitioners and practice nurses about problem-solving in teams
- for newly qualified workers in a neighbourhood to get to know each other
- for doctors and nurses to manage crises in accident and emergency departments
- for primary care teams to devise health education strategies
- to introduce primary care teams to CQI
- about systemic work with families for nurses, social workers and teachers
- for nurses, social workers, police and youth workers, to foster interagency collaboration in child protection
- for pairs of doctors and nurses working with terminally ill patients

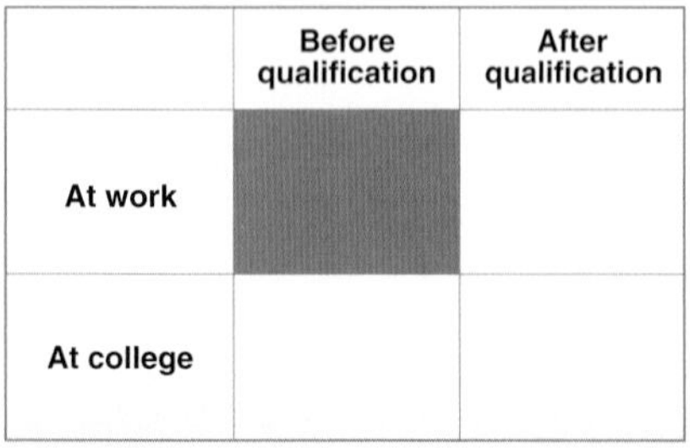

Work-based pre-qualification interprofessional education (Fig. 18.7)

Conventional wisdom long held that interprofessional education was better left until after qualification, by which time participants should be secure in their respective professional identities and have experience to share. No longer: reform of healthcare systems in many countries

	Before qualification	After qualification
At work	██████	
At college		

Fig. 18.7

demands that newly fledged workers must be ready to collaborate from the day that they qualify. Nor is the situation any longer tolerated where negative relationships between professions are reinforced during under-graduate education, to be unlearned later during 'remedial education'.

Clinical practice often seems the least disruptive place to introduce interprofessional education into qualifying programmes, obviating many of the requirements made by academic institutions and regulatory bodies. Some exponents assert that practice learning is the only place to learn col-laborative practice. Seductive though that argument may be, it splits off interprofessional learning from college-based education, which remains wholly uni-professional, with the attendant risk that it continues to induct students into their chosen profession to the detriment of relations with other professions. Students are left to their own devices, to reconcile interprofessional practice learning with uni-professional classroom learn-ing as best they may.

Nor is such practice-based learning the easy option that it first seems. Requirements for practice learning must be respected and reconciled. Assembling the preferred mix of professions at the same time in the same place can be frustrated by different patterns of placement (concurrent or block), of different duration at different stages in the academic year. Imaginative ways have been found to obviate these regulatory and logis-tic constraints. At their most basic, debates, case studies and 'get to know you sessions' are arranged during lunch breaks. Students from different professions in and around Newcastle, England, who happen to be placed concurrently in the same institution or neighbourhood, do better. They meet on Monday to select a patient whose pathway they intend to follow during that week, meeting again on Friday to compare what they have observed and learned. The group assembles similarly in successive weeks, but with a changing composition as new members join and others leave as placements start and finish.

Alternative work-based assignments can also be built in (Fig. 18.8). For example, groups of two or three students visit a patient in her own home. Each sees her through different eyes, focusing on some things according to what they been taught to see, filtering out others. Given skilled facilitation, difference in perception provide many and varied opportunities for interprofessional learning when each pair or threesome reports back to the class.

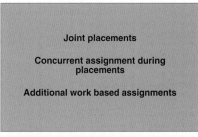

Fig. 18.8 Examples of work-based, pre-qualifying interprofessional education

The Leicester Medical School in the English Midlands has developed a more sophisticated process, originally for medical students, but now extended to include others from nursing and social work. The objective is to give students opportunities to observe and assess patients in the social, cultural and economic context of a deprived inner city neighbour-hood. Three students, one from each of three professions, visit a patient and report back as described above. They return to the neighbourhood to interview the patient's key worker. The complete class then plans an end of semester seminar to present their overall impressions to all the key workers for their observations, although not, so far, to the patients.

Motivating practice agencies to provide enough placements of the required type and quality, as every teacher knows, calls for investment.

Nowhere is this more so than in interprofessional education when it is fishing in the same pool as the professional education programmes with which it is associated.

The Community–Campus Partnership Movement began in the United States to address this problem. It soon spread to Latin America, South Africa and elsewhere in the developing world. As its name implies, it builds mutually beneficial relationships between medical and health schools, on the one hand, and neighbouring communities, on the other. Faculty and student resources are made available by the schools in response to neighbourhood priorities, in the process generating practice learning opportunities.

College-based pre-qualification interprofessional education (Fig. 18.9)

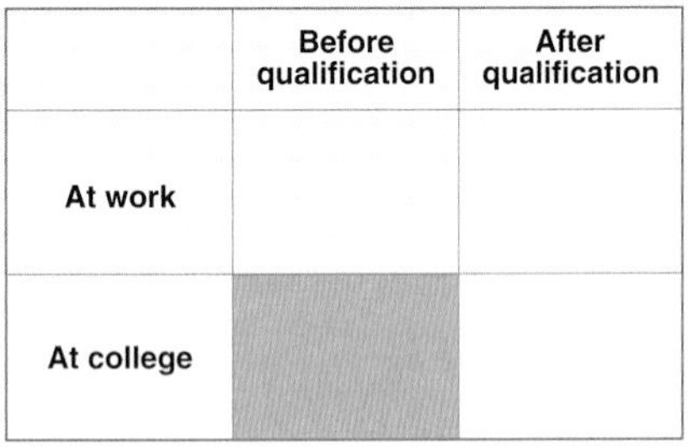

Opinions differ regarding the stage at which interprofessional education should be introduced into pre-qualifying professional education. Some hold that it should wait until the final year, modifying but slightly the arguments that it should wait until after qualification. Others hold that negative attitudes will already have taken root by then, arguing instead for interprofessional learning from the outset.

Students from health and social care professions, including medicine, at the University of Linköping in Sweden have a joint 10-week block of interprofessional study, wholly comprising problem-based learning, before starting their separate programmes. Interprofessional follow up was introduced later when it became apparent that the benefits of the initial block were lost once students became immersed in training for their respective professions.

Experience points to the need to weave interprofessional strands into the fabric of professional education from enrolment to qualification. Viewed thus, it progresses from cultivating a positive disposition towards other professions to the acquisition and testing of teamwork and collaborative skills or competences (Fig. 18.10).

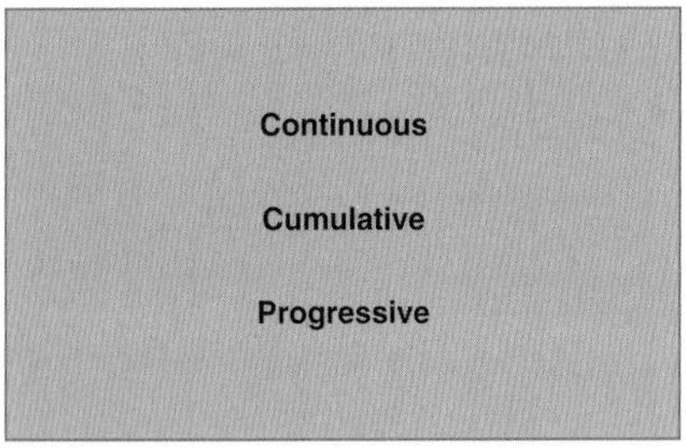

Persuasive though the case is for pre-qualification interprofessional education, profession-specific requirements constrain time and opportunity, exacerbated by pressure to squeeze yet more into an already crowded curriculum. Concern is fuelled by misconceptions about the content of interprofessional learning; some of this may be new and additional, but most of it, in fact, reframes existing curricula for all or some of the constituent professions. The same case study, for example, can be approached from the perspective of one or several professions without additional claims on time.

There is concern too that interprofessional learning will address interprofessional objectives at the expense of professional objectives but this is a false dichotomy. Given that collaborating with others is integral to the role of every profession, interprofessional learning reinforces that role.

Yet another concern is expressed, namely that interprofessional teaching will be pitched at the lowest common denominator for all participant

	Before qualification	After qualification
At work		
At college		

Fig. 18.9

Continuous

Cumulative

Progressive

Fig. 18.10

professions – levelling down, not levelling up. That concern is more appropriately addressed to those who argue for large-scale adoption of common curricula across health and social care professions than to those who make the case for relatively modest amounts of intensive interprofessional learning. The effectiveness of interprofessional education is not dependent on its quantity but on the quality of interaction between the parties, on opportunities to learn as equals in a climate of mutual support and respect in a spirit of cooperative enquiry.

The professions are never likely to spend more than a small proportion of their time learning together during their pre-qualification education in contrast to post-qualification programmes where they may spend the whole of their time together.

Outcomes

Emerging evidence from a systematic review (Barr et al 2005, Freeth et al 2002) indicates that prequalification interprofessional education can, under favourable conditions, modify attitudes for the better and secure a common knowledge base for collaborative practice. It also indicates that post-qualification interprofessional education can, again under favourable conditions, change practice for the better and improve patient care.

These preliminary findings have provoked a predictable reaction, namely that the only effective interprofessional education is in the workplace. This is a naïve conclusion. A work-based project may improve practice in its immediate setting, but evidence is invariably lacking that participants transfer and apply their learning elsewhere to effect comparable improvement.

It is far easier to measure positive outcomes from a quality improvement project where all participants work in the same place than from a college-based programme (before or after qualification) where participants enter or return to different places of employment, so that follow up is difficult. More may be delivered by college-based interprofessional education if it is accompanied by work-based learning which builds in quality improvement. Acting on that belief, Bournemouth University on the English south coast assigned pre-qualification students to interprofessional teams practising CQI, in the expectation that they would learn the method and carry it forward into their future employment. Findings were promising, but widespread extension of the project is impracticable.

It would be needlessly pessimistic to pitch future objectives for pre-qualification interprofessional education no higher than those reported in the past, but the ethics of setting up newly qualified workers as agents of change before they have consolidated their learning are questionable.

Reinforcing one another

Nothing is more invidious than crude comparisons to determine which of the four domains houses the 'holy grail' of collaborative practice. Like is

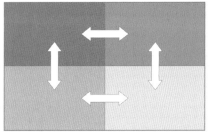

Fig. 18.11

not being compared with like. Each complements the others. Service agencies attuned to interprofessional learning provide fertile ground for interprofessional (and professional) practice learning. Conversely, well-planned and well-supported interprofessional (and professional) practice placements develop, stimulate and sustain a learning culture in an organisation (Fig. 18.11).

Effective interprofessional (and professional) college-based learning depends on effective practice learning in supportive and receptive organisations. In return, it stimulates and sustains learning in those organisations where many of its graduates may choose to work subsequently.

Interprofessional (and professional) education before qualification lays foundations for such education after qualification to which students may progress. Conversely, interprofessional (and professional) education after qualification attracts high quality staff whose expertise contributes, directly or indirectly, to education before qualification.

Getting involved

There are many ways in which, as a medical teacher, you may be invited to help with interprofessional education – by joining a planning group, management committee, teaching team or visiting panel from a regulatory body, or being appointed as an external examiner, programme evaluator or consultant. You might take the lead in launching a new interprofessional initiative. The same principles, guidelines and approaches apply regardless of the challenge.

Planning together

Interprofessional education is best planned by the same professions as those who will participate later. This ensures that the needs of all the professions are taken into account equally and that the programme builds on best education and practice in each. But teachers also carry 'baggage', positive and negative experiences of learning and working with the other professions, which may help or hinder the development and delivery of the programme. They need to share those experiences as they compare their perceptions of interprofessional education, its purpose, form, content, learning methods and realistic outcomes. Much has now been written to help the process, but each planning group must work out its own salvation. There are no quick fixes.

Mixing methods

Teachers from each profession introduce their preferred learning methods. As a medical teacher you may favour problem-based learning, drawing on its well-tried application in progressive medical schools. If so, you will find that it also has an established place in interprofessional education endorsed by the WHO (1988).

Few methods are more potent as a medium for interprofessional learning, but problem-based learning is by no means the only one. Other professions may be keen to introduce other methods such as experiential learning to simulate interprofessional relations in working life, or observational learning to compare perceptions of patients, their circumstances and their treatment (Fig. 18.12). All may unite in subscribing to the importance of practice learning. No one method matches every student, every learning need, or every situation. Imaginative teachers ring the changes when students' interest flags. Effective interprofessional education calls on, develops and synthesises a repertoire of learning methods from its constituent professions within the application of principles of adult learning. The more strongly those principles have been implanted in related professional education, the easier it is to develop a coherent methodology for interprofessional education (Barr 2003a).

Conducting audit

Here are some of the questions that you and your colleagues might well ask at the outset and (amending tenses as necessary) when the time comes to review the programme (Barr 2003b):

- Do the aims as stated promote collaboration?
- How do the objectives contribute towards collaboration?
- Do the aims and objectives contribute to improving the quality of care?
- Are the aims and objectives compatible?
- How is the interprofessional learning built into the programme?
- Is the interprofessional learning informed by a theoretical rationale?
- Is that learning evidence based?
- Is it informed by interprofessional values?
- Does comparative learning complement common learning?
- Are the learning methods interactive?
- Is small-group learning included?
- Will numbers from the participant professions be balanced?
- Are all the professions represented in planning and teaching?
- Are patients and carers involved?
- Will the interprofessional learning be assessed?
- Will it count towards qualification?
- How will the programme be evaluated?
- Will findings be disseminated?

Summary

The interprofessional education river runs wide and deep. Better charted than it was, it still has hidden reefs and treacherous undercurrents to deceive the unwary. It should be navigated with caution in the company of fellow crew members from backgrounds different from your own, who you will learn to trust as the voyage progresses. The strength of your working relationships with them will be plain for students to see, offering a model which, it is hoped, they will emulate in their collaborative practice.

Problem based learning

Experimental learning

Observational learning

Practice learning

Fig. 18.12 Learning approaches that may be adopted in interprofessional education

References

Barr H 2003a, Interprofessional education: today, yesterday and tomorrow. Learning and Teaching Support Network for Health Sciences and Practice, London. Online. Available: www.health.ltsn.ac.uk

Barr H 2003b Ensuring quality in interprofessional education. CAIPE bulletin no 22. Online. Available: *www.caipe.org.uk*

Barr H, Koppel I, Reeves S et al 2005 Effective interprofessional education: argument, assumption and evidence. Blackwell Science, Oxford

Burton J, Jackson N 2003 Work based learning in primary care. Radcliffe Medical Press, Oxford

Freeth D, Hammick D, Koppel I et al 2002 A critical review of evaluations of interprofessional education. Learning and Teaching Support Network for Health Sciences and Practice, London

Freeth D, Hammick M, Barr H, et al 2005 Effective interprofessional education: development, delivery and evaluation. Blackwell Science, Oxford

Meads G, Ashcroft J, with Barr H, Scott R, Wild A 2005 The case for collaboration among health and social care professions. Blackwell Science, Oxford

WHO 1988 Learning together to work together for health. World Health Organization, Geneva

Wilcock P, Headrick L (eds) 2000 Continuous quality improvement in health professions education. Journal of Interprofessional Care 14 (2)

Wilcock P, Campion-Smith C, Elston S 2003 Practice professional development planning: a guide for primary care. Radcliffe Medical Press, Oxford

Chapter 19
Core curriculum and student-selected components

S. Cholerton, R. Jordan

Introduction

The dictionary definition of curriculum as 'a prescribed course of study' offers considerable latitude for interpretation. Some use it in its widest sense to encompass all those processes that contribute to the student's learning experience, while others take a narrower view defining the curriculum largely in terms of the learning content. With few notable exceptions, up until the early 1980s most schools made little attempt to be explicit, relying more on constituent subject groupings to define curricular components. In the absence of any overarching strategic approach to curriculum design, such definitions were almost invariably based on what was perceived as the essential canon of knowledge which characterised the constituent discipline in question. Curriculum design consisted of little more than rationing the available time and sharing it out between the semi-autonomous discipline-based departments jockeying for position to advance their own interests within the overall envelope of the programme as a whole.

Universally recognised in the last quarter of the 20th century, the need to reshape basic medical curricula was neither new nor restricted to any one country. What was different was the will of the professional statutory bodies such as the General Medical Council in the UK, to rethink what should be expected of the newly qualified doctor and to require their constituent medical schools to respond positively to their recommendations.

With the exponential increase in biomedical knowledge, the emergence of new disciplines and subject areas, and a persisting and unrealistic drive for completeness, it was almost inevitable that basic medical curricula should have become intolerably overloaded. In turn, information overload has been identified as the root cause of many of the curricular ills detrimental to student learning including,

- undue emphasis on the acquisition (and examination) of factual knowledge at the expense of other key professional competencies
- stifling of curiosity, enquiry, reasoning and the exploration of knowledge
- poor preparation of graduates for modern practice and the next phase of the medical educational continuum.

"The burden we place on the medical student is far too heavy, and it takes some doing to keep it from breaking his intellectual back. A system of medical education that is actually calculated to obstruct the acquisition of sound knowledge and to heavily favour the crammer and the grinder is a disgrace"

Thomas Huxley 1876

"Education is about filling vessels and lighting fires. In relation to medical education, we have filled the vessel so full, that when the student picks it up it spills over and puts the fire out"

Anonymous, 1992

In the field of education the concept of a core curriculum is not new. However in the first edition of the General Medical Council's *Tomorrow's Doctors* (GMC 1993), its linkage with student-selected components as a strategy to circumscribe the requirements of basic medical education, and in so doing to reduce the curriculum overload, was considered a powerful new idea.

Taking the start of the pre-registration year (equivalent to the intern year in the US) as a reference point, and framing objectives in terms of the essential knowledge, skills and attitudes, all UK medical schools were urged to define a 'core curriculum' that must be satisfied before a newly qualified doctor could assume the responsibilities of a pre-registration house officer/intern. In addition to this 'core' experience, schools were urged to provide opportunities for student-selected study in depth in areas of particular interest to them. The broad purpose of these student-selected components was to supply an experience for students which '. . . *provides them with insights into scientific method and the discipline of research and that engenders an approach to medicine that is constantly questioning and self-critical'*.

Over a decade later, the majority of UK medical schools have made significant progress towards identifying the core elements upon which their basic medical education programme is based and all have introduced student-selected components into their curricula.

Although the second edition of *Tomorrow's Doctors* (GMC 2003) continues to recommend this educational strategy, the educational context of this document is considerably more sophisticated than that of its 1993 predecessor.

Public expectation and demand are now the principal drivers for modernisation. People increasingly want to make informed choices about how to be treated, where and by whom. To meet such public demand, health professionals need to put their patients at the centre of all they do, communicating effectively with them and their carers, recognising and respecting their rights and beliefs, and responding to the diversity of the population. While recognising that pre-registration/ prelicensing education continues to provide the basis for professional competency, in the future it must do more than this. New health professionals need to be adaptable, self-reliant, resilient, and able to learn and work flexibly in interprofessional teams across traditional professional boundaries. They must be prepared to contribute to continuous service improvement through critical and creative reflection on their own practice and competent to evaluate the services they deliver.

In most countries, programmes of basic medical education are prescribed under broad statutory frameworks promulgated by bodies such as the General Medical Council in the UK and the Association of American Medical Colleges in the US. In addition, in England pre-registration medical programmes are, like all other higher education programmes, required to adhere to subject benchmark statements published by the Quality Assurance Agency for Higher Education (2002). The purpose of these is to serve as a blueprint for defining, securing and assuring academic standards.

The term 'standards' has been defined by the Higher Education Quality Council (HEQC 1997) as '*the balance of attributes (types of knowledge, understanding and skills) that are acquired through the study of a particular subject, field or collection of subjects*'. Both the Dearing Report (1997) and the Higher Education Quality Council defined the purpose of standards as yielding information to stakeholders, including faculty and students, but particularly employers, government and the general public at large, about the attainment denoted by awards. So standards refer to the learning outcomes of degree programmes. Thus they are intended to answer the question 'What can be expected of a student who has been awarded the degree X from institution Y?'

Since the adoption of such an outcomes-based approach is one in which the results of learning are expressed in a form that permits their achievement to be demonstrated and measured (see chapter 14, Outcome-based education), it provides stakeholders with clear indicators of attainment. Furthermore it enables medical schools to demonstrate explicitly how they meet three essential 'duties of care':

- Fitness for purpose – the medical school has a duty to articulate and provide learning experiences that meet students' legitimate expectations
- Fitness for practice – the school has a duty to health service employers to ensure that medical graduates are competent and meet expectations of 'employability' in its widest sense
- Fitness of award – the school has a duty to patients and the public generally that its graduates meet appropriate standards.

As the curriculum, that is, the core plus student-selected components, is at the heart of the student experience, it is essential that the design of the modern programme takes account of the ever-changing requirements of society.

While designed to be of use to all medical educators, this chapter is aimed principally at those with institutional responsibility for curriculum design, content and organisation. We explore

- the interrelationship between the core curriculum and student-selected components of the curriculum
- provide working definitions of the core curriculum and student-selected components
- consider the concepts underpinning and the approaches to developing the core curriculum
- discuss the essential role of student choice in enhancing student learning and meeting programme outcomes.

Interrelationship between the core curriculum and student-selected components

Although for pragmatic and practical reasons it may have been useful to consider the core and student-selected components as separate entities within the curriculum, it is essential now that curriculum planners

It is important to recognise that the core curriculum and student-selected components are not mutually exclusive and that some learning outcomes will be achieved as a consequence of opportunities presented in both.

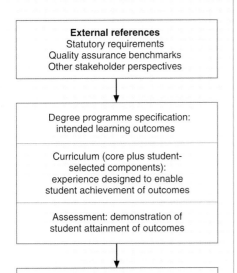

Fig. 19.1

Before considering either the core or student-selected component of the curriculum in any detail, a degree programme specification must be set out.

When the learning outcomes for a basic medical education programme are drawn up, the recommendations of statutory and other relevant professional bodies must be taken into account.

recognise from the outset the intimate relationship between the two. The curriculum of a basic medical education course must be designed to ensure that appropriate learning opportunities are provided to enable the student to achieve the predefined learning outcomes for the programme as a whole. While many learning outcomes will be achieved through the core curriculum, others will be attained through the student-selected components. It is important to recognise that in this respect the two components of the curriculum are not mutually exclusive and that some learning outcomes will be achieved as a consequence of opportunities presented in both.

Working definitions

It is best to consider working definitions of both core and student-selected components in terms of experience. Thus by definition student choice implies that only a proportion of the students will elect to undertake any particular given student-selected topic, while core implies that this experience is undertaken by all, i.e. it is a common experience for the whole cohort. In terms of defining learning outcomes, any outcome which is content-dependent must be addressed in the core curriculum. In contrast any outcome which is content-independent, for example a higher-order process outcome, can be attained through the student-selected component, given that the experience is properly designed. From this it follows that before either the core or student-selected component of the curriculum is considered in any detail, a degree programme specification must be established (Fig. 19.1).

Degree programme specification

In the UK, the concept of a degree programme specification arose from recommendations of the Dearing Report. A programme specification should set out the main purpose and distinctive features of the course of study, and give the intended learning outcomes in terms of:

- the knowledge and understanding that a student will be expected to have on completion
- key skills: communication, numeracy, use of information technology and learning how to learn
- cognitive skills, such as an understanding of methodologies and ability in critical analysis and reasoning
- subject-specific skills.

In drawing up the learning outcomes for a basic medical education programme, heed must be paid to the recommendations of statutory and other relevant professional bodies (e.g. the General Medical Council, the Quality Assurance Agency for Higher Education, the American Association of Medical Colleges), the needs of health service employers (e.g. the NHS), and last but not least those of future patients. The programme outcomes should also be related to the input profile of entrants and the baseline requirements of the next phase of the medical education continuum (e.g. in the UK, the foundation programme for Modernising Medical Careers).

A useful approach to specifying programme outcomes, based upon developing students' professional competence, is that provided by the 'Scottish doctor' project (Simpson et al 2002) which focused the definition of learning outcomes around:

- what the graduate will be required to do as a new doctor
- how the graduate will approach his/her practice
- the personal and professional development of the student, enabling proper preparation as a new doctor, for an appropriate role in the healthcare team.

Upon successful completion of an outcome-defined or driven programme, a student will have acquired a predetermined set of learning outcomes. Some of these will have been achieved by means of a specific component of the curriculum; however, most other outcomes will have been accomplished, often progressively, from multiple learning opportunities in diverse curricular settings and subject areas.

In relation to the curriculum as a whole, in this context it must be defined to embrace all those elements of the student experience enabling the achievement of the specified outcomes. For any educational programme, the curriculum is at the heart and represents the most significant part of the experience designed to enable student achievement of outcomes. In turn the curriculum guides the development of teaching, learning and assessment, and the learning resources strategy. Since the core curriculum, along with student-selected components, contributes to the whole, it is the fundamental part of the experience which must enable students to achieve the essential knowledge, skills and attitudes by the time they graduate.

If one takes the view that standards equate to outcomes, then all outcomes are 'core', and assurance of outcomes is determined by assessment of their attainment. Those outcomes which can only be met through common experience should be attributed to the 'core curriculum', whilst those which are content-independent can be addressed through 'student-selected components'.

The core curriculum

For the institution

The aims of a medical school are mainly dependent upon the health needs of the society which they serve. Other factors which determine the aims of a medical school are current practices in the profession, the cultural beliefs and demands of their local population and society and the prevailing scientific method. At the heart of any local core curriculum is that defined at the national level.

The American Association of Medical Colleges, through its medical schools objectives project, has identified a core set of outcomes for graduate medical education that reflect the essential attributes that clinicians need for effective modern medical practice (AAMC 2000), and in the UK a similar set has been promulgated by the General Medical Council

(GMC 2003) and the Quality Assurance Agency for Higher Education (QAA 2002).

For the subject

For many specialties/disciplines a core curriculum has been defined by their national governing body. For example in the UK, the British Pharmacological Society (2002) has defined core curricula for pharmacology and therapeutics for a variety of educational programmes including undergraduate medicine. In the US, the Society of General Internal Medicine and the Clerkship Directors in Internal Medicine have defined a Core Medicine Clerkship Curriculum Guide (Goroll et al 1995). Although the process which results in the definition of a core curriculum of this nature often takes into account guidelines of the national regulatory body, generally it has not been sanctioned.

There are also examples of individuals taking it upon themselves to define a core curriculum within a particular subject area (e.g. medical statistics, paediatrics).

A word of caution should be given here for institutional curriculum planners. Such externally defined 'core curricula' often emanate from individuals or professional associations with the vested interest of promoting and preserving their own subject area or discipline and its identity. One of the major uses of such initiatives is to support the argument by subject specialists for the maintenance of, or an increase in, curriculum time allocated to their specialty. This is directly contrary to the original purpose of identifying a core curriculum, i.e. to reduce the overburdening of the curriculum.

For basic medical education, it is often better that such inputs from specialties and disciplines be decided at an institutional level, and incorporated into an integrated core curriculum in relation to the learning outcome 'map'.

Methodologies

For an individual school, the first step is to determine a rational basis for identifying the core. In practice the commonest approach is to link determination of core to definition of content.

Careful consideration of the core content is required to guarantee complete mastery of essential competencies. A variety of approaches have been used to enable institutions to identify the core elements upon which their current medical course is based. These include:

- drawing up a profile of desired competencies
- identifying a core index of clinical situations, conditions, problems, cases or presentations
- identifying a set of experiences enabling objectives to be met, e.g. a community-orientated programme
- developing core content around longitudinal themes, e.g. life cycle;
- deriving core from the learning outcomes (although this presupposes the adoption of a rational method for defining the learning outcomes!)

Exercise caution when presented with core curricula defined for a specialty/discipline.

"The core curriculum must be the responsibility of clinicians, basic scientists and medical educationalists working together to integrate their contributions and achieve a common purpose"

GMC 2003

"The core provides the essential knowledge, understanding, clinical skills and professional attitudes which are required by any medical graduate in order thats/he may practise as a PRHO and commence post graduate training"

QAA 2002

Whatever 'wrap' is chosen, the basic aim is to use competencies, clinical situations or experiences as triggers for defining the knowledge base, the performance base and the attitudinal agenda.

The choice of approach to the way in which the curriculum will be delivered can go some way to determining the 'wrap' adopted for defining the core. For example problem-based learning courses tend to define the core curriculum by a series of clinical problems or index cases.

There is little research which relates curriculum content to educational outcome. As such, opinion-based processes tend to dominate when curriculum content is defined. A corollary to this is that the result will depend upon those stakeholders consulted and included in the process; for example a curriculum structured around a list of core clinical cases will depend upon the range and background of stakeholders who contributed to its development. That said, there is general agreement that the involvement of as broad a range of local stakeholders as possible is essential.

- The input of teachers, such as faculty staff (academic and clinical academic), general practitioners, consultants and healthcare professionals, is crucial to facilitating 'institutional' ownership, as these are the people who will have to deliver the curriculum.
- The input of trainers responsible for post-graduation training can provide useful insights into what will be expected of the graduate in the next stage of their medical education.
- The input of consumer groups, including senior students, interns, patients and employers, has much to offer;
- Input of recent product – junior doctors (post-registration trainees) are a useful group in bringing a sense of modern practice, the real world of work, and the level of skills required.

Curriculum planners must never lose sight of the need to constrain the content burden of the curriculum, and the downside of involving a comprehensive range of stakeholders is that it can easily add to that burden! At programme level it is essential that the school has a robust curriculum governance structure in place, including a small, empowered group of generalists who act as the final arbiters of content. This is essential if a balanced curriculum is to be produced and useful in resolving conflicts (which mostly arise from the subject/specialty level).

The question of overall balance is one that should be resolved early in the process: within the purpose of the institutional specification, the balancing of desired learning outcomes, topics for inclusion or exclusion, breadth and depth of content, and the proportion of student effort to be given over to the core curriculum.

Whereas medical education in the last century was mainly focused on the understanding of disease processes as they affect individuals, on their diagnosis and management, the practice of modern medicine demands much more. At the expense of depth the curriculum now must be broader than a purely disease-focused programme, it must be much more patient-focused and also take into account the health of the population.

When attempting to define the core, involve as broad a range of local stakeholders as possible.

Never lose sight of the need to limit the content of the curriculum.

Ensure that the school has in place robust machinery for overseeing the curriculum that includes a small, empowered group of generalists who are the final arbiters of content.

Definition of 'core' content

Levels	Definition	Example
1	Core presentations	Wheeze
2	Core conditions	Obstructive lung disease
3	Core cases	Asthma

Fig. 19.2

Fig. 19.3 Matrix approach for deciding whether or not to include a presentation, condition or case in the core curriculum

Defining the core – an example

A first level of content in a patient-centred curriculum could be clinical presentations, i.e. what patients present in practice. This approach has been adopted already by at least three UK medical schools.

The next 'level' is the core conditions with which patients present. By graduation students should have experienced learning and teaching around all of these conditions, although they may not have had the opportunity to see all of them. Many medical schools have defined a list of such core conditions or problems, and most have used criteria similar to those listed below to justify inclusion:

- commonness
- seriousness
- need to know on qualification
- educational value (i.e. the extent to which one can generalise from the subject to other areas of practice).

In some schools, particularly those which have adopted problem-based approaches, a 'third level' of core has been defined, that of selected ('index') clinical cases indicative of the condition (Fig. 19.2).

If such a three-level model is appropriate to local specification, then defining a core list of presentations will reinforce the patient-centred nature of the programme. Defining core conditions will help determine the core knowledge and skills, while defining core cases will in turn help focus both students' learning and the integration of the programme such that the case list will provide a corpus of illustrative material for use in all stages and strands of the course.

Criteria for inclusion at any level could be based upon two characteristics: commonness and importance. The latter will subsume both seriousness (e.g. conditions which are rare but life-threatening), and educational relevance (e.g. exemplar cases which illustrate key aspects of particular educational significance).

A method for combining these criteria and determining the inclusion or exclusion of any particular example of presentation, condition or case, could be based upon a matrix approach as illustrated in Figure 19.3.

However the approach outlined above, while useful for many topics, is not necessarily comprehensive for all. For example the health of the population is as essential a component of the core curriculum as that of the individual. While the criteria for inclusion and exclusion may prove valuable, the three-level presentation/condition/case method will require modification if it is to be applied to public health.

Besides the obvious need to define a core curriculum, i.e. to limit content to that which is necessary to meet statutory requirements and prepare the graduate for the next stage of the educational curriculum and career specialisation, other advantages of this approach are that it:

- provides the basis of a blueprint for assessment
- enables integration, particularly 'vertical integration', within a spiral model of curriculum design (i.e. enables students to revisit broadly the same problems at various stages in the course)

- provides a basis for better monitoring and evaluation of student experience.

Student-selected components

Tomorrow's doctors (2003) recommends that 'the core curriculum must be supported by a series of student-selected components'. The nature of this support is complex and the relationship actually works both ways.

- The breadth achieved through the core curriculum is complemented by the opportunities for in-depth study associated with student-selected components.
- Student-selected components provide opportunities to study specialist areas in medicine which are not covered in the core curriculum.
- Student-selected components provide opportunities for core curricular learning outcomes to be achieved.
- The core curriculum provides opportunities for students to develop interests which can be pursued in student-selected components.
- A component of the core curriculum can provide the basis upon which a student-selected component can be developed.

Choice

Student-selected components are defined in *Tomorrow's doctors* (2003) as '*parts of the curriculum that allow students to choose what they want to study.*' This essential element of choice has important implications for curriculum planners. In theory the scope of student-selected components should be limitless; however in reality the choice will be constrained.

The range of choice offered will depend first upon a series of high-level factors, such as:

- Resource – the availability of a school's resource, both human and physical, will inevitably constrain the repertoire of student-selected components that can be offered.
- Enthusiasm – the enthusiasm of individual members or groups of staff offering student-selected opportunities is key to their success. Initially staff have to overcome the tendency to believe that student-selected components are in some way less important than core elements. It must be communicated to contributors that delivery of student-selected experiences is both intrinsically rewarding and essential for attaining 'core' outcomes
- Prior learning – the stage in the curriculum at which particular opportunities are offered should be such that the students have had sufficient prior experience to be able to make an informed choice and to benefit from the choice offered by the student-selected component.
- Breadth of experience – measured access to a choice of topics not directly related to medicine may provide students with the opportunity to widen their horizons, and broaden their educational experience, so as to prepare them better for the modern world.

- The organisation of the curriculum as a whole and the proportion of student effort ascribed to the student-selected components will also affect the extent of choice.

While the range of topics offered will be constrained by such policy considerations, it will also depend upon the nature of the experiences themselves, e.g. the opportunity to extend core learning, a chance to explore an entirely new topic or to undertake research.

Broadly, three basic patterns have been used:

- Students select from a broad range of projects that have been suggested by staff.
- Students select a module from a limited range offered, often as an extension to 'core'.
- Students suggest their own topic within the confines of a particular subject, discipline or module.

Student choice first implies a positive selection of a relatively small number of experiences out of a large menu of available options. Conversely, positive selection implies by necessity an opting out from many others. If a student can opt out of an experience that is considered essential to meet the outcomes overall, then by definition such an experience must be included in the core.

Outcomes

Curriculum planners must establish which core learning outcomes can be met by all students irrespective of the content of their selected components. Given the relatively low emphasis placed on the content of the student selected components, it is the acquisition of skills and the development of appropriate attitudes and behaviour that are most likely to be achieved through this part of the programme (Murdoch-Eaton et al 2004).

Examples of core learning outcomes which may be achieved through student-selected components are:

- Communication skills: '. . . clearly present information verbally, visually or in writing and communicate ideas and arguments effectively'.
- Information technology skills: '. . . demonstrate competence in using library and other information systems to access information'.
- Insight into research and scientific method: '. . . demonstrate ability to apply appropriate method of enquiry'.
- Critical thinking: '. . . demonstrate ability to critically evaluate and interpret information'.
- Reflection: '. . . identify one's own strengths and weaknesses'.
- Self-management: '. . . effectively manage time and prioritise tasks'.

Teaching, learning and assessment

Given that range of subject areas, and therefore choice, are key features of this part of the curriculum, some unifying elements must be introduced into the student-selected components to ensure that the core learning outcomes can be achieved and appropriately assessed. A variety of learning activities can be provided to enable students to achieve such

Curriculum planners must decide which core learning outcomes can be met by all students irrespective of the content of their selected components.

"Student-selected study has the aim of stimulating critical thought and developing further generic graduate skills and intellectual attributes underpinning enquiry and critical thinking; it should allow students to acquire research methods and enhance their skills in collection, evaluation, synthesis and presentation of evidence"

QAA 2002

"Student-selected study provides opportunities for study in depth and may extend beyond the traditional medical disciplines"

QAA 2002

defined outcomes. Taking the possible outcomes listed above, some examples of learning activities which may be used in this way include:

- Communication skills – opportunities for verbal and written communication.
- Information technology skills – supervised training sessions to develop information skills and proficiency in the use of communications and information technology.
- Insight into research and scientific method – opportunities to undertake a research project.
- Critical thinking – opportunities for evaluation and interpretation of information from a variety of sources.
- Reflection – use of portfolio or logbook to provide a structured approach to learning through reflection on experiences and performance.
- Self-management – opportunities to manage and prioritise stages of project.

If student-selected components are to be used to enable students to achieve core learning outcomes, then it is essential that reliable and valid assessment methodologies are developed and utilised. This will serve not only to reinforce the importance of this part of the curriculum to the student body, but also to reassure those teachers involved in the delivery of student-selected components of the perceived worth by the school of their contribution to the curriculum. Some examples of methodologies which have been used to assess achievement of the learning outcomes defined above include:

- Communication skills – assessment of an oral presentation for effective communication of ideas and arguments.
- Information technology skills – assessment of a poster for use of information technology skills in ensuring clarity of presentation.
- Insight into research and scientific method – assessment of 'methods' section of a written report for clarity and appropriate use of methodology.
- Critical thinking – assessment of literature review for adequate and appropriate critical appraisal of current literature.
- Reflection – assessment of a piece of reflective writing.
- Self-management – assessment of achievement of a previously agreed set of learning outcomes.

Structure

It is apparent that there is considerable variation in the ways in which schools in the UK have embedded student-selected components into their curricula. Although this is in line with the original concept proposed in *Tomorrow's doctors* (1993), whereby schools were encouraged to demonstrate individuality in how they incorporated student-selected components into their curricula, curriculum planners need to be mindful of the following:

- Student-selected components should be an identifiable 'theme' running through the curriculum which enables students to develop skills and attitudes over an extended period of time.

> If the student-selected components are to be used to enable students to achieve core learning outcomes, then it is essential that reliable and valid assessment methodologies are developed and utilised.

- The purpose of student-selected components should be well defined and made explicit to staff and students alike.
- Student-selected components should not be seen as an 'optional' part of the programme – all students must undertake, complete and demonstrate satisfactory achievement in this part of the curriculum.
- Schools should not use this part of the curriculum as an opportunity for remedial work and resit examinations for those students who have failed elements of the core curriculum.
- Student-selected components should be placed in the overall curriculum in such a way that students have sufficient experience to make real, informed choices about whether to explore a topic of interest in depth, to sample a specialty or subspecialty for career purposes or to add breadth to their experience etc.

Summary

There has been a shift in balance between hospital-based services and the delivery of care in the community, the demography and cultural composition of populations are changing rapidly, the advent of 'new' sciences and technologies are having profound effects upon practice and public understanding of disease and disability has increased dramatically. Consequently expectations of what can and should be achieved through basic medical education are continuing to grow. The changing needs and demands of a wide range of legitimate stakeholders must be taken into account in identifying outcomes and content, and in curricular planning. It must be recognised that curriculum development is an 'organic', continuing process – the curriculum is never finished!

In many respects the original concepts of 'core curriculum' and 'student-selected components' are outmoded. While they focused attention on the pressing need to unburden medical programmes of unnecessary factual information, the 'curriculum' must be considered now as a whole, built around a 'core' set of learning outcomes, which for all practical purposes embody the 'standards' of any single course of study.

Nevertheless the provision of a motivational context, a well-structured framework for learning, opportunity for choice and the promotion of the active involvement of students in their own education, are all desirable factors identified as enhancing attainment and ensuring that basic medical education remains a rewarding experience.

References

British Pharmacological Society 2002 Core curriculum for medicine. Online. Available http://www.bps.ac.uk/education

AAMC Core Curriculum Working Group 2000 Graduate medical education core curriculum (AAMC). Association of American Medical Colleges, Washington, DC

GMC 1993 Tomorrow's doctors: recommendations on undergraduate medical education. General Medical Council, London

GMC 2003 Tomorrow's doctors: recommendations on undergraduate medical education. General Medical Council, London

Goroll A H, Morrison G, Bass E B et al 1995 SGIM/CDIM core medicine clerkship curriculum guide. Health Resources and Services Administration, Washington, DC

Higher education in the learning society, Report of National Committee of Inquiry into Higher Education, 1997 http://www.leeds.ac.uk/educol/ncihe

Higher Education Quality Council (HEQC) 1997 Graduate Standards Programme. Final Report. HEQC, London

Murdoch-Eaton D, Ellershaw J, Garden A et al 2004 Student-selected components in the undergraduate medical curriculum: a multi-institutional consensus on purpose. Medical Teacher 26:33–38

QAA (Quality Assurance Agency for Higher Education) 2002
Subject benchmark statements – medicine. Online. Available:
http://www.qaa.ac.uk/crntwork/benchmark/phase2/
medicine.htm 6 August 2004

Simpson J G, Furnace J, Crosby J 2002 The Scottish doctor –
learning outcomes for the medical undergraduate in Scotland:
a foundation for competent and reflective practitioners.
Medical Teacher 24:136–143

SECTION 4
TOOLS AND AIDS

Chapter 20
Instructional design

A. Stewart

Introduction

In recent years there has been a renewed interest in how teachers teach; the focus has been on teachers' conceptions of teaching (Kember 1997).

Many teachers would argue that, in teaching, the main thing they are doing is 'covering the subject'; others would claim that they are 'imparting information', although some might go as far as claiming that they are 'imparting knowledge'. The emphasis is, essentially, on the content of the subject and their teaching of it. Such teaching could be classified as being *teacher-centred* and *content-oriented*. The teacher is the key person in the session and is concerned, primarily, with the transmission of information.

There are other teachers who view teaching from a different perspective. Their conception of teaching is not about transmitting information or imparting knowledge but about facilitating student learning. These teachers, according to Kember (1997), adopt an approach to teaching that is *student-centred* and *learning-oriented*.

When the emphasis in medical education is firmly on how students can apply their knowledge in solving problems, i.e. on what they can do rather than on what they know, the thrust of teaching has to be on facilitating learning rather than on covering the subject. But, as Light & Cox (2001) point out, teachers have a responsibility which takes them beyond facilitating the 'construction' of knowledge to assisting and supporting the student to develop (or 'reconstruct' themselves) as persons. In achieving this the process of instructional design is significant.

A comprehensive review of instructional design (Dills & Romiszowski 1997) suggests at least 60 models but, at its most straightforward, instructional design can be considered as a process through which we can identify the nature of the learning that is intended to take place, work out an approach to teaching that will facilitate achievement of that learning and administer an appropriate assessment that will determine whether the intended learning has, in fact, taken place.

Learning outcomes

Identifying the nature of learning outcomes is a key aspect of the instructional design process. If we do not identify the learning outcomes clearly it is unlikely that worthwhile learning will, in fact, take place.

Instructional design
- Consider the outcomes to be achieved.
- Organise appropriate instructional events to facilitate learning.
- Determine whether learning has taken place.

As noted in the Introduction, some teachers tend to 'cover the subject' (usually because there is a content-centred curriculum) and the outcome is likely to be little better than that the student will get a sufficient grasp of the subject to be able to answer the questions raised in an examination. Since these examinations frequently require the recall of factual information, gaining a grasp of the subject finishes up as memorising a lot of information. When we cover the aetiology, epidemiology, pathophysiology, etc of any topic, we can, in effect, be passing on factual information, the regurgitation of which is required in an examination which will probably be in multiple choice question format requiring factual recall.

There has been a shift, as noted earlier, towards teaching that is focused on facilitating learning. The student is encouraged to adopt a so-called 'deep approach' to learning and is expected to understand and apply the knowledge acquired. All the evidence regarding how students approach learning, together with our best understanding of how knowledge is built up, certainly suggests that students have to be able to construct their own knowledge, building on an existing knowledge base, and find relevance and meaning in the process.

Relevance and meaning are found through trying to make connections between the ideas that are being encountered and the real world of the practice of medicine. Ideas and practices, the practical application of knowledge, therefore provide the basis for students' learning.

Knowledge

Students who adopt the 'deep approach' to learning try to understand the ideas behind the words; they try to understand the concepts and principles that are involved rather than merely to remember the facts.

Concepts can be thought of as information about objects, events, and processes that allow us to differentiate various things and classes, understand relationships between objects and generalise about events, things and processes. A considerable amount of learning is concerned with the learning of concepts. Lack of understanding of concepts leads to lack of clarity in thinking.

While concepts help us to classify diverse phenomena, principles enable us to predict, explain and control phenomena. Principles state relationships between two or more concepts. In general, principles can be converted into 'if–then' statements. When students have learned a principle they should be able to do more than simply state the principle; they should be able to make some predictions from it and explain appropriate events.

In the structure of knowledge, concepts are combined into principles. A principle is not simply a number of concepts linked in the same sentence. A principle states a relationship between classes of events that enable us to predict consequences, explain events, infer causes, control situations and solve problems.

The acquisition of concepts and principles is, therefore, the key to acquiring knowledge and applying it in practice.

Learning outcomes
Understanding concepts helps us to:
• differentiate between things
• understand relationships
• generalise about events, things and processes.

Learning outcomes
Understanding principles helps us to
• predict consequences
• explain events
• infer causes
• control situations.

Focus on the concepts and principles and the facts will fall into place.

Skills

Learning medicine is not only about acquiring knowledge. Associated with that knowledge there has to be a practical ability to carry out procedures and utilise skills. Such abilities are also key learning outcomes.

Attitudes

Any task that a doctor has to perform will involve knowledge, skills and attitudes. Unfortunately, because attitudes are difficult to define and explain and because they are not easy to measure, we tend to ignore them.

Competencies

According to Gonczi et al (1993) a *competency* is a combination of attributes such as knowledge, skills and attitudes underlying some aspect of successful professional performance. A competency is, however, more than just a set of specific knowledge, skills and attitudes; it involves coordination of a person's cognitive, affective and other resources – and a willingness to use these – in the performance of a professional task. Competence could, thus, be considered as a person's ability and willingness to get their act together, utilising the various competencies they have acquired, with the competencies having been built on the knowledge, skills and attitudes learned earlier.

Competencies arise from the areas of competence that can be identified in an analysis of the roles and functions of a doctor or other health professional. Analysis of the areas of competence leads to identification of the specific competencies, and analysis of the competencies leads, in turn, to identification of the underpinning knowledge, skills and attitudes.

In summary, identification of learning outcomes, that is, areas of competence, their associated competencies, and the prerequisite knowledge, skills and attitudes on which the competencies are built, is a crucial part of the instructional design process (see Fig 20.1).

Topic and task analyses

Because defining attitudes is so difficult, this subject has only recently been included in the identification of learning outcomes. Identifying knowledge and skills outcomes is much more straightforward and is usually done through topic and task analyses.

Topic analysis

Reigeluth and colleagues (1994) examined the implications for instructional design arising from the structure of subject matter. By structure they meant the interrelationships among the components of the subject matter and by components they meant the individual concepts, principles, facts, etc.

They proposed that a content structure, in relation to a learning structure or learning hierarchy, can be represented by a diagram that shows the *learning–prerequisite relations* among the components of the subject matter. The learning structure describes what must be known before some-

Competencies bring together knowledge, skills and attitudes in performance of a task.

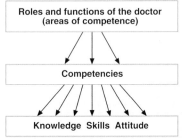

Fig. 20.1

thing else can be learned. For example, the concepts of systolic pressure and diastolic pressure must both be understood before the concept of blood pressure can be learned. Similarly, the concepts of systole and diastole have to be understood before the concepts of their respective pressures can be learned. A learning–prerequisite relation is characterised by the statement: 'A learner must know X in order to learn Y' (see Fig. 20.2).

Two points must be noted here. First, it is important to work out what the concepts are. Second, it is important to work out what their interrelationships are. Since new knowledge has to be built on existing knowledge, absence of prerequisites can mean that new learning does not take place.

Although the term 'hierarchy' is normally used to describe the interrelationships between concepts, other relationships such as those found in concept mapping might be more appropriate and will certainly be equally useful.

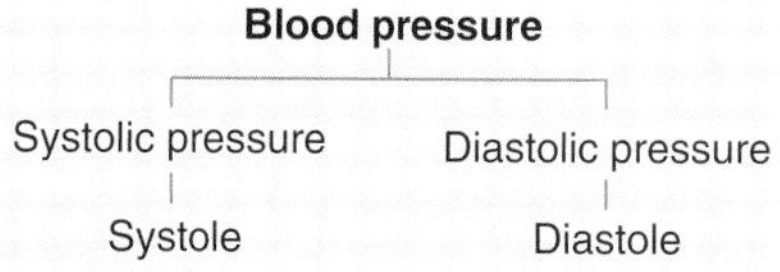

Task analysis

Although the term 'task analysis' is often used to cover what is, in effect, a learning hierarchy analysis, it is really most appropriately used when referring to a job task analysis (Mager & Beach 1967) which focuses on a job description and requires the instructional designer to list all of the tasks in a job and the steps included in each task.

In relation to procedural tasks, Reigeluth and colleagues (1994) proposed that there should be two types of procedural relations. *Procedural–prerequisite relations* are the relationships among the steps of a single procedure (specifically, the order for performing those steps) (see Fig. 20.3) The procedural–prerequisite relation is characterised by the statement 'The performer must do X before he can do Y'.

Procedural–decision relations are the relationships between alternative procedures, and they describe the factors necessary for deciding which procedure, or subprocedure, to use in a given situation. A flow diagram is one way of portraying a decision structure, and the relation is characterised by the statement: 'Given condition A, the performer must do X rather than Y or Z'.

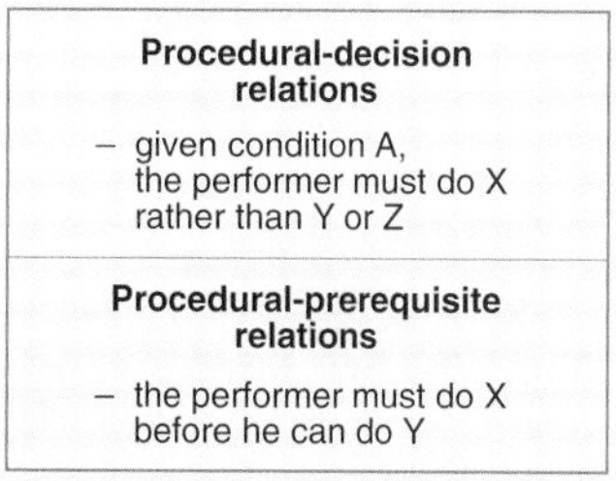

Creating the conditions for learning

In the process of instructional design, the identification of the nature of the desired learning outcomes alone is insufficient; it must be followed up by designing the kind of teaching that is going to take place so that these learning outcomes are likely to be achieved.

Successive editions of Gagne's influential book on instructional design (1985) have followed the evolution from behavioural to cognitive perspectives on learning and have indicated how the student has to construct knowledge rather than merely respond to the stimulus of teaching.

Gagne's model is basically concerned with the kind of learning outcomes to be achieved and the arrangement of specific instructional events which are tailored to achievement of those kinds of outcomes.

Fig. 20.2 Topic analysis: an example of a learning–prerequisite relationship

Fig. 20.3 Task analysis: the two types of procedural relations

Conditions for learning
Arranging external events (external to the mind) that support internal processing (internal to the mind).

Learning outcomes (Gagne 1985)
- Intellectual skills
  - discrimination
  - concrete concepts
  - defined concepts
  - rules
  - problem solving
- Verbal information
  - memory recall
- Cognitive strategies
  - learning how to learn and think
- Motor skills
  - goal-directed muscular movement
- Attitudes
  - mental state influencing action.

Gaining attention	informing learners of objectives	Stimulating recall of prior learning
The teacher	**The student**	
• Provokes interest through statement or question or use of media	• Tunes in to the correct wavelength	
• Makes it clear where the session is going and what should be achieved	• Recalls relevant prior knowledge	
• Refers to earlier relevant learning and indicates its links with the new topic	• Starts to shape up for new learning (creates ideational scaffolding)	

Fig. 20.4 The first three 'events of instruction' in Gagne's approach to instructional design

Presenting the content	Providing learner guidance
The teacher	**The student**
• Concepts and principles presented in organised structured way	• Builds up his/her knowledge structure
• Explanations provided	• Exercises thinking abilities to work things out, find meaning, and build links between ideas
• Links suggested back to other subjects	• Tries to envisage how the new knowledge can be applied
• Links projected forward to application	

Fig. 20.5 The core of the teaching/learning process

The instructional events provide information and interaction that enhance the possibilities of learning.

In essence, creating the conditions for learning is concerned with arranging events external to the mind of the student that support processes internal to the mind of the student. It means that teachers have to organise what they do when teaching in order to influence appropriately what goes on inside learners' minds so that they can learn. What the teacher says, how it is said, the analogies employed, the graphic illustrations and media that are used, i.e. the external events, all have to be designed in a way that triggers cognitive processing in the mind of the student so that learning takes place.

The learning of concepts and principles comes into a category of cognitive outcome that Gagne calls 'intellectual skills', a category that is concerned with complex or procedural knowledge. Other cognitive categories are 'verbal information', which is concerned with memory or recall, and 'cognitive strategies', which are strategies for learning how to learn.

Intellectual skills include five subcategories that range from the basic skill of recognising similarities and differences (discriminations) to skills in the application of learned rules or principles (problem solving). For each of these kinds of learning outcome, a particular strategy of instruction is required.

Events of instruction

The set of events in Gagne's approach to instructional design consists of nine activities carried out by a teacher and learners during instruction.

The first three (gaining attention, informing the learner of the learning outcome, and stimulating recall of prerequisite learning; see Fig. 20.4) collectively prepare the learner for the instruction. The student's attention is stimulated and focused on what is to be learned. Expectations of what is to be learned are clarified and the basis on which learning is to be built is established.

The next two (presenting the information and providing learner guidance) are the core of the teaching/learning process (Fig. 20.5); they must be designed to help the student to make sense of the topic and build up understanding. In this stage, concepts and principles are presented in an organised structured way, explanations are provided, and links with previously learned material and with related subjects are highlighted, so that the student is stimulated to work things out, find meaning, build links between ideas, and envisage how the new knowledge can be applied.

The final four events (eliciting performance, providing feedback, assessing performance and enhancing transfer; Fig. 20.6) are designed to give the student the opportunity to check and enhance learning, correct misunderstanding, monitor understanding, and think about how knowledge can be applied in other contexts.

An alternative approach: the schema model

Knowledge appears to be structured by individuals in meaningful ways which grow and change over time; the way in which it is stored is related to the way it is encoded when it is learned (Romberg & Carpenter 1986). New knowledge is constructed by the learner in a process of building new relationships essential to learning (Resnick & Ford 1981).

One model suggested as an explanation for this 'building' process, is the notion of a *schema* – the building block of cognition (Rumelhart 1980). Activating relevant prior knowledge is, essentially, a schema-activation exercise. When new information is presented in an organised and structured way and appropriate explanations given, the learner engages in a process of schema construction. In a time of summary at the end of the session, the student has the opportunity of refining schemata; what has been learned can be checked against what is being summarised.

Schema activation

In schema activation, existing knowledge relevant to the new material about to be presented is activated. It is unlikely that only one new idea is to be presented in the session. It might be that the new material to be presented will need activation of more than one set of existing knowledge structures. It might mean pulling together previously acquired knowledge from several different areas of experience. This schema activation exercise is probably sufficiently important in the learning experience that teachers need to consider much more carefully how to help learners prepare for the session and how to begin the session to ensure maximum readiness for the new material to be presented.

Schema construction

New information presented is likely to be accepted by students in the form in which we present it and then built into their own cognitive structure. It is important, therefore, that it is presented in a structured and organised way. It is very difficult for students to take amorphous material and make any kind of structure out of it! Some form of topic analysis should be carried out prior to delivery so teachers can see how the different parts of the material relate to each other – what needs to come before what, and where understanding of one concept is dependent on prior understanding of another. Having previously clarified one's thoughts, it is possible to present information in a structured form which will enable students to assimilate it into their own knowledge structures.

In this process of schema construction it is important for the student to be thinking about the material. It is the responsibility of the teacher, as a facilitator of learning, to encourage students to be thinking about the material presented and attempting to relate it to what is already known, to work out what it means in their own context and to think about ways in which it might prove to be useful in future applications and so on. In so doing, students are not only creating meaning and constructing knowledge but are actually strengthening their own learning skills.

The teacher needs to ensure that the teaching/learning session is not given over solely to the providing of information and the building up of knowledge; it is not only knowing *that*, but knowing *how* which is important to the student. The objectives of the course will almost certainly

Elicits performance	Provides feedback	Assesses performance	Enhances transfer
The teacher		**The student**	
• Checks that the students have learned what was to be learned		• Responds to questions by checking his/her understanding	
• Provides corrective/ supplementary guidance as required		• Corrects misunderstanding	
• Confirms that learning has taken place		• Monitors understanding (metacognition)	
• Summarises and encourages thinking about application		• Thinks about how knowledge can be applied	

Fig. 20.6 The final four events of instruction

Schema activation
- helping the learner to 'tune-in'
- encouraging the learner to bring to mind relevant prior knowledge
- assisting the learner to prepare his/her prior knowledge to be the foundation on which new knowledge will now be constructed.

Schema construction
Helping the learner to make sense of the new material by
- linking it to existing knowledge
- making it relevant to learning need
- highlighting its significance to future practice
- presenting it in an organised and structured way
- providing appropriate 'explanations'.

involve higher-order thinking skills and it is these which have to be developed during the session. The student needs to be encouraged, and given the opportunity, to apply acquired knowledge in activities such as analysis, synthesis, evaluation and problem solving. Objectives relating to attitudinal and emotional aspects of the tasks to be performed also need to be remembered; interaction between students in an exchange of views often needs to be fostered by the teacher, so that conflicting views can be considered and resolution achieved.

Schema refinement

Towards the end of the session it is advisable to give the student the opportunity to become involved in refining schemata as the teacher reviews the material and key points covered. Students can then re-examine the nature of the knowledge which has been constructed in their minds and refine as necessary, perhaps modifying it in the light of further consideration at that point. One of the most useful activities for students to undertake may be to make a summary in their own words of the main thrust of the session and to annotate this in relation to previous learning and possible future application.

The idea of a beginning, a middle, and an end has been around for a long time, as has the advice to 'tell them what you're going to say, say it, and tell them what you've said'. What is different is an understanding of how such approaches can, in fact, work. The schema activation, construction, and refinement model for teaching, coupled with encouragement of students to engage in deeper processing and thinking, gives us a credible and robust basis for the design of our teaching.

Instructional design and e-learning

The emergence of the idea of 'learning objects' that can be reused within the context of e-learning has led to a perception that this has become the new design and development paradigm of choice. However, as Wiley (2002) points out, learning objects must be linked with instructional design theory if they are to succeed in facilitating learning. The learning object approach might be of value, but only if it is considered within an appropriate instructional design framework.

Summary

The purpose of teaching is to facilitate learning. The instructional design process is a valuable aid in this task since it involves the identification of the nature of the learning that is intended to take place, the development of an approach to teaching that will facilitate achievement of that learning, and the provision of some kind of assessment that will enable teacher and student to determine whether the intended learning has, in fact, taken place.

The nature of learning outcomes is best identified in terms of the concepts and principles arising from an analysis of the topic or, in the case

---

Schema refinement

- reviewing the topic to give the learner a chance to check his/her constructions
- reviewing what has been presented to let the learner reflect upon what has been learned
- reviewing the topic and projecting forward to situations that let the learner make applications of what has been learned.

of tasks, in terms of steps or stages arising from an analysis of the performance of the task.

Gagne's 'events of instruction' approach provides a systematic way to prepare students for the learning experience, to present new material together with guidance in understanding it, and to check that they have understood the material and can apply the knowledge acquired.

The 'schema' approach provides an alternative framework for activating relevant prior knowledge, building on existing knowledge, finding meaning and relevance in the new material, and checking that the new knowledge is constructed as intended.

References

Dills C R, Romiszowski A J 1997 Instructional development paradigms. Educational Technology Publications, Englewood Cliffs, NJ

Gagne R M 1985 The conditions of learning (4th edn). Holt, Rinehart and Winston, New York.

Gonczi A, Hager P, Athanasou J. 1993 The development of competency-based assessment strategies for the professions. National Office of Overseas Skills Recognition Research Paper no. 8. Australian Government Publishing Service, Canberra

Kember D A 1997 A reconceptualisation of the research into university academics' conceptions of teaching. Learning and Instruction 7(3):255–275

Light G, Cox R 2001 Learning and teaching in higher education. Paul Chapman Publishing, London

Mager R F, Beach K M 1967 Developing vocational instruction, Fearon Publishers, Belmont, CA

Reigeluth C M, Merrill M D, Bunderson C V 1994 The structure of subject matter content and its instructional design implications. In Merrill M D, Mitchell D G (eds) Instructional design theory. Educational Technology Publications, Englewood Cliffs, NJ

Resnick L B, Ford W W 1981 The Psychology of mathematics for instruction. Lawrence Erlbaum Associates, Mahwah NJ

Romberg T A, Carpenter T P 1986 Research on teaching and learning mathematics. In: M.C. Wittrock M C (ed) Handbook of research on teaching, 3rd edn. Macmillan, New York, p 850–873

Rumelhart D E 1980 Schemata: the building blocks of cognition. In: Spiro R J et al (eds) Theoretical issues in reading comprehension. Lawrence Erlbaum Associates, Mahwah NJ, p 33–58

Wiley D A 2002 The instructional use of learning objects. Agency for Instructional Technology and the Association for Educational Communications and Technology, Bloomington, Indiana

Chapter 21
Study guides
J. M. Laidlaw, E. A. Hesketh

Introduction

This chapter deals with study guides and in particular the need for them, their various roles in the continuum of medical education, and the features which can be incorporated to help the learner study more effectively.

A study guide is an aid, usually presented in the form of printed notes or electronically produced, designed to facilitate studies. Not only does the guide give students an indication of what they should be learning, it also informs them how they should best learn and how they can recognise that they have mastered the topic being studied. A guide can also be seen as a management tool which allows doctors to exercise their teaching and training responsibilities while at the same time giving the students and trainees an important part to play in managing their own learning. Rowntree (1986) captured the idea well when he likened a study guide to a tutor sitting on the student's shoulder, available 24 hours a day to offer advice on what to do at any stage of the student's studies.

Why use study guides?

There are several reasons why study guides are becoming more popular with students at both undergraduate and postgraduate levels. Doctors intent on keeping up to date with new techniques and therapies are also making use of study guides especially when they accompany distance learning programmes. We have highlighted overleaf some of the reasons for the increasing interest in this educational tool. You can most likely add to the list from your own experience.

The problem of overload

Students are expected to learn more about medicine today than ever before, but within the same timespan. In postgraduate and continuing education the problem is much the same – doctors have to keep up to date with new treatments and management of diseases as well as trying to tackle new technologies. Clearly all students and trainees need to be selective about the essential information they take on board, and for this reason they need an educational tool that will point them in the right direction.

"A study guide is not a tool which constrains or unnecessarily spoon feeds. Rather it is an instrument which allows students to take more responsibility for their own learning"

Laidlaw & Harden 1990

"A study guide can be updated much more quickly than original materials"

Race & Brown 1995

The knowledge required of a doctor is expanding at more than 14% per year.

A menu of learning opportunities

There are new approaches to learning and a variety of learning opportunities on offer for students and trainees – but which route of study should a learner adopt? Bearing in mind that we all have different learning styles, it is important to try to match the styles and approaches as much as possible, thus ensuring effective learning. No longer are students content to sit passively in the lecture theatre for hours on end to absorb information. Lectures, which can be most effective if they are interactive, continue to remain on most timetables, but the development of clinical skills units and the many resources in ambulatory care, as outlined in chapters 8 and 10, all make up a large menu of exciting learning opportunities for undergraduate and postgraduate students.

A variety of educational approaches

Distance learning, problem-based learning, evidence-based learning, outcome-based learning, service-based learning, task-based learning and blended learning are only a few of the approaches that are becoming more commonplace in undergraduate and postgraduate education. No matter which approach is adopted, learning requires to be facilitated and a guide can help ensure this happens. Harden et al (1996) remind us that 'educators are becoming more aware of the need to develop forms of learning that are rooted in the learner's practical experience and in the job they are to undertake as a professional on completion of training'. Learning 'on the job', for example, has much to commend it for the trainee doctor but too often learning in such an excellent environment is not always maximised due to heavy service commitment. It is a problem which can be addressed to some extent with the use of study guides as they can ensure that the doctor in training uses the tasks being carried out daily as the focus for further study. *Learning paediatrics: a training guide for senior house officers* (Mitchell et al 1998) was developed to support SHOs in new paediatric posts. It focused on everyday clinical problems and provided practical advice and a framework on which to base further study.

Roles for study guides

So how can study guides actually help learners? In facilitating learning they have three specific roles:

- assisting in the management of student learning
- providing a focus for student activities relating to the learning
- providing information on the subject or topic of study.

Given these three roles, it is not surprising that the actual format and presentation of study guides can look very different. From the model shown in Figure 21.1 you can see that guides can be placed at any point in the triangle depending on their purpose. It is more likely, however, that you will find most guides located in the middle, as they will have incorporated all three roles to some extent. We will first look at some of the features of study guides designed to help students or trainees manage their own learning.

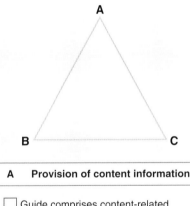

"*People come in many shapes and sizes, so do their ways of learning*"

Beard & Hartley 1984

Blended learning – a mix of e-learning and face-to-face activities – is growing in popularity.

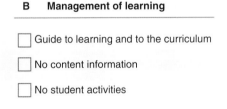

A   Provision of content information

☐ Guide comprises content-related information

☐ No student activities

☐ No help with learning or introduction to the curriculum

B   Management of learning

☐ Guide to learning and to the curriculum

☐ No content information

☐ No student activities

C   Student activities

☐ Guide based on student activities

☐ No content information

☐ No help with learning or introduction to the curriculum

Fig. 21.1 Study guide triangle

"To study epilepsy, you will need a basic knowledge of the anatomy and physiology of the brain. This was covered during your second year, so look back at your notes and handouts"

Medical teacher

"We prefer the term 'learning outcome' since it lacks the narrow behaviourist connotations thst some people give to the term 'objective'. The outcomes belong to the learner"

Ryan et al 2000

"Where you refer to textbooks in your study guide you will help the students enormously if you add the chapter and pages which they should look at and in a sentence tell them why you want them to read the section"

Instructional designer

Managing learning

If the role of the study guide is to help students or trainees manage their own learning then it might contain the components described below.

An overview

This might include the framework for the course, salient points in the study of the topic, some cross-referencing and a scene setter. The scene setter is used to put the topic being studied in the context of the 'bigger picture' so that learners recognise the relevance of the topic. For example, undergraduate students using a study guide to learn more about the thyroid gland need to be aware that this is one of many topics being covered in the endocrine system block. Similarly in a study guide for senior house officers who are learning paediatrics, they need to be made aware that dealing with the breathless child is just one task that might be encountered when managing acutely ill children.

Prerequisites

You might wish to include a statement of the requirements expected of students before they commence their new studies. Some study guides include a pre-test to help students assess their prior knowledge and identify any gaps which need to be revised.

Learning outcomes

All learners need to know what is expected of them – in other words, they need to be informed of the learning outcomes (or objectives). A clear statement of what you hope the learners will achieve on studying a particular topic is essential if you are to keep the learners on track. In specifying learning outcomes it is an added bonus if you can differentiate between the key outcomes and those which the student might wish to master, time permitting. It is certainly important that the outcomes set are achievable.

Learning strategies

Mention ought to be made of the approaches to learning that should be followed. If the student is expected to be a self-directed learner then this information should be highlighted. If the student has a choice in the problem-based learning mode then again this should be stated. There certainly should be a framework or structure for a course of study, enabling students to build upon it and in so doing develop their learning en route.

Learning opportunities

Lectures, small-group teaching, clinical skills teaching, demonstrations and many more opportunities are on offer to undergraduate and postgraduate students. They need to know how best to use these resources to maximise their learning.

A timetable

A guide does not always include a timetable, but there should at least be some indication of the amount of time students should devote to a particular topic. Time is a precious commodity and running out of it does little for morale!

Assessment details

How to prepare for the examinations coupled with the type of assessment tool to be used is perhaps the first thing that a student will read. This is not spoonfeeding students; it is perhaps making life less stressful for them.

Staff contacts

Having a mentor or supervisor is information worth knowing about, but not once the course is over. A name to contact and a note of available hours to make that contact are worth their weight in gold.

Tips or personal comments

It is so reassuring to be given a few words of wisdom from the 'expert' or at least from someone who has years of experience to their credit.

The majority of the components above considerably aid the learning process; however, the self-directed learner also needs to be kept motivated throughout the period of study. This can be achieved by building into the guide some interesting features such as case studies, self-assessment quizzes or scenarios, or simply by highlighting the importance and relevance of the subject. Attention to details such as the layout and design and the style of writing can all help to make a guide a user-friendly tool – and something that will not simply collect dust on a shelf or be thrown in the wastepaper basket!

Providing the focus for learning

Where the guide has been prepared more as a workbook to be used in conjunction with various learning activities and opportunities, there may be instructions for students to summarise, interpret and apply principles to another context. The guide in this situation really becomes the focus for the learning activities to be undertaken. In addition, learners might also be asked to 'think' about an issue, reflect upon a point, and apply their new-found knowledge and skills to practice. In so doing, they are more likely to experience deep rather than superficial learning.

This was exactly the approach adopted in a study guide for doctors starting their surgical training. While studying hypoxia, for example, doctors are invited to: stop and think about the drugs that affect the respiratory centre; reflect on case studies that are used to introduce the topic (Fig. 21.2), and apply the knowledge gained to their own clinical situation. They are also encouraged in this particular study guide to keep a record of these activities in a portfolio. Diaries or logbooks are often used to document learning experiences that subsequently can be formatively or summatively assessed.

Providing information on a topic

To some extent you can say that all study guides provide learners with information about the topic(s) being studied, but if you think back to the model (Fig. 21.1) you will be reminded that some guides, as part of their function, give more core information than others do.

"A mentor is 'someone who has done' helping 'someone who is just starting to do' "

Race & Brown 1993

"Don't hesitate to ask your trainer for advice. Keep in mind that trainers were once new graduates, so they are well placed to steer you in the right direction"

Dental trainer

"Most of the 1,000,000 head-injured attenders at hospital in the UK each year do not need admission, but it is critically important to identify the 10% who do"

Consultant neurosurgeon

Think

Remind yourself of the drugs which affect the respiratory centre.

In case 3, why was Mrs. A. W. hypoxic?

Shallow respiration suggests:
• inadequate reversal of neuromuscular blocking agents
• inadequate recovery from anaesthesia
• opiate overdose

Fig. 21.2 Study guide example of 'think' and 'reflect'

"Portfolios can provide you with the evidence of a learner's ability to meet the standards of your course"

Medical teacher

Be selective with your further references. It can frustrate the student if:
• they cannot easily access them
• they are given too many choices.
Remember that inter-library loans are expensive.

"Remember to check the website so that you can complete the weekly self-assessment quiz"

Tutor

"Each visual should support the learning process by showing something relevant to the content. Otherwise visuals distract learners and complicate the learning process"

Carliner 2002

It is likely that the type of information will fall into the following two categories:

• previously published information – for example, quotations from other texts, an article from a journal, further references
• new information – for example, tips and comments from the teacher/trainer, a glossary, key points on the topic being studied.

You might find, for example, that a textbook does not adequately cover a topic, so by adding your own piece of text you can address the problem; or perhaps information in a textbook is outdated, in which case an up-to-date statement in a study guide might suffice. Then there is the situation where there are differing views on a topic. It is easier to document these views, including your own, in your study guide. Deciding how much core information should be incorporated into a guide much depends on the accessibility to the students of textbooks or journals. If these are scarce commodities then include the pertinent sections; otherwise you will end up with some very frustrated students who have joined the lengthy library queue.

Preparing a study guide

Time spent in the preparation of a study guide is well rewarded. Students are likely to make very good use of guides that really do facilitate learning. There are various strategies which can be adopted to make your guide an effective educational tool. Here are just some inclusions worth considering:

• Use advance organisers. Their purpose is to prepare the learners for new learning experiences. They should take on board what the learners already know and what they need to know to continue successfully with their study.
• Make use of headings which help to provide a structure to your writing and also ensure that the reader more easily assimilates the information.
• Build in some self-assessment exercises but try to make them imaginative and a challenge. Producing endless lists of questions that require a true/false response can thwart stimulation. Too much of a 'sameness' is boring! If you intend the learners to write their responses to the questions in the guide then make sure you leave adequate space for them to do so.
• Incorporate some illustrations. Bear in mind that illustrations can have different functions – the most important being to help your learners better understand a given piece of text. This can be achieved in different ways. Illustrations can be used to break up text and make it less dense to read. They can be incorporated to add some light relief by providing a bit of humour in the hope of keeping your learners 'switched on'. Then, of course, you can use illustrations for the sole purpose of helping learners better visualise a complex concept or remember key points. If you do decide to make use of them be sure that you do just that. Never go to the bother of incorporating an illustration just for the sake of it.

Consider using icons that help the learners to quickly find different types of information, e.g. activities or readings.

Faulkner (1984) gives good advice when referring to the compilation of training manuals and the same advice can be applied to study guides. Here are some of his ideas to get you started:

- Keep sentences short and simple – they tend to be more easily understood.
- Write in the active voice – text is more easily understood.
- Adopt a conversational style – it is much more user-friendly.
- Use familiar words – they are more easily understood and indeed read.

Once you have reached this stage in the preparation of a study guide your job is almost complete…but not quite. We have suggested that you build in features that will facilitate learning. We have highlighted the fact that by keeping sentences succinct and incorporating where appropriate some graphics – be these cartoons, charts, graphs etc. – you can better keep your learners motivated.

Attention to the layout and typography of the study guide are the final points to consider, whether you are producing an electronic or a paper-based study guide. For instance, with printed text it is advisable not to use type smaller than 10 point; otherwise you are in danger of the material not being read. If line lengths are too short you impair legibility. Captions divorced from the figures to which they refer frustrate the readers. Illustrations which appear as 'specks' on the paper are not worth using. This list is by no means complete.

Then we come to the production phase. Here are some questions that should be addressed:

- How many copies of the study guide are required?
  This will help you to decide whether it is an in-house printing production or a commercial production.
- Is colour really necessary or is it just to make the product look nice?
  Think about your budget carefully here.
- What type of paper should be used?
  There is a wide range of paper available. Matt paper can give a very professional finish, and although a glossy look might give a good first impression, if you are expected to write on such a surface your attitude to it will definitely change.
- Are you planning to print on both sides of the paper?
  You need to think carefully about the opacity of the paper. There is nothing worse than an image from a previous page shining through as you struggle to read new information.

Montemayor (2002) outlines 12 tips for the development of electronic study guides. However, before you get carried away with the technology, do ensure that your students will all have access to computers!

There can be no doubt that electronic study guides offer great scope for the creative teacher, but do not be surprised if your students request

"Familiarize your readers with your icon system by explaining what each one means in the introduction of your documentation"

Parker 1997

"There is strong evidence that communicating through text on screen is a new genre in its own right, and that most people are still getting to grips with it. There really are no well established rules"

a downloaded copy of the guide. There is still a place for paper-based materials despite the technological advances.

Summary

The best way to appreciate the key role which study guides play in the field of medical education is to produce a guide and introduce it into your own teaching situation. They are beneficial not only to the learners but also to those doing the teaching and training. They can help you to improve how you plan the learning; select topics for discussions; monitor the learners' progress; coordinate educational activities; plug gaps in content; and integrate theory with on-the-job learning.

So the first decision to make if you are going to produce a study guide is to decide on its role. Will it be designed to:

- assist students in managing their own learning?
- provide a focus for the educational activities relating to learning?
- provide information on the topics being studied?
- address all three of the above functions?

Once these questions have been answered think carefully about the features of guides, and about the educational strategies that you might consider incorporating to make learning more effective for your students.

References

Beard R, Hartley J 1984 Teaching and learning in higher education, 4th edn. Paul Chapman Publishing, London

Carliner S 2002 Designing e-learning. American Society for Training and Development (ASTD), Alexandria VA

Faulkner L 1984 Designing training manuals for the business and industry classroom. Presentation at the Association of Educational Communications and Technology Convention, Dallas TX

Harden R M, Laidlaw J M, Ker J S, Mitchell H 1996 Task-based learning: an educational strategy for undergraduate, postgraduate and continuing medical education. AMEE Medical Education Guide no. 7. Medical Teacher 18:7–13

Laidlaw J M, Harden R M 1990 What is...a study guide? Medical Teacher 12:7–12

Mitchell H E, Harden R M, Laidlaw J M 1996 Towards effective on the job learning: the development of a paediatric training guide. Medical Teacher 20:91–98

Montemayor L L E 2002 Twelve tips for the development of electronic study guides. Medical Teacher 24(5):473–478

Parker R C 1997 One-minute designer, revised edn. MIS:Press, New York

Race P, Brown S 1995 500 tips for tutors. Kogan Page, London

Rowntree D 1986 Teaching through self-instruction. Kogan Page, London

Ryan S, Scott B, Freeman H, Patel D 2000 The virtual university – the internet and resource-based learning. Kogan Page, London

Salmon G 2002 Etivities – the key to active online learning. Kogan Page, London

Chapter 22
Virtual learning environments

D. G. Dewhurst, R. H. Ellaway

Introduction

A virtual learning environment (or VLE) is an integrated set of online tools, databases and managed resources that exist as a coherent system, functioning collectively in support of education. VLEs are increasingly common in all areas of higher education, and in medical education in particular. This widespread use of VLEs is a relatively recent phenomenon driven by the ubiquity of computer-based activities in education, the ever-growing pressures for increasing the quantity and quality of educational efficiency and student support, and the technical opportunities provided by increasingly mature web technologies.

How a VLE is used to support education is, of course, down to the local needs and creativity of the academic and support staff who develop and utilise the features and add the information and content. Irrespective of which VLE system is being used, the goal is to provide students and staff with a range of online services and resources which will enhance the quality of the student learning experience and improve the effectiveness and efficiency of teaching and learning.

In a traditional learning environment students normally use resources such as libraries, teaching rooms, study guides, lectures, tutorials, labs, reading lists, etc. They will also use administrative and logistical systems such as registry, assessment, timetables, and clinical placements and they will receive pastoral support, participate in evaluation and will most probably engage with many of the social aspects of university life.

The VLE will often be developed so as to provide many of the characteristics of a traditional learning environment. The balance between the online and the face-to-face is the essence of the 'blend' and is an inherently situated and locally negotiated equilibrium.

A VLE may, for instance, provide learning and teaching resources such as searchable study guides and lecture materials, computer-aided learning (CAL) materials, (streamed) video, discussion boards (both for general communication and for mediating online teaching and learning), and assessment. It may also provide administrative and logistical systems such as student records, student recruitment (even, maybe, online registration and payment of fees), assessment feedback and results, interactive and personalised scheduling and timetabling information and allocation

"Within less than two student generations, communication and information technology (C&IT) has been repositioned as an integral component of the medical school environment"

Ward et al 2001

"VLEs can become a dumping ground for materials not designed to be delivered on-line"

O'Leary 2002

"Rather than being 'instructional systems', VLEs are designed to act as a focus for learning activities which can either be on-line (in the case of distance learners) or integrated holistically with other forms of (more traditional) delivery in the case of on-campus learners"

Stiles 2000

A key decision (whether at an individual or more likely, institutional level) is which VLE(s) to adopt.

The advantage of the purpose-built approach is that the system precisely meets the needs of the course; the main disadvantage is its cost.

"VLEs are 'components in which learners and tutors participate in online interactions of various kinds, including online learning' whereas an MLE covers 'the whole range of information systems and processes of a college (including its VLE if it has one) that contribute directly, or indirectly, to learning and the management of that learning' "

JISC 2001

and grouping support (for instance for arranging clinical placements or course options and electives).

The key feature of the virtual learning environment is that large amounts of the user's participation can be carried out online, being accessible from anywhere in the world, at any time and at the convenience of the individual user.

VLEs, as entities, come in three distinct forms: off-the-shelf, purpose-built and open source.

Off-the-shelf systems include commercial systems, such as WebCT and Blackboard. These systems are not open to easy modification and are usually configured around a generic optional modular course or programme of study and, as such, are most successful when used in this context.

Purpose-built systems are developed specifically to meet local educational contexts. Many institutions may decide to build their own VLE if their course needs are significantly different from those supported by off-the-shelf systems. This has often been the case in medical education (Cook 2001). The advantage of the purpose-built approach is that it ensures that the system precisely meets the needs of the course context in which it will be used, the main disadvantage being the costs associated with development and ongoing support of such a system.

Open source systems are existing systems whose code is openly and freely accessible so that they can be adapted as needed. This is a relatively new approach and the availability, and hence the use, of such systems is not yet widespread.

Managed learning environments

VLEs do not, or at least should not, exist in isolation from other information systems in their local setting. Any institution will most probably also have systems that serve personnel, finance, student records or business conformance purposes. These systems, along with the VLE(s) in an institution can, in principle, be linked to form a 'managed learning environment' (or MLE).

For instance, a VLE could present timetable information which might coordinate with an external room booking system; data for new students might be automatically loaded into a VLE from the institutional student record system, or a VLE's reading lists might provide direct access to library systems to allow users to check whether particular items are currently on the library's shelves. A VLE in this context can act not just as a system in its own right but also as a portal through which other non-VLE services are delivered and contextualised to specific educational settings, often with previously impossible degrees of granularity and focus.

VLE modalities: on-campus courses and distance courses

VLEs usually exist as web-based applications, allowing users to interact with the system over the internet. The use of a VLE can therefore permit its users to continue their participation in a course despite being physically or temporally distant from their host university or college. For instance a VLE can allow students to continue to communicate with each other using discussion or bulletin boards whilst on clinical attachments contact and submit course work to tutors at a distance and organise their patterns of study in ways that suit their personal lifestyle and circumstances.

VLEs can be used in two relatively distinct learning modalities; distance and blended:

Distance mode – in this modality a VLE is used only at a distance from the institution and the VLE is the dominant or only medium through which course activities are transacted. This use of VLEs is often found in continuing professional development (CPD) in medicine and other healthcare disciplines.

Blended mode – here a VLE is used alongside traditional approaches to teaching and learning to enhance the quality of the learning experience for students. Access may be limited to computers on the university's local network, though most commonly students will have full access to support resources over the internet. The blended approach is that most often found in medical education as it is the approach that best suits the complex and diverse range of experiences, processes and competencies that medical education encompasses.

Participant roles in VLEs

There are a number of key participant roles common to all VLEs.

Students

Despite being the main focus in education, the student's role can be surprisingly varied. Some systems 'process' their students while others provide relatively unstructured 'spaces'. Systems are increasingly able to support a personalised student experience and in subjects such as medicine, online problem-based learning and peer–peer activities can create more equable relationships and blur the boundaries between different user groups of a VLE.

Tutors

As the principal organisers and arbiters of the system, tutors will decide on the content and learning activities that are made available and at what point these will become available to their students. Tutors may also moderate online discussions, set assessments and provide feedback to students on their performance.

Administrators

Medical education carries a much higher administrative burden than other subjects in higher education and, this being so, the role of administrator is more prominent in a VLE supporting medical education. The role of the administrator is to manage processes such as student enrolments, assessments and clinical attachments, making sure they are properly structured and recorded.

"Rather than being 'instructional systems', VLEs are designed to act as a focus for learning activities which can either be online (in the case of distance learners) or integrated holistically with other forms of (more traditional) delivery in the case of on-campus learners"

Stiles 2000

"it is ... impossible for VLEs to be pedagogically neutral. Every decision concerning presentation, navigation and design that is imposed by the VLE will impact on mediated learning"

Harris 2001

Technicians

The role of the technician in a VLE context is to ensure the smooth and reliable functioning of its hardware and software components, to develop and extend the system, where and if required, and to deal with the technical infrastructure on which it depends. This will, in the case of a purpose-built system, also encompass system conception and design.

Irrespective of any intrinsic worth a VLE may have, it is often the case that the success of a VLE may depend on the personnel filling these roles and, in particular, on staff and students acting as advocates, facilitators and champions for the VLE and for the course community using it.

Supporting courses with VLEs

The course support that VLEs may provide falls broadly into the following areas.

Access to primary teaching and learning resources

A VLE may provide facilities for online tutorials, exercises and assessments in support of student learning. These may range from the very basic, such as provision of lecture notes, lecture synopses, and support materials such as PowerPoint slides, to highly developed and structured resource databases linked to the basic course information. Thus, lecture synopses can link to additional teaching materials, such as an animation or interactive graph which will better explain a difficult concept, to articles and publications from the evidence base, to self-assessment questions and to computer-aided learning programs covering specific areas of the curriculum. Resources such as video-lectures, PowerPoint slides accompanied by audio commentary, simulations, case- or problem-based learning activities and self-assessment activities, such as multiple choice questions or collaborative activities, can also be made available. The VLE may also be able to track individual student performance in these interactions either to provide feedback to students or to provide student assessment and performance feedback to staff.

Access to secondary learning resources

Reading lists, links to other sites, datasets, and online reference and textbooks can be made available through the VLE, allowing users to gain easy access to such resources in the course of their studies.

Communication

A VLE may provide its users with asynchronous discussion boards and synchronous chat rooms. Asynchronous forms of communication depend on messages being entered into the VLE and stored so that they accrue over time allowing communication to take place without requiring simultaneous use of the system. These can be extremely powerful aids to teaching if tutors initiate, facilitate and monitor discussion topics. Synchronous forms of communication, on the other hand, do depend on simultaneous access to the system as messages are exchanged in real time.

"it is important that VLEs are not and should not be viewed as 'set apart' from the learning environment in which they are deployed. Indeed the very term VLE can be misleading as there is nothing 'virtual' about such a system; when actively used it has to be a very real part of the broader learning environment in which it is deployed"

Ellaway et al 2003

Synchronous and asynchronous discussions are complementary: asynchronous ones may promote a deeper level of discussion, synchronous ones often provide a higher level of social interaction.

A VLE may also provide messaging or even an email service to its users.

Course information

A VLE can provide course information such as study guides, forms, regulations and workbooks. This can add real value to the documents, in that study guides, for example, can be searchable and rendered in a variety of formats. The use of extensible mark-up language (XML) to provide additional semantic structure can significantly extend these kinds of functions.

By making information available online, not only can print costs be transferred to students (an issue in its own right) but the documents are obtainable independently from the event at which they might have otherwise been made physically available. This is particularly advantageous for lecture handouts and slides, which can be made accessible either in advance of, or after a lecture has taken place.

Scheduling information

A VLE can provide timetables, diaries or calendars of scheduled events for both students and staff. These can be amended to reflect changes in such schedules with alerts and details broadcast to the user community, thus providing a single point around which scheduled activities can be coordinated.

Timetables can also be highly personalised so that students see their personal timetable rather than that of the whole class and, if the appropriate tools are available, they can add their own personal entries.

Individualisation and personalisation

A VLE can help to provide a personalised learning experience for students on the course. When a student logs in to a VLE their previously stored annotations, bookmarks and links can be retrieved; even the ability to change how the system looks may be available to them.

Teaching and learning resources, course information and scheduling information can be highly personalised. Thus, students are presented with resources appropriate to the courses they are studying at that time, and to which they have added annotations, and any additional resources they have discovered. They can annotate their timetables, they receive only notices that are relevant to them or their cohort and they have secure access to their assessments.

Online portfolios are increasingly popular with both staff and students. These may either be formally structured around specific activities and assessments, or act as a reflective log of the student's progress and experiences in the course, or both.

Knowledge base audit and quality assurance

Because VLEs can store so much information about a course and its changes over time they can act as a valuable source of information in the support of quality assurance and audit activities. Archives of the VLE for previous years might be stored in perpetuity, providing detailed information on both what was done and how it was done. This is particularly *"learning cannot be designed: it can only be designed for – that is facilitated or frustrated"*

Wenger 1998

Medical education, unlike almost any other subject area, does not just seek to provide the student with the knowledge associated with medicine but it also seeks to imbue the student with the attitudes and outlook of a medical professional. It is taught, to a large extent, by practising members of the medical profession in real-life settings such as hospitals and clinics. Medicine also has its own social practices and meanings and it has distinct and identifiable interactions with other professions. In these ways medicine can be seen as a particularly coherent community of practice.

"VLEs are about process, and in essence are process reified in a software form. As such, ongoing development is inevitable, as the course itself is subject to continual change and evolution. An effective VLE must be extensible and adaptable to meet these changes and certainly it must not be a force counter to effective change"

Ellaway et al 2003

"a VLE system will never be 'finished' as such, so it is important to appreciate that the development and use of a VLE is an ongoing process, not a project, and as such has no 'end' but is an integral part of the course's life cycle as well as one of its main vehicles for learning support"

Ellaway et al 2003

relevant for students who have to resit a course assessment in that they can be given access to the materials and information for the course that they studied rather than a course which may have been modified over time.

Supporting communities of practice

One of the most notable aspects of medicine is its distinct identity as a 'community of practice' – a 'community created over time by the sustained pursuit of a shared enterprise' (Wenger 1998). A VLE can be a powerful tool in supporting a community of practice. It allows all members of a community to participate in a shared enterprise, to develop and reify shared meanings and values, to participate in mutual engagement and joint enterprise, and to rehearse shared repertoire in a closed and focused way. In this way alone, a VLE can provide particular benefits to medical education, above and beyond that afforded to other subject areas and disciplines.

Object orientation and adaptability

VLEs can, at their most powerful, manage all of the resources, processes, users and events at their disposal in an 'object-oriented' fashion, i.e. it should be easy to assemble, or disassemble and then reassemble, these assets in new configurations, depending on how a course changes over time, how different individuals need to view or use these assets, and on how the assets are to be rendered or presented to the user. This is an important property of a VLE, as educational contexts do inevitably change and any particular system configuration will have a limited shelf-life.

The ability to adapt is even more important in the light of the transforming nature of technology use. It is very likely that using a VLE will change what is valued by its users and, by being able to do new or different things, what is done in future iterations of the course. For instance, the ability to engage with a course at a distance can radically change the levels and forms of engagement between students and teaching staff on clinical attachments.

Security, authentication and identity

Access to a VLE will most probably have to be restricted to legitimate participants in a course, and there will also be a need to identify specific users in order to personalise information or access. For instance, a student should be able to see assessment results only after marks have been ratified and clearly should not have access to the assessment results of fellow students. To that end VLEs should be secured against unauthorised access, whether or not it is malicious, by using individual authentication accounts for each and every user of the system.

The use of login names and passwords allows access to a VLE to be separated from controls associated with a local network, allowing users to participate in the course irrespective of time or location. This is particularly useful in medicine where students commonly move through a series of clinical attachments geographically distant from their base university. Any kind of login is only useful as long as it is not disclosed or otherwise compromised in some way. All users should be aware of the importance of keeping logins safe and secure and the accounts of users who leave the course should be automatically suspended or terminated.

The VLE may also use further security and authentication technologies that could, for instance, encrypt traffic sent between the user and the system or allow users to move from one system to another that shares the same authentication mechanism. This latter facility is an important component in expanding a VLE to a multisystem MLE.

Rules, regulations and policing

Although most staff and students will act in normal and cooperative ways in a VLE, there will inevitably be those who do not share the consensus view of what constitutes appropriate behaviour. Although this is easily recognisable in a face-to-face setting where there are most likely to be rules and regulations to deal with transgressors, this may not be the case for VLEs. Regulations must either be adapted to the needs of a VLE or new regulations drawn up.

For instance the use of discussion boards may lead to some inappropriate messages being posted. Some discussion boards are moderated, that is, when a tutor decides which messages are allowed to be posted. However, this might not be possible for a large student population. An alternative is to let the course community decide what constitutes appropriate behaviour. This second approach can more easily accommodate generational and cultural differences between users than a tutor-controlled approach.

Interoperability and sharing

The section on MLEs outlined the possible benefits that VLEs can bring when they are linked with other systems within an institution. Beyond the institution however, there is an ever-growing number of systems, both national and international, that a VLE could usefully link up with. These include resource repositories, subject hubs and brokering services.

In order for these many and diverse systems to work together and share information and resources appropriately, they need to be able to communicate. In recent years there has been much work by groups such as IMS Global, Advanced Distributed Learning (ADL) and the IEEE (Institute of Electrical and Electronic Engineers) to develop interoperability standards and specifications for common protocols and formats for just this purpose.

A VLE that is able to interact with other systems, using these common interoperability standards and specifications, can easily and rapidly exchange learning materials, learner information and even pedagogical designs and strategies.

A common feature that underlies all of this activity is the importance of metadata; i.e. data about resources rather than data as a resource. When materials and information are moved around their context is often lost;

"technological innovation cannot and should not be regarded merely as an improved means to a pre-selected end because while some technology merely modifies, other technology transforms"

Graham 1999

"Standards are still emerging which will allow educators to migrate content from one VLE to another"

O'Leary 2002

"People want to find content easily wherever it might be on the internet, and incorporate it into their courses; learners want to move between institutions taking their learning records with them; and teachers using eLearning systems want to have good information support from administrative systems...interoperability standards are needed that address all of these areas"

CETIS

The development and use of interoperability standards is a key issue for VLEs. A number of groups, including IMS Global and Advanced Distributed Learning (ADL), are developing interoperability standards and specifications which have direct relevance to both developers and users of VLE systems.

"educators need to recognise that learning is a social process and that providing an effective learning environment which facilitates the active acquisition of subject-specific and general expertise, and addresses the need to adopt a specific subject or professional culture, requires more than electronically delivered course notes and email discussion."

Stiles 2000

"despite the buzz about on-line learning and communities, it can be difficult to form suitably close communities to support learning in cyberspace [... but ...] digital technologies are adept at maintaining communities already formed. They are less good at making them. Hence, paradoxically, technologies may do a better job on the conventional campus than on the virtual one"

Brown & Duguid 2000

metadata ensures that contextual information continues to be associated with an entity as it is passed between, possibly quite different, systems. Metadata can itself be interoperable if its language and syntax is commonly shared. To that end there is an increasing need for, and therefore interest in, controlled vocabularies and other closed semantic and ontological structures, both in medical education and beyond. A VLE that can support and help to manage metadata and controlled vocabularies will have a better chance of interoperability with other systems within and beyond the host institution.

The strengths of VLEs in medical education

The strengths of VLEs in medical education are the ability to:

- provide the means for individuals to interact with a course even when geographically or temporally distant from it
- support personalised learning experiences
- better manage the logistics of the learning process
- better manage the administration of the learning process
- support and extend the essence of a community of practice
- support audit and quality assurance and create a course 'knowledge base'
- provide integration with other systems, either within an institution as part of an MLE, or beyond the institution as gateways to repositories and collections of third-party resources.

Problems associated with using VLEs in medical education

Despite the many benefits they can bring, VLEs do not meet the needs of all areas of medical education. The VLE may indeed provide an encompassing and supportive environment for the many participants involved but cannot replace the intrinsically people-focused nature of medicine. A VLE is most effective when it is used in a blended fashion in support of traditional and new face-to-face methodologies. There are potential problems either when a VLE is overused or when it is underused. Finding the balance in the blend therefore is one of the challenges for those working in this area.

On a more practical note it is also important to realise that VLEs can be expensive, in terms both of purchasing or development and of maintenance and support. Information needs to be kept up to date; hardware and software are needed, not just for the VLE but for all those who are going to use it. Staff training and development will be required and technical support and development expertise retained.

Managing the change from a traditional to a virtual learning environment can also have its problems. Some staff may feel left behind, or worse, ostracised, in the new environment. Traditional skills may become redundant while others increase in importance. Students too may feel distanced from tutors unless the blend is well managed and, on a more practical level, the expectation that students must meet the cost of providing their own computers, internet access and printing, places extra and perhaps unintended burdens upon them. An online working environment can support much faster interactions and rates of change and can therefore significantly affect working cultures as well as individuals. This may be for the best, but either way the change to a VLE-based approach needs to be managed with care.

A VLE can also potentially make the course and its participants more exposed. Securing online environments is therefore a serious matter, particularly in the face of ongoing hacking and virus attacks on computer systems. The occurrence of a software 'bug' although trivial to a programmer may be disastrous to an end-user. Furthermore, data protection and freedom of information legislation is increasing the burden of responsibility for the management of information systems in many countries and regions throughout the world.

Finally, a VLE modality is very likely to constitute a tighter coupling between parts and processes within a course than was present in more traditional approaches. A VLE system failure may therefore have larger, possibly catastrophic, ramifications and affect a wider range of course subsystems than would previously have been the case.

Evaluating VLEs

The evaluation of VLEs has, to date, mostly focused on supporting the selection and procurement of VLE systems for first-time users. However, as the use of VLEs becomes increasingly widespread, and expertise and experience in using them develops, new evaluation techniques are emerging.

Since VLEs encompass so many aspects of the learning environment it is increasingly clear that traditional evaluation techniques are of limited value. For instance, if the focus of an evaluation is solely on the pedagogical efficacy of a VLE then it will inevitably disregard the many other ways that a VLE can help (or hinder) a course, a tutor or a learner. It is therefore important to consider using more holistic techniques that encompass the multifactorial nature of a VLE's interaction with its host course environment.

It is important to distinguish between the VLE-in-abstract from the VLE-in-use. A VLE-in-abstract is the VLE as a software system separated from any specific context of use. Evaluations in these circumstances tend to record or measure the presence of tools and functions, or at best test whether a VLE has the potential to support different educational contexts. An evaluation of a VLE-in-use on the other hand concentrates on how a system is actually being used in a specific context. The same system might be expected to be used differently in different course contexts and, conversely, a course may use different systems in different ways.

Summary

Virtual learning environments are increasingly becoming the norm in medical education. Generic off-the-shelf VLE systems may be purchased,

The VLE-in-abstract (the software system) should be distinguished from the VLE-in-use.

or bespoke systems may be developed from scratch or adapted from other situations. They may be used at a distance from the host institution or most commonly (and effectively) to support on-campus courses as part of a blended approach to teaching and learning.

VLEs can therefore be both a primary medium for the delivery of teaching and perform a scaffolding function in support of face-to-face learning. They can also be used to facilitate communication (both asynchronously and synchronously), provide course information and resources, and manage and provide scheduling information. They can be used to track user activities, in support of both student and staff activities. They can be used to manage learners and tutors, the events and processes they are involved in and the resources they use in support of their activities.

A VLE may also provide unprecedented levels of individualisation and personalisation to its users by supporting user-specific functions such as annotations or portfolios. It may also provide access to secondary learning resources and other information systems, both within the institution and beyond, and act as a commonly available course knowledge base.

However, VLEs are not going to solve all the ills of a course environment. They need significant levels of resources in terms of finance and manpower, they need to be secured against attack and misadventure and their introduction and use raises significant issues of change management for all concerned.

"an electronic learning environment is a social system focused on the permanent development and certification of human knowledge and competencies in a specific domain, in which the subsystems can occur distributed in time and place, and in which ICT ensures integration, representation, personalisation, cooperation and process management"

Koper 2000

References

ADL (Advanced Distributed Learning) Online. www.adlnet.org

Brown J S, Duguid P 2000 The social life of information. Harvard Business School Press, Watertown MA

CETIS (Centre for Educational Technology Interoperability Standards) Online. http://www.cetis.ac.uk/static/standards.html

Cook J 2001 JTAP 623 – The role of virtual learning environments in UK medical education. Institute for Learning and Research Technology. Online: Available at http://www.ltss.bris.ac.uk/jules/jtap-623.pdf

Ellaway R H, Dewhurst D, Cumming A 2003 Managing and supporting medical education with a virtual learning environment: the Edinburgh Electronic Medical Curriculum. Medical Teacher 25:372–380

Graham G 1999 The Internet:a philosophical enquiry. Routledge, London

Harris N 2001 Managed learning. ARIADNE, issue 30. Online. Available: http://www.ariadne.ac.uk/issue30/angel/intro.html

IMS Global Learning Consortium. Online. www.imsglobal.org

JISC 2001 Managed learning environments programme pack. Joint Information Systems Committee, UK

Koper R 2000 From change to renewal: educational technology foundations of electronic learning environments. Open University of the Netherlands, Netherlands

O'Leary R 2002 Virtual learning environments. LTSN Generic Centre Resources Database ELN002:1–5

Stiles M 2000 Effective learning and the virtual learning environment. Proceedings: EUNIS 2000 – Towards virtual universities, IIPP, Poznan, Poland. Online. Available: http://www.staffs.ac.uk/COSE/cose10/posnan.html

Ward J P T, Gordon J, Field M J, Lehmann H P 2001 Communication and information technology in medical education. The Lancet 357:792–796

Wenger E 1998 Communities of practice. Cambridge University Press, New York

Further reading

Schön D A 1987 Educating the reflective practitioner. Jossey-Bass, USA

Chapter 23
Simulators and simulation-based medical education

A. Ziv

Introduction

Medical simulators are educational tools that fall into the broad context of simulation-based medical education (SBME). SBME in its widest sense should be defined as any educational activity that utilises simulative aids in order to enable medical educators to enhance the educational message by simulating the clinical scenario. Simulation devices serve as an alternative to the real patient and permit educators to gain full control of a pre-selected clinical scene without the risk of distressing patients or encountering other harmful aspects of learning on real patients. It must be stressed that SMBE is not an alternative to bedside teaching but rather a valuable, complementary addition.

This chapter will describe the simulation modalities that are presently available for medical education and discuss the driving forces of SBME and the rationale behind the utilisation of simulators in medical education. Furthermore, it will review the different applications of SBME and the various educational environments and delivery models of SBME. The chapter will conclude with a discussion of the challenges the field presents to medical teachers.

SBME modalities

SBME consists of two main families, low-tech and high-tech simulation modalities.

Low-tech simulation modalities
These are characterised by tools which are not computer-driven and serve as models for various educational purposes. This family represents traditional simulation tools that have been in use in medical education for many years.

Simple three dimensional organ models
Heart and lung models, for example, serve educators in anatomy classes.

Basic plastic manikin and simple skills trainers
A wide variety of simple skills trainers and manikins are available for learning life-saving manoeuvres such as basic and advanced life support

☞ Simulation-based medical education is complementary to traditional medical education.

☞ Simulation modalities are categorised as low-tech or high-tech.

☞ Use low-tech simulation models for basic clinical skills training.

(BLS and ALS). These include dummies (e.g. 'Ressusi Anni') which enable simulation of BLS procedures, and more advanced models for endotracheal intubation, defibrillation and more.

Simple simulators are also available for teaching intimate (and embarrassing) physical examination manoeuvres (such as rectal, vaginal and breast examinations) and for several invasive and noninvasive clinical procedures, such as delivery, wound suturing, insertion of bladder catheters or vascular lines, etc.

Animal models

These may be either live models or isolated animal organ models. For example, live animals are utilised in physiology classes or in advanced trauma life support (ATLS) procedural training in tracheostomy and chest tube insertion. Isolated animal gut may be utilised for surgical training in procedures such as bowel anastomoses.

Human cadavers

These are the most realistic simulation of the human body, although without live response, physiology and pathology. Cadavers mostly serve in anatomy and pathology classes.

Simulated or standardised patients

These individuals represent the ultimate alternative to live patients. They may be volunteers or actors who are trained in standardised role-play of different psychological and physiological aspects of patients, for the purpose of structured training and assessment of clinical skills such as history taking, physical examination and communication (see chapter 8).

High-tech simulation modalities

Such modalities are characterised by models operated by computers, utilising advanced hardware and software technologies to enhance the realism of the simulation experience and to increase the anatomical and physiological validity of the training tools.

Screen-based simulators

These are computer-based software based on the personal computer (PC); these simulators reflect sophisticated advances in technology and the software includes multimedia and virtual reality components. Screen-based software is readily available today in almost any clinical or basic science domain in medicine and plays a central role in medical education. The screen-based simulators range from simple noninteractive computer programs to advanced fully interactive teaching medical software. These programs enhance cognitive knowledge, clinical reasoning and decision making.

An example of such simulation application is the field of anatomy, where many medical schools have replaced cadaver-based anatomy classes (traditional simulation) with advanced screen-based simulation software. Another example of clinical application of screen-based simulation is the comprehensive multimedia curriculum in cardiology that integrates auditory and visual clues in order to simulate a comprehensive program for medical students.

Standardised patients serve as the ultimate simulation modality for communication skills education.

High-tech simulators are computer-driven advanced hardware and software.

Ensure that screen-based simulation programs are accessible for students as self-tutorials.

Realistic, high-fidelity procedural simulators (task trainers)

A new generation of state-of-the art computer-driven realistic simulation devices has expanded the armamentarium of tasks and procedures that can be applied for education, training, assessment and research. These tools, mounted on powerful software, invest static models with advanced audio-visual and tactile interactive cues and create a simulated 'cockpit' for procedural and diagnostic tasks in multiple clinical domains such as radiology (ultrasound simulator), clinical cardiology (auscultation simulator) and invasive cardiology (catheterisation or pacemaker insertion simulators). Also available are endoscopy simulators in the fields of gastroenterology urology, pulmonology, gynaecology, ENT, orthopaedics, and so on, as well as several minimally invasive surgery simulators for procedures such as cholecystectomy, hernia repair, arthroscopic surgery, etc.

Important common features that characterise this family of simulators include the following.

- Advanced endoscopic and surgical training simulators offer learning experiences in a near-authentic environment, catering for all levels of training from the novice to the expert.
- An extensive library covering a broad spectrum of diseases and scenarios is available online.
- Post-procedure debriefing and performance assessment are valuable additions to the inherent learning process.

Realistic high-fidelity task trainers are best utilised for residents' training in minimally invasive procedures.

Realistic high-tech interactive patient simulators

Computerised, realistic patient simulators (RPSs) were first introduced in 1966 by Abrahamson for anaesthesia training. Two decades later Gaba and Gravenstein independently led the way in the development of RPSs as we know them today.

RPSs are advanced in the number and detail of their features and in the wide range of programs and trainee types they support. Common features include a realistic, full-size manikin, a computer workstation, and interface devices that actuate manikin signs and drive actual monitors.

RPSs have eyes responsive to light, an anatomically correct, dynamic airway, patient voice, arm movement, heart and breath sounds, and exhalation of carbon dioxide. Additional features include chest-tube insertion capacity, monitoring of neuromuscular transmission and provision of dynamic physical cues mimicking extremity compartment syndrome. Physiological computer models of ventilation, gas exchange, and cardiopulmonary function react, like patients, to drugs and fluids. RPSs may be controlled via direct or wireless means, as well as 'at the bedside'. Patients can be 'designed' on the computer interface using many variables such as weight, blood volume, and indices of heart function.

Lifelike, realistic, hi-tech patient simulators simulate multiple clinical conditions and situations that are fully designed and controlled by the medical educator.

RPSs have been installed in a variety of flexibly staged, low- to high-fidelity immersive clinical environments (emergency room, intensive care unit, office-based setting, operating room) limited only by imagination, resources and training objectives.

To enable team simulations, RPSs have been integrated with standardised patients, simple simulator tools, and complex task trainers to create actual environmental microsystems.

Applications of realistic patient simulators (RPSs) are varied and include individual and team training as well as integration with other simulative methods.

Define the aim of the simulation experience.

Virtual reality (VR) has been defined as 'a system that enables one or more users to move and react in a computer-simulated environment' (Encarta Online Encyclopedia 2000).

Medical teachers should adopt SBME as an educational approach contributing to patient safety.

The aim is to accustom trainees to cope with ambiguity, time pressure, changing workload, interpersonal issues, and to foster adaptability in problem solving. Myriad RPSs have gone into use worldwide since their inception in 1994.

Virtual reality (VR)

The trend in VR is for maturing technologies to be first combined in hybrid approaches with simulation methods, moving to completely digitally represented worlds. The Virtual Human Project (Oak Ridge National Laboratory) is expected to create the human simulation environment of the 21st century – an integrated system of biological and biophysical models, data and computational algorithms, supported by advanced computational platforms.

The progress in VR technology models will eventually enable the creation of 'customised simulation environments' where medical data (derived from MRI or from other imaging modalities) from a particular patient could be downloaded into VR simulation platforms, so that physicians could practise on the virtual patient before actually operating on the real one. Such simulation is expected to have both clinical and educational applications that will radically change the face of medical training.

Driving forces of medical simulation

SBME is now recognised as an increasingly powerful complementary teaching methodology in the medical profession. It is driven by a combination of the following forces:

- *The patient safety movement* – is the most powerful driving force behind the demand to find means that will increase the competence of health professionals and reduce the grave phenomena of medical errors.
- *Objective structured clinical examinations (OSCEs)* are a development that have been strongly endorsed by accreditation bodies and professional boards worldwide. Many of these bodies have already introduced simulated-patient based exams into their formal certification requirements, recognising the unique advantages of simulated environments for evaluation purposes.
- *Patient rights movements and patient ethics issues* have contributed to the growing recognition that medical education should optimise the use of simulation-based education prior to jeopardising patients or even discomfiting them.
- *Animal rights movements* have a stronger voice these days as they demand lesser use of animals for procedural training purposes. The American College of Surgeons (ACS) has recently acquiesced to certain of these demands.
- *Risk management and the medicolegal atmosphere* demand accountability and high safety and quality standards even in a training environment.
- *Economic forces* reduce patient accessibility and decrease the training opportunities in traditional medical education.

- *The simulation industry* is responding to the growing demand for incorporating new technologies and providing educators with more (virtually) realistic, high-fidelity training devices than before.

Benefits and rationale of medical simulation

The rationale for incorporating simulation into medical education lies on solid educational and social grounds:

- Medical simulation is a safe environment where trainees can learn from their errors without the risk of harming a real patient. The very notion that SBME is 'mistake-forgiving' provides educators with a unique opportunity to take advantage of the fact that such mistakes have the potential to be very powerful educational tools in saving human lives.
- Simulation offers a trainee-centred environment that can provide full attention to his or her individual needs, pace, strengths and deficiencies. It enables controlled, proactive clinical exposure of trainees to gradually more complex clinical challenges, including the more uncommon, life-threatening 'nightmare' scenarios.
- Simulation is a 'hands-on' (experiential learning) educational modality, acknowledged by adult learning theories to be more effective.
- Simulation provides unique opportunities for team training; this is seldom addressed in traditional medical education, and lack of such training is increasingly recognised as a major factor in system errors and safety failures in medicine.
- SBME provides a reproducible, standardised, objective setting for both formative assessment, that includes debriefing and feedback, and summative assessment, via testing.
- Simulation provides a unique opportunity to expose trainees to the concept and experience of debriefing – an inherent component in every SBME program; an important value message to convey to all trainees is that debriefing should become a norm in everyday medical practice.
- SBME can assist in increasing public trust in a medical profession that has been increasingly accused in recent years of being weak and deficient in its safety practices and culture.

SBME applications

SBME by its very nature is suited for multiple educational applications with almost unlimited potential as computer knowhow expands.

- Most experiences involve 'hands-on' skill training that can be basic or advanced and serve for clinical training or as a means to enhance cognitive knowledge.
- SBME is destined to serve as a superior continuing medical education (CME) platform, which will provide experienced health professionals with an opportunity to be introduced to new devices and clinical

Errors and mistakes are great teaching opportunities; SBME is the art of learning from mistakes in a safe environment.

Use simulation as a way of exposing trainees to life-threatening 'nightmare' scenarios.

Use simulation for team training.

Simulation introduces new assessment methods.

Use simulation as a means to teach trainees the art of debriefing.

Integrate simulation into continuing medical education courses.

procedures or hone their skills, in today's rapidly changing medical and technological environment.

- Simulation allows for focused exploration of areas of deficiencies in competencies and skills of health professionals, as well as providing a powerful interventional tool to enhance skills of those identified as needing such training.
- SBME can be set up to introduce medical devices and technologies to the health profession in a structured and safe manner.
- Patient safety applications focus on error reduction and may include teamwork and system training, quality assurance and risk management models and issues regarding malpractice insurance.
- SBME provides the medical industry with an opportunity for safe and valid research and development where human factors and the human–machine interface can be explored.
- The ultimate application for SBME may relate to licensing and certification; when this is endorsed as a standard for medical education, it will signal maturity of the health profession and its acknowledgement of a safety culture as appropriate to the high-risk and high-stakes medical field.

Simulation-based teaching environments

Simulative teaching can take place in a broad range of set ups, ranging from traditional classrooms, clinical departments and home PCs to ultra-advanced multimodality/multidisciplinary medical simulation centres. The multimodality and multi-application nature of simulation-based training challenges medical educators to select the appropriate simulation modality and the optimal environment for each educational task.

Traditional environments
Classrooms can host SBME as part of a clinical demonstration, utilising a task-oriented simulator or a simulated patient. Similarly, simulators can be placed within clinical departments where they are accessible to residents and students who may practise different clinical tasks in their own free time, or at fixed times.

Clinical skills laboratories
These have evolved as a common site of simulation-based training. They differ from the more comprehensive multimodality, multidisciplinary model in that they usually focus on a single simulation modality and serve a single profession or a narrow professional branch. Although these centres seldom gain an extensive expertise in the full range of simulation modalities, they achieve an in-depth expertise in their specific educational field.

Multimodality/multidisciplinary medical simulation centre
This new paradigm of simulation centres is based on unique multidisciplinary and interdisciplinary principles. The centre serves all branches of the medical profession (horizontal integration) and is capable of providing

Involve patient safety and human factors experts in simulation-based team training and simulation-based interventions aimed at error reduction.

Simulation-based training can take place in a wide range of teaching environments. Adjust the appropriate simulation modality to your educational goals.

Consider which simulated experiences can be introduced into traditional environments.

In clinical skills laboratories, strive for in-depth expertise in your specific educational field.

Direct simulation activities to all medical professionals, at different stages of their training and careers.

superior cross-professional training (teamwork). Furthermore a centre of this kind incorporates simulation-based education at all training levels (vertical integration), from undergraduate studies, through residency training and into CME levels.

The centre simulates multiple clinical environments, utilising a variety of simulation modalities, depending on the features of the experiences required. Simulated emergency rooms and operating rooms with sophisticated manikins, and clinics with standardised patients are examples of near-authentic environments. These simulated environments mostly serve in scenario-based training and entail extensive pre-scheduling of logistical and educational support.

This model, the ultimate platform for SBME, if initiated and implemented in a centralised (regional, or national) manner is envisioned to have great potential to induce change in the training and safety culture, while improving cost-effectiveness and utilisation rate. A centre of this kind is functioning with great success in Israel as a National Medical Simulation Center and fulfilling its potential.

Unique challenges and strategies related to SBME

SBME presents challenges for medical educators on many fronts.

Medical and safety culture

Overcoming resistance to change
Medicine is a conservative field that has been based for generations on apprentice methods. When the culture of training is changed by the introduction of proactive SBME, resistance from both conservative educators and trainees is encountered.

Creating a constructive atmosphere
For trainees to appreciate the advantage of learning by means of and from mistakes, it is essential to create an environment that will feel safe, and to carefully plan experiences that will be constructive. A well-designed curriculum should convey and stress the importance of patient safety and error reduction.

Educational

Recognising limitations of SBME
Teachers need to be fully aware of the limits of SBME and that it is complementary to hands-on training on real patients.

Selective use
One of the most challenging demands upon medical educators is to match the appropriate simulation modality to the correct educational goal for a specific target population.

Simulators should be used selectively, with attention paid to cost-effectiveness. Many important procedures for beginners may be learnt using simple inexpensive manikins, whereas experts often need high-cost cutting-edge equipment.

Adjust simulation modalities to the features of the required experience.

Consider the great potential of centralised centres.

Convey messages regarding patient safety and error reduction in a constructive manner.

Select simulation modalities best suited for the educational goal and target population.

Combine simulation modalities to increase effectiveness.

Trainers' courses should develop educators' expertise in multiple relevant domains.

Debriefing is central in SBME.

Developing and applying innovative testing and evaluation tools will raise medical education standards.

Empirical evidence is needed regarding the effectiveness of SBME.

Valid performance measures are essential for assessment.

Combine simulation modalities

Medical educators should strive to develop expertise in multisimulation scenarios and combine simulation modalities to enhance the realism and effectiveness of the training experience.

Incorporating SBME into the formal curriculum

A crucial aspect of the acceptance of SBME as a legitimate and valuable teaching tool is the incorporation of SBME programmes into health professional schools and CME curricula.

Faculty development

Train the trainer

SBME faculty should be trained as SBME trainers and raters, through instructors' courses and raters' workshops, as a prerequisite to their participation in SBME programmes. They should develop expertise in testing and evaluation of clinical competencies, performances and human characteristics.

Debriefing

As debriefing is a key element in SBME, faculty should also gain expertise in audiovisually based transparent debriefing. Teachers should also convey the value message of debriefing as a take-home skill for the trainees to be implemented in real-life practice.

Expertise in testing and evaluation

It is essential that educators using SBME gain basic knowledge and understanding in assessment principles and methods, both formative and summative. Furthermore, it is important for medical educators to join forces with national and international psychometric bodies in order to increase their understanding of the assessment domain, jointly develop new assessment tools and ultimately enhance educators' power to penetrate the certification field (in the spirit of 'assessment drives education').

Research and development

SBME is a rich environment for research in medical education and assessment.

Validation

Teachers of SBME are challenged to provide evidence beyond face value of its effectiveness, in the spirit of the BEME initiative (Best Evidence Medical Education), by pursuing studies that will explore validity aspects, such as the predictive values and transferability and sustainability of skills acquired through SBME.

Performance measures

Educators need to develop and validate measures of performance of health professionals as the key for meaningful formative and summative assessment. New sets of skills must be developed, taught and then tested in parallel with the inevitable expansion of SBME.

Curriculum-driven research and development

Medical educators should take the lead in driving the simulation industry to meet curricular needs, rather than vice versa.

Delivery models of SBME

Cost-effectiveness and educational justifications are major driving forces behind the emerging multidisciplinary/multimodality training centre model. These revolutionary facilities raise a few more considerations.

Multidisciplinary educational and support staff

These are a basic requirement of an effective SBME environment. Dedicated, multidisciplinary staff with educational and clinical expertise across a wide spectrum of health professions, as well as experts in human behaviour, performance measurement and curriculum development, must be thoughtfully recruited. In addition, support staff with expertise in logistics, audiovisual and simulation technology, biomedical engineering, business development, accounting and so on must be mobilised.

Sustainable business model

The high visible short-term costs of simulators and simulation centres, as well as the heavy dependency on educational and support staff, demand that medical educators create a sustainable business model for SBME. Furthermore, evidence must be presented to confirm SBME's significant long-term cost benefits, including safety outcomes in terms of patient mortality and morbidity and medicolegal consequences.

Endorsement by regulators

Medical educators should involve regulators at different levels and in the early stages of SBME programmes, aiming towards eventual acceptance of this modality as a routine and obligatory component of medical education and certification.

Summary

SBME is gaining a central role in medical education, a trend that is expected to expand as social, educational, regulatory and technological changes proceed.

Ongoing technological progress in the simulation and virtual reality industries continuously allows for new cutting-edge simulators to become available, with higher fidelity and at lower cost. Customised simulation models will enable health professionals to practise on simulators tailored to data from individual patients. The delivery models of SBME will refine and emphasise the more cost-effective models such as those serving multidisciplinary/multimodality regional centres.

SBME will become an integral part of the medical curriculum, across all medical professions and throughout medical careers. It will be incorporated as the leading standardised performance assessment method of health professionals' competencies. Regulators at all levels will endorse SBME as an integral part of individual and institutional certification,

Prepare a comprehensive SBME business plan.

licensing and malpractice insurance. Finally, safety, ethical and social considerations will continue to force a major culture change in the way medicine is taught and practised. As this process is irreversible and just, medical educators must endorse it proactively rather than react to external forces.

Further reading

Gaba D M, Howard S K, Flanagan B et al 1998 Assessment of clinical performance during simulated crises using both technical and behavioral ratings. Anesthesiology 89:1–2

Gordon J A, Oriol N E, Cooper J B 2004 Bringing good teaching cases 'to life': a simulator-based medical education service. Academic Medicine 79:23–27

Issenberg S B, McGaghie W C, Hart I R et al 1999 Simulation technology for health care professional skills training and assessment. JAMA 28:861–866

Kneebone R 2003 Simulation in surgical training: educational issues and practical implications. Medical Education 37:267–277

Kohn L, Corrigan J, Donaldson M (eds) 1999 To err is human – building a safer health system. Institute of Medicine–National Academy Press, Washington, DC

Maran N J, Glavin R J 2003 Low- to high-fidelity simulation – a continuum of medical education? Medical Education 37(Suppl 1):22–28

Satava R 2001 Surgical education and surgical simulation. World Journal of Surgery 25:1484–1489

Ziv A, Berkenstadt H 2004 Multidisciplinary, multimodality medical simulation center – the Israeli model. In: Dunn W (ed.) Simulators in critical care medicine and beyond. Society for Critical Care Medicine (SCCM), Chicago

Ziv A, Small S, Wolpe P 2000 Patient safety and simulation-based medical education. Medical Teacher 22:489–495

Ziv A, Wolpe P, Small S, Glick S 2003 Simulation-based medical education – an ethical imperative. Academic Medicine, 78:783–788

Useful links

BEME Collaboration. Issenberg S B, Gordon M S, Gordon D L et al. Systematic review of high fidelity simulation in medical education. Best Evidence Medical Education. Available: http://www.bemecollaboration.org/topics.htm

Oak Ridge National Laboratory. Virtual human project. Available: http://www.ornl.gov/sci/virtualhuman/

Chapter 24
E-learning

D. Davies

Introduction

For many readers e-learning will have become in recent years part of their remit as a medical teacher. They will be addressing issues such as the integration of e-learning into their teaching and learning programme to help students achieve the expected e-learning outcomes, the sourcing of resources to allow them implement e-learning and the development of e-learning content of an appropriate quality. Other readers will have yet to explore the possibilities offered by e-learning. Whatever the reader's personal position on the subject, however, there is no doubt that e-learning is a subject that is attracting increasing attention and recognition.

In the past few years there have been scores of books written on the topic and an increasing number of academic journals devoted to the subject. Of the 900 or so papers submitted for the AMEE 2004 conference, organised by the Association for Medical Education in Europe, almost 20% were on e-learning. This represents a dramatic increase from about 4% only a few years ago. A policy discussion paper from the Australian Government (1997) suggested that:

> The traditional view that higher education services are best provided on a campus, to a student body resident nearby, via a narrow set of delivery methodologies...will come under increasing scrutiny.

This chapter defines e-learning, identifies some of the associated myths and highlights the issues that are likely to become increasingly important in the successful use of e-learning in medical education.

What is e-learning?

The term e-learning describes the use of the new electronic technologies including the internet to facilitate learning. It includes

- the online delivery of course content
- discussion forums
- online tutoring or mentoring
- bulletin boards
- synchronous communication and instant chat
- online assessment
- offline resources such as CDs and DVDs.

"The spread of the Internet and new information and communication technologies (ICT) has transformed the way people communicate, the way industries operate, the way government interact with their citizens, and, significantly, the way people learn"

European Commission 2003

"I skate to where the puck is going to be, not where it has been"

Wayne Gretzky

"E-learning includes both content (that is information) and instructional methods (that is technology) that help people learn the content"

Clark & Mayer 2003

"Arguably the most important consequence of the new digital media for higher education is that they make major innovations in education possible"

Farrington 1999

"The reality is that technology is playing, and will continue to play, a critical role in teaching and learning"

Phipps & Merisotis 1999

E-learning is not just about informing goals, it is also about performing goals.

It should be emphasised that the use of information and communication technology (ICT) is not itself the goal of e-learning. For e-learning, ICT has to be an integral part of the overall educational approach, so-called blended learning.

In many ways the educational principles underpinning e-learning are no different from the principles underpinning learning more generally. What is new is the powerful synergy that exists in e-learning between education and technology. This has the potential of achieving educational aims which, in the past, one could only dream about. The potential of the new learning technologies to impact on education is almost without limits. Visions which e-learning can make possible include

- the adaptive curriculum where learning is customised or personalised to the needs of the individual student
- learning made available at the optimal time and place for the learner
- access by learners to teachers and resources not only from their own school or institution but from experts and the best institutions worldwide
- learners, as part of a community of learning, working together more closely and more meaningfully than is possible even with groups of students in traditional problem-based learning
- access to interactive content not possible with any other medium
- learning through simulations, the ability to rehearse complex real-world scenarios and procedures in a risk-free environment.

Myths about e-learning

There are a number of myths about e-learning (Harden 2002).

- 'E-learning is just a passing fad.'
  Not true: e-learning is establishing itself as a mainstream approach to education.
- 'E-learning is only about knowledge transfer.'
  Not true. E-learning can address the range of learning outcomes including those relating to clinical skills, communication skills, decision making, ethical issues and the personal development of the individual and their role in healthcare.
- 'Online learning is ineffective and inefficient.'
  Not true. There is abundant evidence now that e-learning represents a powerful and effective tool for learning.
- 'The isolation of the student prevents serious learning.'
  Not true. Increased attention is being paid in e-learning to the value of communities for learning and peer-to-peer learning.
- 'Teachers will become redundant.'
  Not true. There is a need for teachers as learning facilitators, information providers, assessors, curriculum developers, role models and resource developers. All these roles, however, are unlikely to be encapsulated in the same individual. As suggested by Sloman (2001) 'Three distinct functional specialisms for trainers will evolve: design, delivery and learner support.'

- 'Technology is king.'
  Not true. An appropriate educational strategy is essential, with collaboration between content experts, educators and technologists.
- 'E-learning is an unrealistic dream.'
  Not true. Today there is no doubt that e-learning is not some sort of disguised science fiction. It is fact. It is not a dream, it is a reality. 'Adopting new approaches to the provision of education and training, including the utilisation of new learning technologies' suggested Inglis and colleagues (2002) 'is not an option – it is an imperative.'

Content development

E-learning brings with it new approaches to content development. Highlighted below are some of the emerging trends.

Reusable learning objects

One of the most important aspects of e-learning is the development of new approaches to instructional design incorporating 'reusable learning objects' (RLOs). These are small discrete chunks of learning resources and may range from a single diagram or illustration to a sequence or aggregation of such resources including a learning context, such as learning outcomes or teacher commentary. To create a course, RLOs can be linked or aggregated together in the same way as small pieces of Lego can be assembled to create a structure such as a castle. As with Lego blocks, the same RLOs can be reused to create other courses.

This approach to instructional design has been adopted in the International Virtual Medical School (IVIMEDS) a collaboration of 37 member institutions worldwide (Harden & Hart 2002). The use of RLOs facilitates the flexible and easy retrieval, customisation, refiguration and re-use of learning materials and the sharing of existing high quality learning and teaching.

The semantic web

The semantic web is a vision for the future development of the internet where web-based materials, including e-learning resources, can be automatically linked together or associated in some way as a result of their context. This context is provided by not only the content of the resource itself but also by data that describes that content, so-called metadata. In a learning scenario, a student browsing a web page describing the electrical activity of the heart could easily find images of the relevant heart anatomy regardless of whether the teacher had explicitly created these links. Researchers round the world are now working to implement such technologies.

Semantic web technologies will allow more intelligent searching of the web and allow students to more effectively retrieve and share relevant information from the web. It will also facilitate online collaborative learning between students who are geographically and culturally separate and will allow students to share learning experiences more efficiently and effectively.

"There is a danger of becoming seduced by the functionality of the technology, rather than concentrating on its use"

Sloman 2001

"The instructional technology called learning objects currently leads other candidates as the technology of choice for the next generation of instructional design, development and delivery"

Wiley 2002

Similarly, teachers creating web resources to support student learning can locate material from across the internet to rapidly create customised e-learning materials to meet local curriculum needs.

Open content, traditional publishing and intellectual property rights

Academic institutions, professional bodies, individuals and publishing companies are all actively involved in the creation of e-learning resources. This raises problems relating to intellectual property rights (IPR) and business models for digital rights management (DRM), which have not yet been resolved. The future e-learning marketplace will almost certainly see a mixed economy of pay-per-use, fee-based courses and free-access materials.

New approaches to e-learning

We are now far removed from the concept of the computer as a mechanical page-turner with the transmission of knowledge as the aim. Three potentially valuable instructional methods associated with e-learning (Clark & Mayer 2003) are

- practice with automated personalised feedback
- integration of collaboration and peer-to-peer learning with self-study
- use of simulation to accelerate expertise.

The development of new strategies and a better understanding of what works in e-learning will help to identify the most useful educational approaches suited to different learning contexts.

Issues of accessibility and inclusion

E-learning, because of its characteristics of accessibility, affordability, adaptability, reusability, durability and interoperability can be seen as a positive response to the pressure for widening participation in learning including home learners, disability and accessibility to learning materials.

Institutions need to establish technology-enabled 'joined-up learning' to meet the needs of a continuum which includes lifelong learning, support for alumni, continuing professional development, shared e-learning with schools and colleges as well as higher education and workplace learning.

An e-learning marketplace

There are local, national and international marketplaces for e-learning resources. 'With greater interaction between physicians of many countries, the concept of a global profession of medicine with its core values and specialised knowledge and skills comes into sharp focus' suggested Schwarz (2001). When individuals within an institution create e-learning materials, they automatically add to the accumulating e-learning materials available at that institution and, if viewed as a commodity, to trade with other institutions, to a wide marketplace. This is facilitated by collaborations such as the IVIMEDS.

"What can be done in a Web-based learning environment is limited only by the imagination of the designer and the available resources. For the most part the range of possibilities is almost endless"

Jolliffe et al 2001

"An educational free market will emerge. As e-learning and e-commerce get together, a global free market will develop. Suppliers with highly effective courses and other knowledge products will thrive"

Horton 2001

Technology-mediated assessment

New approaches to assessment are possible with e-learning, which include learner profiling, more sophisticated forms of questions and encouragement for the learner to take more responsibility for assessing their own competence. Increasing use will be made of electronic portfolios for assessment and other purposes, developing in the student higher-order competencies and reflective thinking.

Managing e-learning

A number of issues relating to the management of e-learning are likely to be increasingly important if e-learning is to be successfully adopted in medical education.

Effective change management to allay fears about new technologies and to incorporate e-learning into mainstream teaching and learning

The transition to e-learning models for learning activities and course delivery requires an effective change strategy. There is a need to establish an appropriate learning culture, to find and leverage champions, to recognise, reward and disseminate best practice and to create sound communications about the developments (Rosenberg 2001).

It is essential that teachers and students have the skills and knowledge to successfully engage in e-learning initiatives. The development of new skills on the part of both teacher and learner is a key part of developing successful e-learning.

Providing timely and relevant training should be part of an effective change-management strategy. This will become easier as more experience is gained with e-learning and the results of research into the cost–benefit and effectiveness of e-learning become available. Learners will need to develop the high-level critical appraisal skills that are necessary to navigate the increasingly complex range of e-learning materials and courses on offer.

Finally, it is important to ensure that adequate resources are available to support e-learning both in the short and long term.

The development of a strategy for blended learning, identifying the role of different teaching methods

The buzzword of the moment is blended e-learning. This seeks to recognise that e-learning alone is not going to lead to successful learning. Finding the place of e-learning alongside more traditional forms of learning opportunities is likely to generate the most success. In this process there will be an increasing convergence between e-learning and traditional learning.

Managing the convergence of content management, virtual learning environments and knowledge management system

At the level of the institution, decisions need to be made about the technical aspects of e-learning including systems interoperability, and the shift to new ways of delivering functionality including component-based archi-

"The people who define and constitute institutions are caught up in a transition between eras that can lead to widespread confusion, alienation, anger and, in some cases, apathy. It can also have the effect of excitement and challenge, sparking creativity and the development of approaches and strategies"

Inglis et al 2002

The readiness of an institution to accept e-learning and the reasons why some individuals may be resistant to the approach needs to be identified and understood.

"If you are going to introduce e-learning be sure that the technology is adequate to make the experience worthwhile rather than painful"

Rosenberg 2001

tecture and web services. Decisions about investment in commercial or open-source systems will need to be taken. It will be important to avoid technology 'lock-in' as e-learning vendors develop proprietary solutions. A central issue will be the portability of learning materials from one system to another when the institution upgrades systems. Virtual learning environments are discussed further in chapter 22.

Development of an antiplagiarism strategy

Attention has been drawn in education in recent years to problems of cheating and plagiarism. The development of an antiplagiarism strategy is important as e-learning becomes more prevalent. This involves a clear institutional policy on the topic, which has been agreed with students in the institution. Software is now available which can be used to detect plagiarism of web-based materials.

Quality control of e-learning

Increasing attention will be paid to the quality of e-learning. The process will include review of material by subject experts, instructional designers, educators and peers.

The review will help to identify material that is out of date, incorrect or badly designed and presented. Such reviews will be made readily available to potential users.

Summary

E-learning is almost certainly one of the most important developments in the delivery of medical education. It is not simply a method which uses information communications technology to deliver a more effective and streamlined education system. It is a tool for transforming medical education. For its potential to be realised, however, there has to be a close partnership between technology, educators and content specialists. New approaches to instructional design, such as the use of reusable learning objects, should be considered.

The process of change to e-learning must be carefully managed and should involve an institutional commitment to e-learning and this should include staff training.

"Universities that do not transform courses and degree programs so that they can be delivered over the Internet will not survive long into the next century"

van Horn 1996

Use e-learning not only to do better what you are already doing but to do something different.

References

Australian Government 1997 Higher education review, learning for life: review of higher education financing and policy. A policy discussion paper. Australian Government Publishing Service, Canberra.

Clark R C, Mayer R E 2003 e-Learning and the science of instruction. proven guidelines for consumers and designers of multimedia learning. Wiley, San Francisco.

European Commission 2003 eLearning. Better e-learning for Europe. European Communities, Luxembourg.

Farrington G C 1999 The new technologies and the future of residential undergraduate education. In: Dancing with the devil: information technology and the new competition in higher education. Katz R N and Associates (eds). Jossey Bass. p 73.

Harden R M 2002 Myths and e-learning. Medical Teacher 24(5):469–472.

Harden R M, Hart I R 2002 An international virtual medical school (IVIMEDS): the future for medical education. Medical Teacher 24(3):261–267.

Horton W 2001 Leading e-learning. American Society for Training and Development (ASTD), Alexandria VA. pp. 130–131.

Inglis A, Ling P, Joosten V 2002 Delivering digitally, managing the transmission to the knowledge media. Kogan Page, London. p 20

Jolliffe A, Ritter J, Stevens D 2001 The online learning handbook, developing and using web-based learning. Kogan Page, London. p 7

Phipps R, Merisotis J 1999 'What's the difference?' Institute for Higher Education Policy, Washington DC

Rosenberg M J 2001 E-learning. Strategies for delivering knowledge in the digital age. McGraw Hill, New York.

Schwarz M R 2001 Globalization and medical education. Medical Teacher 23(6):533–534.

Sloman M 2001 The E-learning revolution. From propositions to reality. Chartered Institute of Personnel and Development, London.

Van Horn R 1996 Technology, Phi Delta Kappan, 77 (February):796.

Wiley D A 2002 The instructional use of learning objects. Association for Educational Communications and Technology, Bloomington, Indiana.

SECTION 5
CURRICULUM THEMES

Chapter 25
Basic and clinical sciences

P. McCrorie

The traditional approach

It is widely agreed that, for doctors to be competent, they need an adequate knowledge of the sciences underpinning medicine. There is much less agreement over the quantity of science required, how and when it should be learnt, who should teach it and even how to define it.

Traditionally, when there was a clear pre–clinical/clinical divide in undergraduate medical education, the four basic sciences, anatomy, biochemistry, pharmacology and physiology (together with genetics, histology and embryology), were taught in blissful isolation from each other, using curricula laid down by the heads of each discipline. The so-called behavioural sciences, statistics, psychology and sociology, were taught alongside them. All of this so-called 'education' took place during the first two years of undergraduate medical course with little involvement of anything clinical, apart from the odd clinical demonstration. The clinical sciences, histopathology, medical microbiology, clinical chemistry, immunology and haematology were taught, again independently, in the subsequent two years, either alongside, or in interspersed lecture-filled chunks between clinical attachments on the wards. Often the attachments themselves were accompanied by a programme of lectures dealing with clinical aspects of disease including diagnosis and treatment.

Splitting up the teaching in this way had a number of consequences, mostly adverse, as described below.

Repetition

There was much repetition of material, e.g. concerning hormones, muscle or the autonomic nervous system, with students being taught topics three or even four times, admittedly from slightly different perspectives. While repetition is a good thing, there is a limit! There was little logic to the overall teaching programme with the same topics or systems being covered in different terms by different disciplines.

Factual overload

With control in the hands of departments, staffed mainly by nonclinical scientists, a substantial amount of material that students were expected to know was unnecessary for prospective doctors. In fairness, this was more an issue about the level of detail students were expected to memorise, rather than the inclusion of topics that had no place in a medical course. Thus an insistence that students should know details of biochemical pathways, including structures of intermediates and names of enzymes, the names of every muscle in the body and the names of every drug on the market, was a complete waste of time, encouraged rote-learning and led to massive over-cramming of the curriculum – 'curriculum hypertrophy' (Abrahamson 1978). It was surely better to ensure that students understood the purpose of pathways, the functions of the clinically important muscles and the modes of action of classes of drugs, the individual names of which would have changed by the time they qualified anyway.

Lack of relevance

With little input from practising clinicians into the design of the curriculum, the material presented to students was set in a discipline context, rather than a clinical context. Setting teaching in a clinical context facilitates learning and improves retention of knowledge.

Lack of integration

Many opportunities for integrated teaching, both horizontal and vertical, were missed. Departments were in competition in those days and interdepartmental cooperation was actively discouraged. Changed days! Separating normality from abnormality was believed to be educationally sound, hence the delay in studying pathology until third year. There was no attempt to introduce clinical skills teaching into the early part of the medical course, merely surface anatomy.

Emphasis on teaching rather than learning

In addition, the style of teaching was highly didactic, with a very strong emphasis being on teaching rather than learning: there were lectures, lectures and more lectures; hours and hours of anatomy dissection; and endless pointless and costly practicals. Clinicians constantly complained that the students they helped to select had lost all motivation by the time they reached them in third year. The preclinical years were seen as a test of endurance, a painful hurdle students had to overcome before they were allowed to get near a patient. Yet nothing changed; the discipline-based lobbies refused to yield their power. In the UK, change did eventually come in 1993 when the General Medical Council, responsible for the validation of all UK medical courses, insisted on a radical transformation of all medical school curricula. Such a change has been slow in coming elsewhere, particularly in Europe, where the disciplines still maintain their stranglehold on the medical curriculum.

The modern approach

The first thing to say is that there is no single best approach to designing a modern medical course to cover the basic and clinical sciences. This variety in style is important. Different students want different things. Some are fascinated by science and can't get enough of it. Some want to be researchers. Others are only interested in people. Some come into medical school with a science degree already. Some even have a PhD. Others enter medical school with a degree in history, or philosophy, or law, or economics and with only a basic understanding of science. Some

Recognise that variety in curriculum style among medical schools is a good thing. Different people learn in different ways.

Accept that students will learn more if they enjoy their learning.

like learning in groups. Others like to work on their own at their own pace. Some want to have everything handed to them on a plate. Some only learn what they perceive as relevant or practical while others like to take time to reflect and like to understand the theory behind everything they have to study. Therefore it is only appropriate that students should be able to select the school that suits their particular needs.

One option is to make a BSc or BMedSci compulsory for all students, either as an entry requirement or as an integral part of the course; that's fine for those with a strong interest in science. But medicine is an art as well as a science. Shouldn't we be encouraging students with an arts background to apply for medicine as well? The integral BSc is also a demanding option requiring a project to be found for each student which may be made more expensive if the project involves laboratory work. If they don't involve laboratory work, why do them? Student-selected components in the medical course where students spend a short period of time engaged in research that interests them, may be a better and cheaper solution.

But what should be taught in the basic and clinical sciences, how and when should it be taught and, most importantly of all, who should make these decisions?

The curriculum committee

Avoid curriculum hyperplasia.

The only way to avoid dictation of curriculum content by disciplines is to create a new committee, outwith department control, which is given the responsibility for curriculum design. At this stage it is often called the 'curriculum development group' or 'curriculum steering group', but after the course is developed, to ensure implementation of their ideas, it is transformed into a 'curriculum management committee'.

It is crucial to get the membership of the committee right at its inception. It needs to be chaired by someone committed to change, who is high up in the university hierarchy, such as the dean of undergraduate medical education (preferably a clinician). The criteria for becoming a member of the committee – and why not get people to apply for membership rather than be invited on to it? – should include a demonstrable interest in medical education, backed up with evidence, enthusiasm, and a willingness to change. The fewer professors on the committee the better. The lower the average age group the better.

Ensure the curriculum is designed and managed centrally, with full support and authority from the top.

It is crucial to have a balance between basic and behavioural scientists, hospital clinicians (the less specialised the better), general practitioners and others such as public health physicians, non-university hospital clinicians, medical educationists and administrators. Recently qualified doctors, students and community representatives have proved welcome additions to such committees. Since the purpose of undergraduate medical education is to produce doctors, clinicians should hold the balance of power in the committee. The more generalists on the committee, the more rounded the curriculum will be.

Devolving the details

Create a series of design groups to take responsibility for particular areas or aspects of the curriculum from first year to final year.

While the above committee oversees the curriculum development process, subcommittees need to be set up to design the nitty-gritty details. Such groups should be systems-based, not discipline-based and, most importantly, should be responsible for curriculum design for the entire course. Thus a committee set up to design a module in, for instance, the respiratory and cardiovascular system, should include a physiologist, an anatomist, a pharmacologist, a histopathologist, a chest physician, a cardiologist, a cardiothoracic surgeon, a general practitioner and a public health physician at the very least.

This module committee needs to design and oversee *all* the learning and teaching around a particular system, from first year to final year. There is no point in designing a course a year at a time: that leads to disintegration and ignorance among the teaching staff about what the students have learnt and have still to learn. The committee's first job is to select the core cases for their module. These cases could be core presentations, such as chest pain, shortness of breath, haemoptysis, hypertension, or core clinical diagnoses such as myocardial infarction, asthma, pulmonary embolism, abdominal aortic aneurysm. They then have to decide what learning could arise from each case and put the cases in some sort of logical order to make learning easier and more structured. Thus chest pain, due to coronary heart disease (CHD), could help students learn about the functional anatomy and physiology of the heart and its circulation; haemoglobin and oxygen transport; atherosclerosis; cardiac enzymes; the pharmacology of drugs used in the treatment of CHD; the psychosocial sequelae and prevalence of CHD, and the risk factors for, and prevention of, CHD, not to mention the surface anatomy of the heart, the clinical examination of the heart, taking a chest pain history and talking to patients with CHD. Straight away the next issue that arises for the module planning group is how to deliver the course. In fact this issue is so important that it needs to be centrally decided by the curriculum steering group.

Learning and teaching methods

From the above discussion, it is clear that an integrated case-based approach to learning and teaching is an apt way forward. This can be done in two basic ways:

- *Approach A:* start, in the time-honoured way, with the basic and clinical sciences and illustrate (i.e. bring them to life) with case-based studies.
- *Approach B:* start with the cases and out of them learn the sciences needed to understand them.

Approach A

The more traditional approach, this maintains the inherent logic of the disciplines concerned and might, to continue with the CHD example, involve lectures and practical sessions from anatomists on the anatomy of the heart and the circulation; lectures from physiologists on the physiology of the heart (Starling's law, autonomic nervous system etc); lectures from pharmacologists on the mechanism of action of cardio-effective drugs; and lectures, and possibly histology practical sessions,

Ensure each group is appropriately balanced in terms of staff input, the balance of power being held by generalist clinicians.

Decide whether to establish a curriculum based on lectures but illustrated by case scenarios or a curriculum based on case scenarios but illustrated by lectures. If the latter, decide whether to develop a problem-oriented curriculum or a problem-based curriculum.

from histopathologists on atherosclerosis. There might be a whole-class clinical demonstration involving a patient who has recovered from a previous myocardial infarction. There might also be some self-directed learning exercises around patients with CHD. Here the teaching team will have prepared some brief case scenarios with some carefully thought out questions designed to bring out key principles of the basic sciences underlying the condition(s) under discussion.

There is nothing wrong with the above approach, but it does still mean that the material given to the students, much of which is delivered in a didactic and passive way, is at the behest of the anatomy, physiology, pharmacology and pathology lecturers. The topics and concepts are probably important, but the level of detail delivered may well be excessive. Perhaps a better example would be diabetes. Here there is a high risk that the biochemists go to town on metabolism. After all, without insulin, much of intermediary metabolism is affected. That means that students have to learn the whole of intermediary metabolism, including the often-quoted dreaded Krebs cycle! Ask any clinician if the Krebs cycle has ever entered their thought process since passing their biochemistry examination and you'll get a scornful and very direct answer 'No!'. Now that doesn't mean that medical students don't need to be aware of the existence of the cycle and understand what its role is, but they most certainly do not need to know the names of the intermediates, and especially they don't need to know the names of the enzymes involved. Hence the importance of clinicians in course planning, right down to this level of detail. Pruning undergraduate medicine down to a manageable core is not so difficult at the topic and concept level; indeed most medical schools would probably be in reasonable agreement with this. Where the disparity occurs is at the level of detail required within each of these core topics, and that is where Approach B wins hands down.

Approach B

In this approach the first thing the students get is the case scenario, be this on paper (most common), video, or clinical demonstration. The ideal learning method to adopt is *problem-based learning* (PBL). Here a group of seven or eight students is presented with a clinical case, either a short summary (McMaster/Maastricht model; Schmidt 1983) or a much longer progressively released version (Harvard/New Mexico model; Kaufman et al 1989). The students decide themselves what they need to learn (although it has been carefully thought out in advance what learning issues are triggered by each PBL case), undertake their learning using the resources available, and feed back their findings to the group after 2–3 days' study. In this way, only topics that specifically arise out of the case are researched. Extraneous and irrelevant material is therefore selected out. The biggest problem for students on all PBL courses is working out the level of detail required – and I sadly, but realistically, have to add this – to pass their exams. To a certain extent this is up to each student: some will enjoy going into a great deal of detail and others will go to any length to avoid it. The key to this, as hinted, is assessment.

Assessment

Assessment drives learning. This is a well-known tenet of medical (or indeed any other) education. Therefore, no matter how much freedom students are given to direct their own learning, it always comes back to the same thing. If it's in the assessment, students will learn it; if it's not, they won't – a truly sad reflection on higher education. But it can be turned to the advantage of the course planners. Design the assessment which produces the kind of learning you want, and you're on a winner. Get the wrong people designing the assessment, you're on a loser. Just as it is crucial for the curriculum to be designed and controlled centrally, it is equally essential that the assessment is designed and controlled centrally. If you ask for a lot of detail in assessment questions, that will encourage students to memorise a lot of detail. If you want students to *apply* their knowledge, rather than regurgitate it, then create questions that require them to do just that. If students learn through cases, it is appropriate to assess through cases. Minicases, modified-essay questions, extended-matching questions and case-based single best answer multiple-choice questions will fit the bill. What is pointless is learning by PBL and being assessed by memory recall true–false multiple-choice questions. Get the assessment right, and the rest will follow.

Learning resources

Integral to the learning process is the adequacy of the learning resources. Traditionally, learning resources were confined to lecture notes, handouts, cadavers, practical reports and textbooks. Nowadays much more is available to the student. Many medical schools have stopped using cadaveric material. Certainly little dissection is carried out any more, although many schools do still use prosected specimens. Models and plastinated specimens have taken over from cadavers stinking of formalin as it is still important for students to obtain a three-dimensional perspective of the human body. The biggest change is, of course, in information technology (IT) capability. A wide range of learning material is now available, at the touch of a button, on the internet. Of course, not all of this material is scientifically sound, but simply by recommending specific approved websites, this problem can be easily overcome. Many medical schools store information on CD-roms for student use, much of it in an interactive form. While this is good practice, it is not best practice. Best practice makes use of web delivery and uses specially designed, password-protected intranet sites. The problem with CD-roms is that they can only be used by one person at any one time (or possibly a small group), and usually only in one place (e.g. the library). Putting material on an intranet site allows everyone access whenever and wherever they want. Most medical students possess, or have access to, a personal computer. Some medical schools supply their students with a laptop. Some supply their students with a personal digital assistant (PDA). With all these advances in technological knowhow, and with more to come no doubt, universities need to respond to this IT revolution and not ignore it (see chapter 22, Virtual learning environments and chapter 24, e-learning).

The other important point to make about IT resources is that there really is no point in using them just for pages and pages of text. That's

Use assessment to drive learning.

Design all assessments centrally, involving only staff who understand and support the philosophy of the course.

Offer students the most up-to-date technology for their learning, especially for image-based resource material.

what books are for. Computer-based learning (CBL) has two major advantages over book-based learning:

- it can, and should, be image-based, not text-based
- it can, and should, be interactive.

CBL is ideal for learning anatomy, histology and histopathology, for example. Moving images or drawings can be used, for instance, to show how DNA replicates, or how proteins are synthesised. Video material can be included showing patients being interviewed about their condition or demonstrating a laboratory technique. Self-assessment is easy with CBL, for example by labelling diagrams; pointing an arrow at a site on a diagram or photographed cadaveric part; or by using multiple-choice questions to check understanding and reasoning. Not that I'm suggesting that sitting in front of a computer all day long is the way future doctors should be trained. It is always essential to use an array of learning methods in any course. The most important thing is to decide which method to use for which learning outcome.

Who delivers the basic and clinical science teaching?

There is a belief among some scientists that it is their right, and only their right, to teach their own discipline. This is no longer acceptable. The sciences underlying medicine should be taught by whoever is the most appropriate in the context and stage of the student learning. And indeed, it may be that no-one teaches much of it, but that it is left up to the students to learn it for themselves. The role of the teacher is then to prepare the materials (e.g. PBL cases) that will trigger the appropriate student learning, to provide a small number of overview and summary lectures and to attend an expert forum. An expert forum is where one or more experts in a particular topic stand in front of the students and simply answer questions that the students put to them. This is a teaching technique that satisfies everyone. The students are satisfied because they get an answer to the questions that have been puzzling them, and the teachers are satisfied because they are being allowed to demonstrate and show off their expertise: a win–win situation.

Summary

Understanding the basic and clinical sciences underlying medicine is vital. Rote-learning masses and masses of facts is not. The key to success is to ensure that students have a thorough grasp of concepts and principles; that they know how and where to fill gaps in the knowledge; that they appreciate that medicine is not a static discipline, and that keeping up to date with medical advances is a lifelong process; and that learning is interactive, exciting and, above all, in context. Who teaches it, where and when is not relevant. It is how the students learn that matters. Instead of putting effort into imparting detailed information, effort is far better spent in creating high quality learning resources, be they self-directed learning exercises, PBL cases, web-based material or workbooks, and limiting the didactic input to overviews, summaries and difficult topics, plus of course the much lauded expert forum.

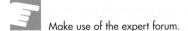
Recognise that the basic and clinical sciences do not have to be taught by basic and clinical scientists – indeed much of their material can be self-taught.

Make use of the expert forum.

References

Abrahamson S 1978 Diseases of the curriculum. Journal of Medical Education 53:951–957

Schmidt H G 1983 Problem-based learning: rational and description. Medical Education 17:11–16

Kaufman A, Mennin S, Waterman R et al 1989 The New Mexico experiment: educational innovation and institutional change Academic Medicine 64:285–294

Chapter 26
Communication skills

D. Snadden, J. S. Ker

"Communication skills are not an optional extra; without appropriate communication skills our knowledge and intellectual efforts are easily wasted"

Silverman et al 1998

"To do good and to communicate forget not"

Hebrews ch 13, v 16

The word 'communicate' comes from the Latin, 'to impart, to share'.

Introduction

There is growing evidence that good communication has a positive effect on patient outcomes. The evidence that doctors are not all good communicators and that communication skills can be taught is well established (Simpson et al 1991).

What are communication skills?

In a comparison of generic skills required for the workplace, reports from the USA, Australia and the UK identified communicating ideas and information as a key competence for effective participation in the changing patterns of work and work organisations. In medicine, communication skills are needed for forming and maintaining relationships, to gather and share information, to gain informed consent, to support problem solving, to provide reassurance, to alleviate distress and to make best evidence-based decisions. Communication is about how doctors and patients talk with each other in a search for mutual understanding and shared solutions to problems.

Communication skills also include interaction between colleagues and other professionals involved in health and social care. A variety of media are also influencing the development of communication skills. In addition to written patient records, telephones and electronic written communications such as e-mail and text messaging are increasingly being utilised within the healthcare services. With the role of the doctor becoming more diverse and accountable, skills in communicating with legal services, the media and press and with students as a teacher are also required. However, the doctor–patient interaction, which lies at the heart of medical practice, will be our focus in this chapter.

Why are communication skills important?

Having identified what communication skills are for, in both a medical care context and as a key generic skill for the workplace, it is essential to highlight their central importance to clinical practice. It is well established that patients prefer clinicians who are warm and sympathetic, listen to what they say and ask questions which are precise and easily understood. Doctors who communicate well are more likely to:

- make an accurate diagnosis especially in relation to psychiatric conditions
- have their patients manage their medicines better
- encounter fewer malpractice claims.

In addition and perhaps in the context of this chapter there is established evidence that communication skills can be learnt and that those who need to improve such skills can do so.

Communication models

A number of models of communication for clinical practice now exist and each of these is well described in the literature with appropriate instruction on how to teach the model (Neighbour 1992, Pendleton et al 1984, Stewart et al 1995). They all emphasise the importance of understanding not only the patient's disease process but also their thoughts, beliefs, feelings and expectations in helping to determine the best course of action for each person (a more patient-centred approach). In addition the models share similar approaches with regard to the basic skills elements of a successful consultation. These basic skills focus on five key areas of the consultation described by Silverman et al (1998) as:

- initiating the session
- gathering information
- building the relationship
- explanation and planning
- closing the session.

More advanced communication skills are required for areas such as breaking bad news or dealing with anger or sadness, while examples of difficult situations for communicating might include where there are language and cultural differences, communication through an interpreter and where there are medical problems such as dementia, a sensory deficit or drug addiction.

It is better to think about which model suits the purpose of your particular context, whether it is a small teaching unit or an entire medical school. What is important for learners is that they apply the same model in different settings, particularly at the start of their clinical experience.

How to teach communication skills

One of the challenges in education for communicating in clinical practice is how to empower the learner to analyse and evaluate their own skills in one specific patient setting and then to transfer this learning to another patient setting. In addition, in structuring education and training in communication skills, it is essential to plan the progressive development of these skills in the context of other learning.

All patient-centred models emphasise the importance of appreciating the patient's context; communication skills teachers need to find ways of helping students to develop ways of understanding the context of each patient they talk with.

Concentrate on core skills before special skills. The core skills are:
- initiating the session
- gathering information
- building the relationship
- explanation and planning
- closing the session.

"The lists of medical questions memorized during training are often interpreted as 'to do' lists by inexperienced students with poor understanding of how to discriminate based on relevant patient context"

Martin 2003

Be prepared to lead by example and hold demonstrations of your own consultations for your students to criticise constructively. Do not ask your students to do anything that you have not done yourself or are not willing to demonstrate to them.

The communications map

Concepts of communication skills all sound very grand, but the teacher has the task of finding a means of allowing students to appreciate the issues in a way that actually helps them develop sound basic skills and build on them, as well as understanding their relevance to clinical practice. Despite training, working with simulations and getting feedback, students seeing patients for the first time can appear nervous and clumsy and default into asking disorganised rote-memorised questions.

Martin (2003) argues that the current patient-centred frameworks do not easily lend themselves to interpretation by students and in response to this has developed and tested, over 10 years, a 'communication map' which attempts to help students to begin to organise their clinical communication encounters. It draws on concepts within most of the current communication models and tries to order them in a way students can relate to. The map is based on three principles: the patient's turn is first, then the doctor's and finally there is a closing period to ensure some mutual understanding. Within these three broad areas, subsets help students organise their communication effectively.

Martin's paper challenges educators in the following terms: 'How do we make communication skills education relevant for students?' 'How do we offer complicated concepts in a way that students can understand and relate to?' 'How do we help them put these into practice in an organised way?'

It may be worthwhile ensuring, as a teacher, that you yourself have experienced the teaching methods; if you are expecting students to be viewed on video, it is better if you have had this experience yourself. It is often helpful for students to see their teachers on video or in role play from time to time if these are the methods in which the students will participate.

Feedback

It is difficult to see how students can improve their communication skills without practising them in safe settings and receiving feedback on their performance. There are a number of models of how to give feedback on communication skills, including Pendleton's rules (Pendleton et al 1984) and the SETGO method (Silverman et al 1998). Effective feedback is one of the cornerstones of effective communication learning and needs to be:

- *Clear* – if you are vague you will not be understood. 'Well, I don't know if this matters or not, it might not be relevant, but the patient seemed a bit more upset after seeing you.'
- *Owned* – the feedback you give is your own perception but comments such as 'I think the way you handled that situation was very clever' can be positively helpful.
- *Regular* – feedback will be more useful if it happens regularly and is given close to the event in question and in a way that an individual student can use to make changes. For example, 'Do you want to think about trying out some ways of stopping the consultation effectively and we'll discuss it next time?'

- **B**alanced – feedback can be perceived by students as being negative, but constructive feedback is about discussing strengths as well as weaknesses.
- **S**pecific – generalized feedback can be harder to learn from. 'You can be frustrating' may be less useful than 'I get frustrated if you are not talking about problems that occur around prescribing.'

Medicine is a knowledge-based profession and it is very challenging to be learning how to share information when you are unfamiliar with the information. As communication skills are something that doctors use every day in practice, teaching will be more effective if it contains practical experience and feedback as well as theoretical material.

Preparation for delivering the experience

In preparation for a communication skills teaching session you need to take account of the following:

- type of resource best suited to the clinical experience of the learners
- links to other curricular outcomes
- maturity of learners
- context of learning opportunity
- expected outcomes for the session
- assessment process.

Demonstrations

Demonstrations can be created on videotape, on audiotape or as role plays, to show students examples of good and poor communication or to give them practice at understanding, analysing or evaluating various models. Taped consultations can be real or simulated. These can illustrate diverse medical settings, such as the hospital ward, the outpatient department or a primary care setting. Such demonstrations can be used in discussion groups and seminars to help students understand core concepts.

Simulations

Simulated consultations (see chapter 8, Teaching in the clinical skills centre) can be created using members of the teaching team, volunteer patients or professional actors. They have the advantages that the same people can be used in different situations and they can be used for repeated practice by learners. The disadvantages are that all simulated patients require training for their roles and in how to provide feedback. The cost of professional actors is also considerable.

Simulations can be particularly powerful when the student meets the simulated patient in a one-to-one encounter and receives feedback on performance, either at once or later if the consultation is video- or audiotaped.

In addition, simulations can be developed in complexity from patient consultations to ward simulation exercises, where communication with patients, colleagues and other healthcare professionals can be

"Basic interviewing skills can be learned at undergraduate and postgraduate level, providing effective methods are used. These include demonstration of key skills, practice under controlled conditions, and audiotape or videotape feedback of performance by a tutor within small groups. More complex skills can also be learned but may not be used or maintained without ongoing training and supervision"

Maguire 1990

"Having the opportunity to take histories from simulated patients and get feedback on how you've done, gave me more confidence to go on to the wards and speak to real patients"

Medical student

observed. Such observation of students in action in a safe, simulated work environment can provide evidence about communication within the healthcare team.

Observation

Observation of students can take place in any setting where they meet patients. It is best if the observer has a check sheet to write down observations during the consultation to ensure accurate feedback is given.

Video- and audiotaping

Students can make video- or audiotapes of their consultations with real or simulated patients. They can then bring them to meetings with a tutor or a learning group. Videorecording of student–patient encounters is increasingly common in family medicine settings where students can go over the consultations with their supervisor afterwards and receive positive and constructive feedback. Videotaping has advantages over observation in that the student can see and hear themselves and can revisit the consultation. Videos allow students to analyse their use of body language during a consultation or the type of eye contact used. In the UK videotaping to provide evidence of communication abilities is now mandatory for all postgraduate family medicine trainees prior to their final certification.

One-way mirrors

Some teaching centres use one-way mirrors to observe students with patients. Although mirrors allow a consultation to be viewed in real time, they have some disadvantages over videotaping. Firstly the students cannot see themselves, and secondly a dedicated observation room is needed. However, these devices allow others to observe the consultation process without participating in or influencing it.

Role play

Students may take on the roles of patient and doctor and carry out a simulated consultation.

This can be a very useful introductory step in learning communication skills where students are able to explore the patient's perspective. In addition, for remedial training, taking the roles of patient, doctor and assessor can contribute to students' awareness of their own learning needs.

Role play has a number of advantages in that consultations can be stopped and parts of them revisited, or different approaches can be tried to find different solutions to various communication issues. Role play can evoke powerful feelings and must be used in a supportive environment. It is extremely important to 'de-role' those involved at the end of the session.

Role play consultations are now used in a number of educational settings to evaluate communication skills as part of professional accreditation exams, such as those of the College of Family Physicians of Canada.

"The thought of being videoed was scary, but once you got into the consultation you forgot the camera was there"

Medical student

'De-roling'

One way to 'de-role' is to say to those in role that the role is now over and they now have to think themselves back to who they are. This might be about publicly acknowledging their return to themselves. This is particularly important if the role involved breaking bad news or where the role player was asked to exhibit anger or other emotions.

Explaining theoretical material

Demonstrations of examples of communication relevant to clinical settings can be used in large- and small-group settings to generate and link knowledge concepts. Such demonstrations can either be live, using role play with experienced role players, or prerecorded using videotapes to trigger discussion.

Students need to consider the effect of the set-up, the use of nonverbal communication, timing of recording information and the layout of the consulting room. (Figs 26.1–26.4).

Providing experience

Practical experience of communication can be provided to students in a variety of ways, by role play with one another or by simulations using faculty members, patients or actors. Initially this could be based on the core skills of communication, leaving more difficult and complicated situations until later. It is essential to provide opportunities for analysis and discussion of experiences. Whichever practical method is to be used key issues regarding consent, the 'ground rules' for the session, and feedback must be addressed.

Consent

If real patients are involved, their informed consent must be obtained, particularly if video or audiotapes will be used.

Ground rules

It is best to develop ground rules with the learners at the start of any teaching session, to ensure ownership. Some students find communication training threatening, particularly where they are seen to be 'performing' by their peers. For this reason the learning session must be made safe for them. One way of doing this is to encourage students to express their anxieties and concerns which allows the development of ground rules with which they are comfortable. If a group stays together over a period of time they can use the same ground rules or modify them as time goes by.

Feedback

If a tape is to be used, reach agreement on how it will be discussed and how constructive feedback will be given. It is important that a climate is established in which it is safe and supportive for individuals to discuss difficulties openly and receive feedback on how to tackle them. This can only be done in one-to-one or small-group settings.

Ground rules for feedback may include:

- how the feedback will be given
- what will happen to any material collected during the teaching session
- total confidentiality about what happens in the session.

(See Appendix for an example of the type of script used for role play or simulated consultation.)

Practising communication skills in a safe environment and giving effective feedback are at the heart of teaching communication skills.

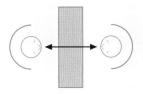

Fig. 26.1 If the patient and doctor face each other across a desk, this can create a barrier to effective communication

When real consultations are video taped, informed consent is essential:
- Give a written information sheet and a consent form to sign before the consultation starts.
- The information sheet must say what the tape could be used for, who might see it and how long it will be kept.
- Patients must feel free to say no.
- When the consultation is finished patients should sign once more to show that they still consent to the tape's use for teaching purposes.

Giving feedback on communication is important, but the feedback needs to value the opinions and feelings of learners, as well as being constructive in helping them to improve. Ways of doing this include
- asking the learners what they were trying to achieve in the communication session
- asking the learners what they think went well
- asking the observers what they think went well
- asking the learners what didn't go so well or what they would do differently next time
- asking the observers what didn't go so well or what could be done differently next time.

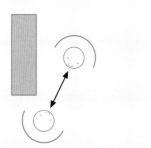

Fig. 26.2 Facing each other across the corner of a desk provides a less threatening setting and may facilitate communication

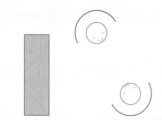

Fig. 26.3 Having no desk may feel too informal for some doctors or patients

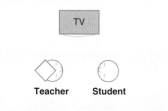

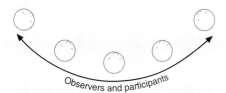

Fig. 26.4 Role play with learner and teacher and small group around them

Providing experience for specific communication skills

Nonverbal communication

Non-verbal communication is an important aspect of communication skills training. It is important for students in learning to build attitudes that express empathy, and for them to be able to relate to the nonverbal cues that patients may demonstrate. This can be done following a similar framework to that outlined above. Firstly students can be given some information about nonverbal communication followed by examples which may be from role play or from video. They can then use some of these examples in discussion groups. They can also, during teaching sessions, have some feedback and discussion on the nonverbal communication in their own consultations. Video is particularly useful for this as students can examine the nonverbal cues given during a consultation. It is often worth trying to get a group of students to analyse a consultation with the sound turned off. Understanding nonverbal communication is an important prerequisite for dealing with some of the difficult communication issues mentioned earlier.

This is also a good opportunity to discuss where the patient and doctor sit in relation to each other. In general the consultation is less confrontational if patient and doctor face each other across the corner of a desk rather than directly across a desk (Fig. 26.2).

Special situations

Once students have mastered basic communication skills there are a number of special situations which merit further learning:

- breaking bad news (Buckman 1994)
- dealing with distressed patients who are angry or upset
- dealing with ethical dilemmas
- dealing with patients who have communication difficulties through sensory impairment
- communicating across language or cultural differences
- communicating through an interpreter
- giving lifestyle advice
- communicating using the telephone.

Teaching about communication in such situations again requires preparation, patience and tact. It is difficult to arrange for students to experience these in the course of their clinical practice. If they do meet these situations they are usually only able to observe experienced doctors handling them. Real learning often comes from trying things out yourself so simulations and role play are often the best methods. These particular situations can provoke a lot of emotion in those involved in acting out the scenario. For this reason scripts need to be carefully created, everyone involved has to be well briefed, and there must be plenty of time for discussion, debriefing and feedback afterwards. Well-trained simulated patients are very helpful in this situation as, if things are not going well, the consultation can be stopped, the problem discussed and the student can try again. Particularly in these situations teachers need good skills in facilitation and counselling. The sessions can be most effective in small-group or one-to-one situations.

Assessing communication skills

Continuous self-assessment

For assessment of communication skills evidence about all aspects of communication has to be sought from throughout a clinician's practice. The learner's evaluation of his or her progress should become the main focus of the assessment process. However most curricula still include both formative and summative elements.

Formative assessment

Feedback on a student's performance can be given using observation or audio or video tapes. With communication skills in particular, it is not what the student knows that is important, it is what the student does in practice. Therefore formative assessment is best carried out as close to the real clinical situation as possible.

Formative assessment focuses on constructive feedback about the student's performance. Records of teaching sessions and formative feedback comments can give an indication of progress over time. It is, however, important that formative assessments are used to support learning. If they count towards summative assessment they can reduce experimentation and real exploration of weaknesses and inhibit learning.

Summative assessment

Communication assessments can be built into examinations such as the objective structured clinical examination (OSCE) where simulated patients can be used for standardised consultations. Standardised instruments for assessing communication skills now exist and can either be used as they are or further refined in different settings (Campbell et al 1995, Stewart et al 1995). More complex assessments have been developed using simulated surgeries (Rashid et al 1994). The latter are costly in terms of time and resources and may be more applicable in the post-graduate setting.

Barrier exams

In the undergraduate setting it is imperative that robust assessments of student performances are devised, so that students only qualify after they have mastered and demonstrated certain core communication competencies. This then leads to the question of whether students should have a barrier exam. As communication is at the heart of the practice of medicine, there is a powerful argument that students should not graduate without demonstrating competence in communication. In remediating communication skills after a summative assessment, a focused period of study with good student communicators has been shown to be effective in addressing those students with problems (Dowell et al). The effect of peers on the development of progress in communication skills can be very positive in a supportive simulated environment.

Teaching the teachers

Communication training requires sensitive dedicated teachers who are themselves excellent communicators and role models. It is very important that those who are teaching medical students communication skills have had adequate training and have experienced the teaching methods that will be used. They will also need effective feedback on their own performance as teachers.

Summary

Effective communication skills can be taught at undergraduate and post-graduate level.

Knowledge alone is insufficient to make an effective doctor, as doctors have to be able to communicate with patients, colleagues and staff.

Basic communication skills are most effectively taught using a recognised communication model in small groups or one-to-one situations. Effective teaching methods may involve role play, simulated patients and real patients, with video or audio recording or direct observation being used to support constructive feedback to the student.

Teachers of communication skills need to be well trained and themselves excellent communicators and role models.

Good communication skills are at the core of the doctor–patient interaction. They are not an addition or an option but central to the effective practice of medicine.

Acknowledgments

We are grateful to Mary Thomas for help with the CORBS feedback model, and to Jon Dowell and Cathy Jackson for their work on remediation of communication skills.

References

Buckman R 1994 How to break bad news. Papermac, London

Campbell L M, Howie J G R, Murray T S 1995 Use of videotaped consultations in summative assessment of trainees in general practice. British Journal of General Practice 45(392):137–141

Dowell J, Dent J, Duffy R. What to do about medical students with unsatisfactory consultation skills? Medical Teacher, (in press)

Maguire P 1990 Can communication skills be taught? British Journal of Hospital Medicine March 43(3):215–216

Martin D. 2003 Martin's Map: a conceptual framework for teaching and learning the medical interview using a patient centred approach. Medical Education 37:1145–1153

Neighbour R 1992 The inner consultation 3. Kluwer Academic, London

Pendleton D, Schofield T, Tate P, Havelock P 1984 The consultation: an approach to learning and teaching. Oxford University Press, Oxford

Rashid A, Allen J, Thew R, Aram G 1994 Performance based assessment using simulated patients. Education for General Practice 5:151–156

Silverman J D, Kurtz S M, Draper J 1998 Skills for communicating with patients. Radcliffe Medical Press, Oxford

Simpson M, Buckman R, Stewart M et al 1991 Doctor patient communication: the Toronto consensus statement. British Medical Journal 303:1385–1387

Stewart M, Brown J B, Weston W W et al 2003 Patient-centered medicine. Transforming the clinical method. Radcliffe, London

Appendix

Here is an example of the type of script which can be used either for role playing or for simulation.

Simulated-patient instructions

The student seeing you will have a limited time to speak to you. Please spend some time thinking yourself into the role. The student has been asked to explore your reasons for visiting the doctor today.

You are a 26-year-old male/female named Jones. You are at university in the second year of a PhD in biochemistry. For the last 6 months you have been getting a cough at night. When the student asks you why you have come, say that you have 'been getting a cough at night' and wait and see what he or she asks you next.

It is likely you will be asked more about your cough. This wakes you up sometimes and you have been feeling a bit tired because of lost sleep. The problem has gradually worsened.

Give the following information if you are asked directly or if the student encourages you to talk with open-ended questions:

You are in the university swimming team and train regularly. Training nights are Tuesdays and Fridays. Your times have not been so good recently and during training you are feeling unduly short of breath and develop a sensation of tightness across your chest. Last Tuesday this got pretty bad and scared you – that is why you are here – your chest was making funny wheezy noises. This settled eventually but you had a really bad night with coughing.

You have no personal or social problems. You are happy as a student. Your only past history of note was eczema as a child. Your brother has hay fever; otherwise there is no relevant family history. Your parents are alive and well.

You think it is asthma because the swimming coach told you. A quick suck on an inhaler (salbutamol) belonging to a team-mate sorted you out; you will only admit to this if asked what you think is happening to you, what you think is wrong with you or some similar question.

If you are asked anything else make it up!

Notes for the student

This patient is consulting you as a doctor for the first time. Elicit his or her story. The patient is Mr/Mrs Jones. The patient is 26 years old – despite how old he or she may look! You will be given feedback on the types of question you ask, your listening skills and how you acquire information.

Chapter 27
Ethics and attitudes

M. G. Brennan

"*Students should acquire a knowledge and understanding of 'ethical and legal issues relevant to the practice of medicine' and an 'ability to understand and analyse ethical problems so as to enable patients, their families, society and the doctor to have proper regard to such problems in reaching decisions'* "

GMC 2002

Introduction

To be a doctor is literally to be a teacher. One of the most valuable lessons doctors can impart to their students is how to be a 'good' doctor, an ethical practitioner. Like all areas of medicine, this is a complex lesson, best learnt by hard work, application, reflection and experience. For the lesson to be successful it needs to be relevant, credible and well delivered; there must be prior planning and preparation. For the teachers of ethics to be successful they also need to be credible, to be able to 'walk the talk', and to know how to plan, prepare and deliver the teaching.

This chapter provides a practical introduction to the teaching of medical ethics and attitudes. It uses a case study to illustrate recent innovations in the teaching of medical ethics, and focuses on some of the factors which have precipitated such developments. Above all, it is intended to show how ethics can be taught in a way that is enjoyable and effective for the lifelong learner in medicine.

How it has been

Sir Lancelot Spratt lives on in medical education. He first appeared over 50 years ago as an eminent consultant surgeon in *Doctor in the house* (Rank 1954), the film inspired by Richard Gordon's books. Sir Lancelot's attitude towards medical ethics was best displayed in the classic ward round scene. In this, he drew a long incision line across a patient's abdomen and then said 'Don't worry, my good man, this has got absolutely nothing to do with you,' having first told him that 'you won't understand our medical talk.' Since then, he has made his mark in numerous hospitals and medical schools worldwide. Medical ethics for Sir Lancelot and some of his generation could be summed up as not seducing your patients, avoiding too much alcohol on duty and not advertising your services.

Fortunately, times are changing. Most doctors and medical students have high ideals and aspirations and want to practise medicine in an ethical way. At the very least, they are keen to avoid complaints by their patients and colleagues, or being sued for malpractice; this might be described as the default position. Medical litigation has increased exponentially over the past few years and seems set to continue its rapid growth. With this background, it is actually not very difficult to capitalise on the willingness of doctors and medical students to practise medicine in an ethical way.

New curricula have been developed in medical schools across the world over the last decade; in many of them, the study of medical ethics has taken its rightful place at the centre of the curriculum. At a postgraduate level, there are very few medical training schemes or specialties prepared to neglect medical ethics in their provision of education, training, discussion and debate.

Moving forward

The dictionary defines ethics as 'moral principles or codes', and ethical as 'conforming to a recognised standard'.

But medical ethics involves more than these definitions might suggest, encompassing the way a doctor lives his or her life and practises the art of medicine. In an episode of the US television sitcom, *Frasier*, the eponymous radio psychiatrist is resisting his father, Martin's, attempts to persuade him to do something which he disagrees with. Frasier says: 'Dad, you taught me about ethics; you taught me that ethics is what you do when no-one else is watching.' This seems an excellent definition of ethics for all of us working in healthcare, highlighting as it does the need for good behaviour and the exercise of integrity – internalised or personal ethics – rather than over-reliance on external rules and regulations.

It used to be assumed that, if one was taught by 'good' doctors (like the 'well disposed physician' described by the ethicist Len Doyal), one would become a good doctor oneself: ethics would be acquired almost by a process of osmosis. Of course, this ignored the fact that there might be considerable variability in how good the teacher actually was at imparting the skills, qualities and precepts that enable a doctor to engage with medical ethics. In a typical British medical school in the early 1990s, medical ethics teaching might have amounted to a 1-hour lecture out of 5 years of teaching. There was no structure, little coordination and very little relevance to everyday practice.

Medical ethics teaching in UK medical schools has been in a state of flux since the Pond Report in 1987. The recommendations of the General Medical Council on undergraduate medical education (GMC 1993) provided additional impetus for an increase in the teaching of medical ethics as part of the core curriculum to be implemented in every UK medical school. A survey in the *Journal of Medical Ethics* (Fulford et al 1997) reported that although the majority of schools in the UK were able to provide ethics teaching in one form or other, there was a wide variation in the quality and quantity available across the country. The report identified a number of key problems, including a lack of teachers, teaching materials and library resources.

In 1998, the *Journal of Medical Ethics* and the *British Medical Journal* published a consensus statement, agreed by a number of British teachers of medical ethics (consensus statement 1998). This provided a minimal 'core curriculum' in ethics and law which it was hoped medical schools would be prepared to incorporate in their undergraduate

"With purity and holiness I will live my life and practise my art. Into whatever houses I go, I will enter them for the benefit of the sick, and will abstain from every voluntary act of mischief and corruption. Whatsoever I see or hear in the life of men which ought not to be spoken of abroad, I will not divulge, as reckoning that all such should be kept secret"

Hippocrates 460–377 BC

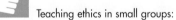

Teaching ethics in small groups:
- Use cases and vignettes
- Create a safe environment
- Use students' names
- Set out ground rules
- Encourage discussion
- Allow experiences to be shared
- Aim to develop:
  - tolerance
  - the ability to cope with ambiguity
  - the ability to appreciate different views.

curricula (Gillon & Doyle 1998). Since the publication of these documents, there has been a significant increase in the number of academic staff employed by the UK medical schools to teach or coordinate the teaching of medical ethics and law. Ethics is now an integral part of the curriculum in nearly all of these British schools as it had been for some time previously in other parts of the world, notably North America and Australasia.

Organising medical ethics teaching – a case study

At an undergraduate level, ethics has often been taught in a variety of places in the curriculum by a wide range of teachers. This variety, though good in its way, has sometimes lacked coordination and lost educational impact as a result. The following describes the development of medical ethics in one medical school, where coordination and collaboration were critical factors in achieving a successful contribution to the curriculum.

The Bristol approach

At Bristol medical school in the UK the development of ethics teaching was given considerable impetus by the inaugural appointment of Alastair Campbell to a chair of ethics in medicine. Campbell, who is now an emeritus professor of the University of Bristol, was a highly respected academic who had previously held senior appointments at the universities of Edinburgh and Otago. He became the founding director in 1997 of Bristol's new Centre for Ethics in Medicine. This led to the introduction of a structured and incremental approach to the teaching of ethics at the Bristol Medical School. Medical ethics became a vertical theme running all the way through the curriculum, which required considerable collaboration with preclinical and clinical colleagues. A core group of ethics teachers was formed (several of whom were from outside the university), whose roles in contributing to the overall curriculum came to be described as either sole, joint or advisory. This group comprised full- and part-time academic specialists in medical ethics as well as clinical and preclinical teachers who had a long-established interest in the subject.

A nodal expansion of ethics throughout the curriculum was planned which would allow students to develop their understanding of ethics as their scientific and clinical grasp of medicine increased. Three major teaching nodes were built into the 5 years of the curriculum with additional teaching taking place in clinical and specialist attachments. The teaching comprised core material, special study modules and an optional intercalated BSc in bioethics.

Ethics teaching at Bristol started in the first week of the first year of the medical course. A session on the doctor–patient relationship was followed by a session jointly taught with anatomy teachers and the university chaplain. This took place before the students entered the dissection room to begin their study of anatomy and aimed to provide a gentle introduction to what can be a somewhat traumatic experience for some. Both of these early sessions relied on accessing the students' views, opin-

---

Teaching ethics to large groups:
- Keep the session interactive
- Use video clips and other media
- Set up an ethics debate
- Divide the students into 'buzz' groups
- Team-teach with others
- Vary the style and pace.

"As part of its full integration into the curriculum, teaching in ethics and law should feature in the students' clinical experience, consistently forging links with good medical and surgical practice. Each clinical discipline should address ethical and legal issues of particular relevance to it and its students should be subject to assessment as they would be for any other teaching in that specialty. Students should be encouraged to present problems which they have personally encountered in their course"

Consensus statement 1998

ions, fears and aspirations at the point of entry to the medical profession. An exercise was conducted in which the new students devised a list of core ethical values with which they identified as doctors-to-be.

In the second term of year 1, the students underwent several afternoon sessions of ethics teaching spread over consecutive weeks. This core teaching formed part of the 'human basis of medicine' unit. Considerable reference was made to their visits to general practice in their first term as medical students. Topics covered included:

- the patient's values
- the patient's narrative
- going into hospital
- professional obligations
- the individual and society
- justice and healthcare.

These afternoon sessions took the form of a plenary presentation followed by small-group tutorials. Tutors were drawn from a range of disciplines and included nurses, hospital doctors and general practitioners. Assessment was by the submission of an essay at the end of the course, and an integrated examination paper at the end of the first year.

In year 3, an ethics symposium was held when the students returned from their first clinical attachment in secondary care. This day comprised small group tutorials and large group discussion of the ethical issues encountered by the students in hospitals, followed by plenary sessions on a range of ethical dilemmas.

Joint teaching also took place during a number of clinical attachments, including obstetrics and gynaecology, where the use of ethical cases and dilemmas was tailored to the relevant clinical situation.

In year 5, further ethics teaching was provided, enabling the students to enter the preregistration year with a renewed sense of confidence. This teaching focused on the demands and realities of the preregistration year, and provided a further opportunity for the students to discuss their fears, concerns and experiences within a safe setting.

Postgraduate teaching in medical ethics

The teaching of medical ethics now extends into postgraduate training and education for doctors and dentists; as in undergraduate curricula, ethics is often taught under an umbrella heading of professionalism and personal development. This title covers a variety of broader topics including: communication skills; professional duties and responsibilities; the avoidance of plagiarism and cheating; personal presentation; the importance of punctuality and good time-keeping; reflective practice, and teamwork and leadership.

One example is the Developing Professional Skills programme, offered since 2001 via the postgraduate deanery in the south-western region of England for doctors, dentists and other health professionals (South Western Medical Postgraduate Deanery). The author and Professor Colin Coles teach two of the components in this programme,

 Key points of the Bristol approach:
- student-centred teaching
- patient-centred ethics
- structured and incremental
- case-based
- grounded in theory but applied to clinical practice
- inclusive and humanistic approach
- team-teaching wherever appropriate
- interactive and nondidactic
- opportunity for discussion within a safe environment
- positive critique employed throughout.

 Why it was possible to develop ethics teaching at Bristol:
- a clearly visible senior academic leader
- dedicated academic and support staff
- a physical focus for ethics teaching in the form of the new centre
- policy documents which strongly emphasised the requirement for medical ethics teaching
- synchronicity of a major process of medical curriculum change across the UK
- a remit to coordinate and improve ethics teaching across the curriculum
- the enthusiasm of fellow teachers and students to embrace the teaching of medical ethics.

namely the core and ethics modules. Both modules provide an opportunity for clinicians to discuss ethical, legal and professional issues, and to discuss situations of uncertainty or ethical dilemmas which they have themselves faced. Many participants on these modules have commented on the benefits of stepping out of the clinical environment for a short while in order to consider the nature of professionalism in medicine and the challenges of ethical practice.

Another example is presented by the postgraduate workshops on medical ethics and law run by the Medical Defence Union in the UK (MDU). These workshops aim, *inter alia*, to prepare doctors (many of whom qualified overseas but are now working within the National Health Service) for the ethical questions they are likely to face in postgraduate job interviews or membership exams set by the medical Royal Colleges. These take place at a number of locations around the UK.

'Walking the talk'

The development of appropriate attitudes is implicit in the teaching of medical ethics. Attitudes are developed in a number of ways, and the example set by doctors, health professionals and senior medical students is an especially powerful form of teaching. The most commonly used visual aid in clinical teaching is the patient. Frequently patients are used as the subject of a clinical teaching session without being asked for their consent, without their being involved in the discussion or being referred to at all except in an offhand way. This is obviously unacceptable, and the GMC have made it clear in *Duties of a doctor* that doctors must:

- make the care of the patient their first concern
- treat every patient politely and considerately
- respect patients' dignity and privacy
- listen to patients and respect their views.

Many medical students and doctors will be aware of teaching situations, primarily in hospitals, where these rules have not been observed and where they have often felt acutely embarrassed to be present. Medical teachers have a duty to act as appropriate role models to junior colleagues in medicine and to other health professionals.

Just as bullying of students and juniors is still an unfortunate part of medical education in some places, so the humiliation of patients is present too – and it is up to all of us to change it! Nowhere is it more important that doctors display appropriate attitudes and ethical behaviour than in clinical teaching. This might be called 'walking the talk'. This does not mean that even the most conscientious doctors should expect always to get it right; the most credible clinical teacher is probably the one who admits to occasional mistakes, errors of judgment and lapses of concentration. Where he or she is prepared to admit to students, juniors or peers what they have learnt from such situations, and discuss possible remedies and solutions for similar problems which may occur in the future, there is the possibility for excellent practical teaching of ethics and professionalism to occur.

Giving praise and developing collegiality

Good medical teachers remember always that people respond much better to praise and constructive criticism than to criticism that is merely negative and destructive. Some medical teachers, principally in hospital and academic medicine, seem to believe that humiliation and constant negative criticism are acceptable and even successful teaching approaches. This is patently not so, and a change in this aspect of medical culture is required. Positive critique in which the emphasis is on what has gone well and what can be improved can have significant effects on the learner's self-esteem and confidence. Medical teachers sometimes underestimate the power of their words, both positive and negative; criticism which is made without thought and care can have a profound and lasting effect.

The development of collegiality in medical education, that is, treating student doctors and juniors with the respect, kindness and consideration with which one might treat one's peers, is vital. One occasionally comes across doctors whose bedside persona is exemplary, yet whose 'offstage' behaviour towards their colleagues, juniors, students and other health professionals is appalling. Ethics teaching should include this aspect of professionalism in its remit.

Sources of reference

Teaching materials for medical ethics abound. Perhaps the first resource to use is the experience of fellow medical teachers, students and patients; much of the best medical teaching starts from an anecdote, and this strongly applies to ethics. Students rate very highly ethics teaching which is directly applied to clinical situations, and which accesses their own views, ideas and opinions. Discussions and video clips can help to draw out these experiences, and CD-ROMs, videos and DVDs are freely available which can assist this process. New books on medical ethics are published regularly. The *Journal of Medical Ethics* and *Bioethics* are perhaps the best-known journals, containing topical articles and academic papers. The main medical journals invariably contain papers or correspondence on ethical issues.

In the UK, the General Medical Council publishes a number of pamphlets that are made freely available to doctors and medical students; these are also available online via the GMC website. Among these is the regularly updated set of booklets, *Duties of a doctor*, which includes *Good medical practice*. Medical regulatory bodies in other countries will usually have their own set of guidelines for incorporation into the ethics curriculum where appropriate. The *Oxford Practice Skills Course Manual* (Hope et al 1996) is an excellent source of materials for ethics teaching, containing as it does cases, vignettes and handouts. The Medical Defence Union (MDU) has provided each medical school in the UK with a teaching pack, *The MDU Introduction to Medical Ethics*, which contains materials and student handouts on consent and confidentiality (Brennan & Schutte 1997). Versions of the pack have also been produced for use in GP vocational training and dental schools. As with the other defence organisations, the MDU also provides members with publications containing advice on ethical practice.

An obvious (but sometimes underused) resource is the nonmedical media, the output of which can help immeasurably to keep teachers and students informed about medical ethics in practice. TV and radio, newspapers and magazines often present medical stories from the patients' or public's point of view; medical students and doctors need to appreciate this perspective. Every day there is a news report or media discussion of an ethical dilemma in medicine and health care. This coverage, wherever it is found, often provides the perfect material for discussion of ethical issues. Much of this material is available online.

Summary

A good understanding of medical ethics is central to the practice of good medicine. The study of ethics can act as the cement that binds the medical curriculum together, promoting the integration of preclinical and clinical teaching. Ethics teaching is able to benefit from the synthesis of many approaches and the involvement of many practitioners from the arts, humanities and law, science, technology and medicine.

All medical teachers have the responsibility to develop knowledge, skills and attitudes in 'tomorrow's doctors'. Teaching medical ethics provides a fine opportunity to help them develop their humanity. There can be no better reward or stronger incentive for a medical teacher.

Acknowledgments

Many thanks are due to my partner Sîan and my family for all their support. Thanks also to those who have taught me about ethics, law and professionalism. Most of all, I thank the students, doctors, dentists, health professionals and others with whom I have been privileged to work over the years. To all of you, I owe a great debt and express my deep appreciation.

"Patients must be able to trust doctors with their lives and wellbeing. To justify that trust, we as a profession have a duty to maintain a good standard of practice and care and to show respect for human life"

GMC 1998

References

Brennan M G, Schutte P 1997 The MDU introduction to medical ethics. Medical Defence Union, London

Consensus statement 1998 Teaching of medical ethics and law within medical education: a model for the UK curriculum Journal of Medical Ethics 24:188–192

Fulford K W M, Yates A, Hope T 1997 Ethics and the GMC core curriculum: a survey of resources in UK medical schools. Journal of Medical Ethics 23:82–87

GMC 1993, 2003 Tomorrow's doctors. Recommendations on undergraduate medical education. General Medical Council London

GMC 1998 Duties of a doctor. General Medical Council, London

Gillon R, Doyle L 1998 Medical ethics and law as a core subject in medical education. British Medical Journal 316:1623–1624

Hope T, Fulford K W M, Yates A 1996 The Oxford practice skills course manual. Oxford University Press, Oxford

MDU (Medical Defence Union). Online. www.the-mdu.com

Pond D 1987 Report of a working party on the teaching of medical ethics. Institute of Medical Ethics, London

South Western Medical Postgraduate Deanery. Online. www.swndeanery.co.uk

Further reading

Baxter C M, Brennan M G, Coldicott Y G M 2002 The practical guide to medical ethics and law. Pas Test, Knutsford, Cheshire

Brennan M G, Coles C 2003 Developing professional skills. The Lancet 362(9394):1506

Campbell A V, Gillet G, Jones G 2001 Medical ethics. Oxford University Press, Oxford

Hope T, Savulescu J, Hendrick J 2003 Medical ethics and law – the core curriculum. Churchill Livingstone, Edinburgh

Kennedy I, Grubb A 2000 Medical law, 3rd edn. Butterworths, London

Kultgen J 1998 Ethics and professionalism, University of Pennsylvania Press, Philadelphia

Kushner T K, Thomasma D C 2001 Ward ethics. Cambridge University Press, Cambridge

Schwartz L, Preece P A, Hendry R A 2002 Medical ethics – a case-based approach. Saunders, Edinburgh

Wear D, Bickel J 2000 Educating for professionalism – creating a culture of humanism in medical education, University of Iowa Press, Iowa City

Useful links

Centre for Ethics in Medicine, University of Bristol, 73 St Michael's Hill, Bristol BS2 8HW, UK
Tel: 0117 928 9843; www.bristol.ac.uk/Depts/Ethics
General Medical Council, 178 Great Portland Street, London W1N 6JE, UK
Tel: 0207 915 3568; fax: 0207 915 3599; email: standards@gmc-uk.org; www.gmc-uk.org
Medical Defence Union, 230 Blackfriars Road, London SE1 8PJ, UK
Tel: 0207 202 1500; email: mdu@the-mdu.com; www.the-mdu.com
South Western Medical Postgraduate Deanery, 1st Floor, Academic Centre, Frenchay Hospital, Bristol BS16 1LE, UK
www.swndeanery.co.uk

Chapter 28
Preparing for practice

M. E. T. McMurdo, M. D. Witham

"Medical education is not completed at medical school: it is only begun"

William H Welch 1850–1934

"I embarked on my career as a doctor brim-full of textbook learning and realised by lunchtime of the first day that I was as useful as a chocolate tea-pot. I knew all the sub-types of glomerulonephritis, but did not know how to organise an urgent CT scan, or how to tell a young wife that her husband had died"

A junior doctor

"I was a keen medical student among the top dozen in my year, but it still took me four or five weeks in post as a junior doctor to learn the ropes. With hindsight, I am sure that my medical school could have done more to have me better prepared"

A junior doctor

Introduction

The student–doctor transition

The purpose of undergraduate medical training is to produce newly qualified doctors who are well prepared for the responsibilities of their first year of practice. Medical curricula have been justifiably criticised in the past for having produced inadequately prepared graduates. The aim should be to provide a smooth transition of experience between undergraduate and doctor, rather than a step change.

Problems with conventional undergraduate teaching

Too often in the past, medical graduates have stepped onto the wards on their first day as a doctor only to discover themselves ill-equipped for the task in hand. This disconcerting experience can be a shattering one for the young doctor, but also means that the quality of clinical care delivered falls short of the high standard to which all physicians aspire. There is a need to ensure that students qualify having demonstrated competence in key skills and arrive armed with sufficient insight and prior experience of life as a junior doctor to function as a productive member of the clinical team from day one. The concept of the 'steep learning curve' for the new graduate is undoubtedly true, but our students (and their patients) will be better served by some progress along that curve prior to qualification.

What areas may be lacking?

Undergraduates must be trained to recognise that, although in their early student years it may take an hour to derive a history and examine a patient, this process has to be refined through experience to be rapid, efficient and thorough. It is at the point of graduation that newly qualified doctors must learn to trust their own clinical skills and become adept at distinguishing the sick from the well. Good communication with colleagues, focused evaluations, knowing what elements of assessment can be deferred, and knowing when to seek senior help are all essential to the survival of any junior doctor. This is even more vital in today's clinical environment, where reduced hours of working are leading to changing work patterns worldwide, with fragmented care the potential result.

Several areas may require further practice or experience before skills are attained:

- Streamlined and efficient history and examination. Most students can take a history and examine a patient, but the art of doing this rapidly under pressure of time and with frequent interruptions is a key skill for junior doctors.
- Requesting investigations and obtaining results. This is one of the main functions of junior doctors and requires good time management, familiarity with the role of other professionals, and a sound grasp of diplomacy.
- Management of common medical and surgical emergencies. All junior doctors should be confident in the management of patients with chest pain, breathlessness, overdose, an acute abdomen and cardiac arrest.
- Competence in core practical skills. By the time they reach their first job students should feel they have had sufficient supervised practice at common procedures such as venepuncture and bladder catheterisation.
- Time-management skills and an ability to prioritise tasks. One of the surprises of life as a junior doctor is how frequently your bleep sounds while you are in the middle of one task, which you may then have to leave to deal with a more pressing clinical problem. A clear mind, good note-taking and an ability to rank tasks in order of clinical need are essential. An ability to anticipate problems is the hallmark of a good junior doctor.
- Effective written and oral communication with patients, relatives and colleagues. Good documentation is an essential part of good clinical care and can provide an effective response to clinical complaints. Knowing what to write and what not to write, and meticulously recording discussions with relatives are important skills. Changes in junior doctors' hours means that the clear handover of clinical information from one shift to the next is crucial. The effective exchange of information between all members of the multidisciplinary team is based on an understanding of one another's roles and respect for the contribution of non-doctors to patient care.

"it is the embracing of responsibility and accountability that matures the clinician"

Smith 1996

Opportunities to rectify these problems

Reorientation of the undergraduate curriculum

Some recent recommendations on changes to the undergraduate curriculum have been made specifically to prepare young doctors better for clinical practice. Opportunities exist in revising medical courses to identify the elements of core clinical knowledge which all graduates should possess and generic skills in which graduates should be proficient. Good problem-solving and clinical reasoning skills are the foundation for learning effectively. An emphasis on teaching students how to acquire and evaluate information and on self-directed learning will also prepare graduates for lifelong learning.

Job shadowing

As an integral part of their training, medical students should spend some time shadowing a junior doctor. Ideally this experience should be in the hospital in which they will undertake their first post after qualifying. This offers considerable potential benefits:

- familiarisation with the day-to-day working of the unit, including management protocols
- familiarisation with laboratory services and request systems
- meeting future nursing, medical and paramedical colleagues
- spending time shadowing the individual whose job they will be doing
- the senior staff having a vested interest in ensuring that the students:
  - have a positive experience
  - demonstrate appropriate clinical judgment
  - participate in the work of the unit
  - identify and rectify any deficiencies in skills or behaviour.

Job shadowing should involve defined responsibilities for both day-time and night-time duties, acute receiving, clerking, ward rounds, scrubbing up and assisting in theatre, as well as gaining an insight into the role of other members of the multidisciplinary team.

In conjunction with the unit consultant, students should draw up and agree a timetable for each week which should include targeting known areas of weakness. Progress towards these targets should be reviewed midway through the attachment and activities redirected as necessary. Performance during job shadowing attachments may usefully be assessed jointly by both senior nursing and medical staff. Nursing staff often have considerably more day-to-day contact than consultants with both students and junior doctors, making their perspective invaluable. Part of the assessment process should include review of a logbook of cases, procedures witnessed or performed, and other experiences (see Work-based assessment, chapter 36). These should be countersigned by the member of staff who supervised them.

Induction days and handovers

Formal induction days are recommended for all junior doctors when arriving for their first medical post. Induction 'fairs' have been used successfully in some hospitals when information on key aspects of the young doctor's work can be presented to the entire cohort of new doctors.

Programmes should include:

- opportunities for discussion with key medical and nursing staff
- consultant and junior doctor views of the role of the new doctor
- teamworking with nursing staff
- time for a formal handover with the outgoing doctor
- duties of the doctor
- management of the dying patient
- pain relief
- cardiac arrest code and team
- medicolegal issues of consent, certification, reports to coroner
- dealing with complaints.

This introductory day should ensure the rapid integration of the new doctor into the working environment. It is, however, simply the beginning of what should be an ongoing process of education and information provided for junior doctors during their first year in practice.

Handbooks

For reference purposes, junior doctor handbooks can be very helpful. They should contain key information, including for example:

- list of useful contact phone numbers for laboratories, local doctors, accident and emergency
- details of which blood tubes are required for which tests
- practical procedures for arranging investigations within and outside normal working hours
- arrangements for resuscitation training
- the educational programme for the hospital
- local guidelines on the management of common presentations
- local drug formularies
- domestic arrangements such as accommodation, catering, security
- how to request annual and study leave
- on-call rotas.

Preparation courses

An alternative approach is to dedicate a portion of the final year of the undergraduate course to preparation for practice. Logically this should be timetabled near the end of final year when the impending realities of life as a junior doctor serve to concentrate the mind wonderfully. Such a course should not be seen as a 'stand-alone' item, but rather as an opportunity to polish those clinical and practical skills acquired throughout the curriculum which are necessary to function as a junior doctor. This provides an opening for interactive sessions, derived from the students' own experiences, on:

- medical ethics – informed consent and refusal of treatment, confidentiality, death pronouncement and certification, dying and palliation, transplantation
- teamworking and relationships with other colleagues
- defusing complaints, dealing with angry relatives, negotiation skills
- personal skills – time management and dealing with stress.

Presentations by junior doctors in post are greatly valued, and there is no doubt that this 'front-line troop' perspective is appreciated by students. Likely topics include:

- prioritising
- when to ask for senior help
- relationships with nursing staff
- incident and accident forms
- arranging admissions
- discharge arrangements
- the function of the junior doctor on the ward round

"The education of the doctor which goes on after he has his degree is, after all, the most important part of his education"

John Shaw Billings 1838–1913

Try to include only essential information in the junior doctor handbook. The longer you make it, the less likely it is to be read. Keep it short.

"I thought that I had done a good job talking to this patient's relatives about her prognosis. I was stunned when my attending physician received a letter of complaint about it from the family. This has shattered my confidence."

An intern

Junior doctor preparation should give priority to avoidance of life-threatening mistakes and illegalities.

"It was only when the coroner telephoned me two hours before the cremation that I realised I should have reported that the patient's death was the result of a road traffic accident"

A junior doctor

- what to write (and what not to write) in case notes
- night-time rounds
- on-call rotas.

There is scope at this point for students to discover the role of their professional bodies in their future lives: for example, the medical defence unions, medical associations, and registration authorities such as the General Medical Council.

Most students will also appreciate a brief overview from personnel services on:

- contracts
- hours of work
- pay and conditions
- annual leave entitlement
- grievance procedures
- counselling services.

Students may be helped to organise their knowledge in preparation for practice by working through examples of common 'nurse calls'. None of the material should be new; for example, all students will have covered the subject of 'pyrexia' during their course. Consideration of this material in the context of a clinical scenario with which they are certain to be faced in practice – 'Doctor, your patient has a temperature' – requires a subtle but crucially important change in thinking.

A session on practical therapeutics may be appropriate and should certainly cover prescribing for common conditions and the use of analgesics, laxatives and hypnotics. It should include:

- the need for clear and unambiguous prescribing
- the use of generic names
- nurse prescribing
- warfarin/insulin/steroid/fluid charts
- prescription review and discharge prescriptions
- the legal implications of failure to comply with good prescribing.

Part of the time of a junior doctor is spent undertaking practical procedures. Medical students should qualify with confidence in their ability to complete these tasks. Ideally competence should be demonstrated in a group of core practical procedures prior to graduation. This may involve devising a practical procedures checklist carried by the students through their clinical years, specifying which tasks are required, how frequently each should be performed and what level of competence is required. The signature of a clinician is necessary to confirm that the task has been performed to the expected standard. Examples of such practical procedures include:

- venepuncture
- giving an intravenous injection
- peripheral cannulation
- running through a drip
- setting up a syringe driver

"I vividly remember starting work as a junior doctor being asked to prescribe a laxative. I thought, hold on, I know four different types of dopamine receptor, but for the life of me, I couldn't come up with the name of a laxative. The staff nurse eventually told me what to write up"

A junior doctor

When considering the content of a preparation course, ask your own junior doctors what they wish they had known and what additional skills they wish they had possessed when they started.

- arterial blood sampling
- suturing
- recording an ECG
- basic cardiopulmonary resuscitation, and advanced life support including defibrillation
- bladder catheterisation (male and female).

For students who have failed to achieve these target skills or for others who simply wish to improve their technique, simulations involving models and manikins are now widely available. The ideal environment in which to practise and master such basics without the distraction of a patient is the clinical skills centre (see chapter 8). There is an expanding role for more complex simulation-based training, not only in the context of managing cardiac arrest, but also for recognising and instituting basic management of critically ill patients.

Continuing professional development

During the first year of medical practice new doctors will gain respect for and learn from the knowledge and skills of their senior colleagues. Wise new doctors will be acutely aware that they do not 'know it all', and nor are they expected to. They will know when to ask for senior advice. The rapid rate of expansion of medical knowledge means that a commitment to continuing professional development is vital. Ample opportunity for attendance at block release training courses and educational meetings should be an integral part of each junior doctor's post. In addition, the emerging role of senior colleagues who act as educational supervisors and mentors for junior doctors is welcomed.

Summary

There has been much debate in recent years about appropriate curricula for undergraduate medical education, with a specific concern being that the essential skills required by the graduate at the beginning of the junior doctor year are lacking. A variety of programmes and resources may be used to ensure that medical graduates 'hit the ground running'. Probably the most effective of these is job shadowing, undertaken ideally in the hospital in which the student will work during his or her first post after qualification. This usually works well as senior medical and nursing staff also profit from ensuring that the student develops appropriate skills and attitudes during the attachment.

Induction days and handovers are recommended for all junior doctors arriving for their first medical post. This should include time for a handover with the outgoing doctor, and ensure the rapid integration of the new doctor into the working environment.

Handbooks can be helpful reference guides, but should be kept concise. A dedicated preparation course is the alternative. It should incorporate interactive sessions on medicolegal topics and interpersonal skills, and should provide opportunities to practise key practical procedures.

"An inquiring, analytical mind; an unquenchable thirst for new knowledge; and a heart-felt compassion for the ailing – these are prominent traits among the committed clinicians who have preserved the passion for medicine."

Lois DeBakey

Where possible junior doctors should be involved in delivering the course as their front-line perspective is highly regarded by medical students. The course should not be seen as a 'stand-alone' item, but rather as the opportunity to hone the clinical and practical skills acquired throughout the entire curriculum. The first year in practice is a challenging period of rapid learning and professional growth but a variety of educational opportunities are available to ease the transition between medical student and junior doctor, and to ensure that medical graduates are better prepared for life in practice.

References

Smith L G 1996 First year of practice: a year of rapid learning. Academic Medicine 71:580–581

Further reading

Consensus Group of Teachers of Medical Ethics and Law in UK Medical Schools 1998 Teaching medical ethics and law within medical education: a model for the UK core curriculum. Journal of Medical Ethics 24:188–192

Cooper N 2003 Medical training did not teach me what I really needed to know. BMJ 327:s190

English W A, Nguyen-Van-Tam J S, Pearson J C G, Madeley R J 1995 Deficiencies in undergraduate and pre-registration medical training in prescribing for pain control. Medical Teacher 17:215–218

Frain J P, Frain A E, Carr P H 1996 Experience of medical senior house officers in preparing discharge summaries. British Medical Journal 312:350–351

GMC 1993 Tomorrow's doctors. General Medical Council, London

GMC 1997 The new doctor. General Medical Council, London

Goldacre M J, Lambert T, Evans J, Turner G 2003 Preregistration house officers' views on whether their experience at medical school prepared them for their jobs: national questionnaire survey. BMJ 326:1011–1012

Smith G B, Osgood V M, Crane S 2002 ALERT – a multiprofessional training course in the care of the acutely ill adult patient. Resuscitation 52(3):281–286

Chapter 29
Informatics

F. Sullivan, E. Mitchell

Introduction

We live in an information age. The emergence of digital computer technology has made it easier than it has ever been to store, collate, access and analyse data. Computers permeate every aspect of our lives and healthcare is no exception. That being the case it seems obvious that undergraduate medical education should be more firmly supported by informatics skills and evidence-based practice. The challenge for us as teachers is to meet the needs of students and to exceed their expectations. Encouraging students to identify and use information from a wider range of resources than their lecture notes and single textbooks demands more effort on their part to integrate information and it is more likely to result in deep learning.

Patients already acquire, process, and use healthcare-related evidence from a variety of sources including the press, television, radio and the internet (Fig. 29.1). Such patients will expect their physicians to be aware of everything that they know, and to be able to add further insights based on their understanding of the issue from more diverse sources. Patients may also begin to demand more computer use from their physicians as they realise that supported decisions are often better decisions (Coiera 1998).

Of course, informatics and evidence-based practice are not new concepts: an ability to interpret data, apply logic and manage uncertainty was taught by Hippocrates. However, the implications of the digital age are so profound that these have become important themes which ought to run throughout the undergraduate curriculum. The Conference of Heads of Medical Schools in the UK published a report identifying four informatics-related areas, derived from the General Medical Council's *Duties of a doctor*, *Tomorrow's doctors* and *New doctor* (CHMS Joint Working Group 1998). These are:

- record keeping
- ethical and legal imperatives
- professional communication
- education and research.

Various outcome attainments can be categorised in these areas.

Four areas of informatics

Record-keeping

Medical records serve a variety of functions. A definitive report on quality assessment in general practice suggests that records are more than an

"It is a very sad thing that nowadays there is so little useless information"

Oscar Wilde, novelist and playwright, 1854–1900

"Informatics is the study of the acquisition, processing and use of knowledge"

Friedman & Wyatt 1997

"Knowledge is of two kinds. We know a subject ourselves or we know where we can find information upon it"

Samuel Johnson, essayist and lexicographer, 1709–1784

"It is astonishing with how little knowledge a doctor can practice medicine, but it is not astonishing how badly he may do it"

W. Osler, *Aequanimitas*, in Bryan 1906

"The medical record is the link to accountability to the outside world"

CHMS 1998

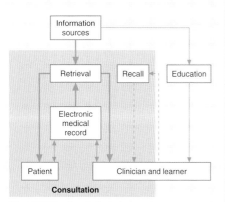

Fig. 29.1 Learning in an information age consultation

aide-memoire to the doctor or nurse and, furthermore, that good quality record keeping is an 'essential aspect of care' (Roland et al 1999). Completeness of information is an integral part of that quality along with legibility, accuracy and relevance of the information (Dick & Steen 1991).

The practice of keeping accurate and contemporaneous patient records can be emphasised by clinical skills courses. Indeed, taking a careful history and expertly eliciting physical signs may be negated by a poor record of the encounter. The use of simulated patients presenting the same challenges to several students allows learners to compare themselves with their colleagues. Tutors who ask to see the written records which students keep about every patient seen will encourage good record keeping. Patient records currently exist in various forms and using paper or electronic formats to emphasise the structure of a record may be helpful, especially in the early phases of the clinical apprenticeship.

In addition, some introduction to the alphanumeric coding systems used to standardise data recording, including the International Classification of Diseases (ICD), the Systemized Nomenclature of Medicine (SNOMED) and the Read Clinical Classification (for general practice) might also be of benefit.

Ethical and legal imperatives

The relative ease of access to patient information which has been created through the use of technology has resulted in the issuing of several pieces of guidance. In the UK, the Data Protection Act (1998) requires consent for the use of identifiable data relating to a person's health, whilst a subsequent government statute sanctions the use of such data if it is of 'substantial public interest' and does not cause 'substantial damage' or 'substantial distress' (Data Protection Statutory Instrument No. 417, 2000). The General Medical Council originally planned to discipline any doctor who provided patient data to a disease registry, but now takes a more moderate view of access to data (GMC 2000). But given the ambiguity of the guidelines, it is unsurprising that there is still confusion surrounding access to patient data (Mitchell 2003).

Briefing and debriefing of students may be used to direct attention to issues of security, confidentiality and the legal implications of what is recorded and stored about patients. Universities with a traditional forensic medicine 'course' need to supplement this with a 'right thing to do' theme as implemented in the University of Glasgow's problem-based learning (PBL) curriculum. This can run throughout the curriculum and involve ethicists, moral philosophers, lawyers and medical defence union staff. Specialist contributors may be used to teach directly and also to prepare teachers for the issues which arise in almost every encounter.

Professional communication

Recent initiatives and the drive towards clinical governance have placed increasing emphasis on patient information and its exchange within and across healthcare sectors. This is in keeping with the UK government's vision of an 'NHS information superhighway' (Department of Health 1997), to facilitate improved coordination of care through the safe flow of patient data between healthcare sectors. In Scotland, this has resulted in the establishment of the Electronic Clinical Communications Implementation (ECCI) programme. Communication between primary and secondary care is aided through a variety of ECCI functions, including electronic outpatient booking, use of email to solicit consultant opinion, ordering tests and receiving results through online links with laboratories, electronic clinic letters and discharge summaries and electronic referral letters containing all relevant information.

Thus, keeping colleagues and others informed about issues which are relevant to patient care can now be addressed in a variety of ways. Writing referral letters and discharge summaries is one method often used. Tutorials might also include completion of electronic letters based on clinical scenarios. Group discussions could include the development of a 'minimum dataset' to ensure that all relevant information is presented, as well as discussion on the implications, for both the patient and the practitioner, of missing information. Role play, with medical undergraduates adopting the role of other professionals, may be useful in prompting a deeper understanding from an alternative perspective. In other situations, shared learning may be appropriate, e.g. learning resuscitation with nurses (see Interprofessional education, chapter 18). Comparisons between medical and nursing records on ward rounds or in practice may be useful, as may attendance at multiprofessional case conferences. Asking students to record what they told the patients emphasises the importance of this skill. Whatever approach is used to develop these communication skills, it will increasingly involve computers.

Education and research

In Oxford, David Sackett integrated education and research by asking learners on ward rounds to summarise 20 things about the patient in less than two minutes, including something that they did not know about the patient but needed to know. Access to clinically useful information is increasingly straightforward using portals like TRIP or the National electronic Library for Health (NeLH) and resources such as Bandolier and GP Notebook. Searching these resources, or the primary literature, forms the basis for critical appraisal of the relevant evidence, which can then be stored as a critically appraised topic (CAT). Software to facilitate this process may be found at the website of the centre for Evidence-Based Medicine (CEBM).

Encounters with individual patients and communities could be used to build on this method more widely. Student-selected components (SSCs) provide additional scope to combine education and research. One example is for students to develop an educational tool for their peers. This might involve reviewing the literature to identify existing evidence on a particular clinical topic and using this to develop an electronic algorithm, stored in a simple office programme such as Access or PowerPoint, which can then be used by other students as a learning resource.

The 'virtual clinical campus': an ideal scenario

In an ideal situation, undergraduate students would be provided with educational challenges in the optimal sequence and at the most appropriate

"I find that a great part of the information I have, was acquired by looking up something and finding something else on the way"

Franklin P. Adams, Journalist, 1881–1960

rate for their learning needs (Friedman 1996). They would have easy access to patients, patient data, laboratories, libraries and teachers, wherever they were. Their assessment processes would emphasise the importance of applying the best evidence to meet the needs of their future patients. This is technologically feasible and, increasingly likely due to economic pressures, maturing technology and better infrastructure within the community. One of the key issues for educators will be to ensure that our students are able to critically appraise what they find in their literature searches (Jadad & Gagliardi 1998). Why does complete curricular integration of this theme not occur universally already? Several studies have identified financial, practical and educational issues which impede progress, but there are reports of innovative methods which can be used to overcome the barriers.

Staff development

Although few medical teachers have had the benefit of information technology (IT) training, most use a wide range of information resources in their scientific and/or clinical activities. This provides a sound basis for effective teaching in the four areas of informatics. However, some teachers have a narrower range of skills than they, their colleagues or their students might wish. The inevitable expansion of electronic educational resources means that we will all have to enhance our existing knowledge and skills in order to benefit our students. Responsibility for upgrading our capabilities should not only rest with individual teachers and the occasional journal article. Until the technology becomes easier to use, staff training and development needs to be provided by the medical school or university centrally.

Basic skills for students

When it comes to informatics, undergraduates, like their teachers, might describe themselves as 'nerds', 'norms' or 'phobes'. Nerds, self-evidently, need no training at all and may be useful resources for other students (and teachers). Norms need only an introduction to the facilities available but they may need some encouragement and support. Phobes may never have touched a computer and may not wish to do so. Gentle but firm reassurance that they will be able to cope may be required as well as extensive introductions to the facilities. Some medical schools have gone further by insisting that all new students buy a computer and a few have supplied the students with a palmtop PC (Oswald & Alderson 1998).

However, students are becoming more technologically adept before they even reach university. We recently carried out a questionnaire survey with over half of the first-year medical students attending the University of Dundee (n = 96; 54%). Almost all had used a computer before starting university and 94% had been using one for more than 3 years. Almost two-thirds of the students (62%) had at some time received training in computer use. Cheaper hardware and software mean that IT resources are now readily available to the majority of medical students in the developed world.

Develop the teachers.

Supply basic skills (and equipment) for those students who require them.

Vertical integration

Skilled teachers who wish to facilitate deep learning will direct students to a wide variety of computer-assisted learning resources held on compact disc (CD), digital video disc (DVD) and internet technologies. Many schools link these resources throughout the campus and some, such as Stanford in California, link learning resources for undergraduates and postgraduates via a simple search of high quality, integrated knowledge resources and paper versions following electronic information. The University of Sydney has structured its graduate programme around web-based multimedia. The International Virtual Medical School goes one stage further and links medical schools worldwide to provide a 'meta-campus' with a comprehensive, blended curriculum (IVIMEDS). Not only will this provide better access to medical education, but it will also allow students to experience learning through a variety of media and shared learning resources.

Internet-supplemented ward rounds, outpatient clinics and general practitioner surgeries are additional ways of enhancing the experience of the early years in medical school. PBL is a method which is particularly suited to informatics integration within curricula. Students in PBL curricula will expect to go beyond the material presented by patients and teachers, to retrieve more information and bring it into subsequent teaching sessions. Some useful websites for teaching have been identified and can be found at the end of this chapter.

Good use of resources

New forms of information technology are constantly being introduced into professional practice worldwide. In the UK, the NHS Information Management and Technology strategy states that,

> . . . information should be person based; systems should be integrated; management information should be derived from operational clinical systems; data should be secure and confidential; and data should be shared across the NHS.

> (Leaning 1993)

This policy can only serve to enhance educational opportunities. Rapid access to electronic laboratory data as well as to inpatient, ambulatory and community records is becoming possible via initiatives like ECCI. Subject to security concerns being addressed, it is likely that the technology employed by current, innovative sites which permit this in health maintenance organisations (HMOs) in the USA will become generally available.

Assessment in informatics

Any curriculum theme which is not examined will remain undervalued by the majority of students. Objective structured clinical examination (OSCE) stations could require students to review a patient record and decide whether a particular drug may be used safely. The Medical Independent Learning Examination (MILE) and the 'triple jump' are

Ensure vertical integration of informatics as a theme.

"On the internet no-one need know you're a dog"

Cartoon in *New Yorker* 1997

Make good use of resources, both existing and new.

"In 2021 computers will collect histories...together with the results of physical examination and special investigations. They will suggest diagnoses and therapy, taking into account previous experience and existing state of the art"

McManus 1991

Assess informatics skills, for example by emphasising project work.

methods of presenting students with a challenge which requires an initial review of a patient problem to be followed by critical appraisal of the literature and a second phase of examination based on the increased knowledge derived from the search (Smith 1993).

In addition, informatics can be used as a method of assessment in itself. A wide variety of assignments can be set using internet technologies and returned by students to their tutors via e-mail. These assignments and other aspects of the curriculum or its content can be discussed more widely by all students in electronic discussion groups. Internet technology also allows online evaluation, whereby students complete web-based questionnaires, the results of which can be automatically entered into a spreadsheet for analysis. DMS-online, the virtual learning centre of Dundee University Medical School, facilitates such informatics-based assessment in addition to providing learning resources for each year of the medical curriculum.

Essential skills

Ten essential clinical informatics skills have been identified by the University of Sydney Medical School. Students need to be able to:

- Understand the dynamic and uncertain nature of medical knowledge and be able to keep personal knowledge and skills up to date.
- Know how to search for and assess knowledge according to the statistical basis of scientific evidence.
- Understand some of the logical and statistical models of the diagnostic process.
- Interpret uncertain clinical data and deal with artefact and error.
- Structure and analyse clinical decisions in terms of risks and benefits.
- Apply and adapt clinical knowledge to the individual circumstances of the patients.
- Assess, select and apply a treatment guideline, adapt it to local circumstances, and communicate and record variations in treatment plan and outcome.
- Structure and record clinical data in a form appropriate for the immediate clinical task, for communication with colleagues, or for epidemiological purposes.
- Select and operate the most appropriate communication method for a given task (e.g. face-to-face conversation, telephone, email, video, voicemail, letter).
- Structure and communicate messages in a manner most suited to the recipient, task and chosen communication medium.

One further method of assessing students' informatics skills is to require them to conduct project work such as carrying out an audit (Morrison & Sullivan 1997) (Fig. 29.2). This has the added advantage of encouraging students to work at the higher levels of Bloom's cognitive taxonomy, integrating information from multiple sources (Bloom et al 1971). One example involves students on a four-week general practice attachment being briefed about an evidence-based audit project and sup-

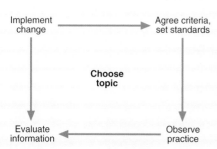

Fig. 29.2 The audit cycle

ported in the different phases of the project by departmental staff and tutors trained in evidence-based practice skills. The topic to be studied may be chosen on the basis of a critical incident during the early days of an attachment, a personal interest or a practice concern. Students need evidence-based resources to decide which criteria should be studied in that topic, what level of performance denotes high quality care, and what changes need to occur. The type of evidence used in projects by final year undergraduate students may include published studies, guidelines, policy statements and local protocols. This approach integrates many of the aforementioned practical methods of ensuring that informatics skills are employed to encourage evidence-based practice. Moreover, students and teachers seem to enjoy it.

Summary

Medical teachers need to obtain and transmit informatics skills and to rely upon evidence to a greater extent than ever before. As the technology to sustain this change becomes more widespread, the task will become more straightforward. We should embrace the opportunities to integrate informatics and evidence-based practice throughout the curriculum to improve the quality of teaching and make it even more enjoyable.

"A worthwhile exercise in information gathering and communication with the primary healthcare team"
"It is very satisfying to be involved in something that the GPs could make use of"

Students commenting on an evidence-based audit project

References

Bandolier. www.jr2.ox.ac.uk/bandolier

Bryan C S 1906 Osler: inspirations from a great physician. Oxford University Press, Oxford

Bloom B S, Hastings J T, Madaus G F (eds) 1971 Appendix. Condensed version of the taxonomy of educational objectives. In: Handbook on formative and summative evaluation of student learning. McGraw-Hill, London

CEBM catmaker (Centre for Evidence-Based Medicine). www.cebm.net/catmaker.asp

Coiera E 1998 Medical informatics meets medical education. Medical Journal of Australia 168:319–320

CHMS (Conference of Heads of Medical Schools) Joint Working Group 1998 Informatics in medical and dental undergraduate curricula. National Health Service Executive, London

Data Protection Act 1998 HMSO, London

Data Protection (Processing of Sensitive Personal Data) Order 2000 Statutory instrument 2000 no. 417. HMSO, London

Department of Health 1997 The new NHS. HMSO, London

Dick R S, Steen E B (eds) 1991 The computer based patient record: an essential technology for health care. National Academy Press, Washington DC

Friedman C P 1996 The virtual clinical campus. Academic Medicine 71(6):647–651

Friedman C P, Wyatt J C 1997 Evaluation methods in medical informatics. Springer, New York

GMC 2000 Confidentiality: protecting and providing information. General Medical Council, London

GP Notebook. www.gpnotebook.co.uk

IVIMEDS (International Virtual Medical School) www.ivimeds.org

Jadad A R, Gagliardi A 1998 Rating health information on the Internet: navigating to knowledge or to Babel? Journal of the American Medical Informatics Association 279(8):611–614

Leaning M S 1993 The new information management and technology strategy of the NHS. British Medical Journal 307:217

McManus I 1991. How will medical education change? Lancet 337:1519–1521

Mitchell E 2003 Invited commentary: patient derived data, so why not patient determined access? The Journal on Information Technology in Healthcare 1(1):46–48

Morrison J M, Sullivan F M 1997 Audit in general practice: educating medical students. Medical Education 31:128–131

NeLH (National electronic Library for Health). www.nelh.nhs.uk/

Oswald N, Alderson T 1998 Basic medical education in primary care. The report and evaluation of the Cambridge community based clinical course 1993–8. GP Education Group, School of Medicine, University of Cambridge, Cambridge

Roland M, Holden J, Campbell S 1999 Quality assessment for general practice: supporting clinical governance in primary care groups. National Primary Care Research and Development Centre, Manchester

Smith R M 1993 The triple jump examination as an assessment tool in the problem-based medical curriculum at Hawaii University. Academic Medicine 68:366–372

TRIP. www.update-software.com/scripts/clibng/html/tripusernamelogon.htm

University of Glasgow. PBL curriculum http://www.gla.ac.uk/generalpractice/routemaps_home.htm

Useful links

Educational websites

Bristol Biomedical Image Archive. Around 8500 images, including medical and dental, donated by academics around the world for the purposes of teaching and learning. www.brisbio.ac.uk/index.html

Centre for Evidence-Based Medicine. www.cebm.net

GHIFT (Gateway to Health Informatics for Teaching). A database of information and resources to support education and training in informatics in the UK. www.chime.ucl.a.ac.uk/resources/GHIFT

Guide to Medical Informatics, the Internet and Telemedicine. www.coiera.com

OMNI (Organising Medical Networked Information). This project is a UK initiative which acts as a gateway to sources of biomedical information. http://omni.ac.uk

The Risk Files. A free publication dedicated to informing healthcare professionals about the internet and related issues. It is compiled and issued monthly by Ahmad Risk and delivered by email. www.cybermedic.org

The Virtual Heart. Descriptions of cardiac function and pathology with audio and visual clips. http://sln.fi.edu/biosci/heart.html

Free Access to Medline

PubMed. The National Library of Medicine's search service of over 16 million citations in 9000 journals since 1967, based in Bethesda USA. Very fast. www.ncbi.nlm.nih.gov/PubMed

Chapter 30
Evidence-based medicine

C. Heneghan, P. Glasziou

Introduction

Doctors and other healthcare workers must not only keep pace with the rapid changes in medical knowledge, they must assimilate new relevant and valid research into their clinical expertise, and appropriately alter their clinical practice and organisation. The practice of evidence-based medicine (EBM) is a process of lifelong, self-directed learning, in which caring for our patients gives rise to clinically important questions and information about diagnosis, therapy, prognosis and other aspects of healthcare. The methods of EBM aim to provide skills that help clinicians to rapidly assimilate new evidence and ideas and put them into practice.

We can summarise the EBM approach as a five-step process (Sackett et al 2000):

- asking answerable clinical questions
- searching for the best research evidence
- critically appraising the evidence for its validity and relevance
- applying the evidence to groups and individuals
- evaluating your own self-education performance.

To be able to teach these well you should first reflect on your own practice. How well are you keeping up to date? How often are you finding answers to the questions that arise in your practice? If you don't currently feel proficient, then you might consider one of the many available courses in practising and/or teaching EBM (for example, see the website of the Oxford Centre for Evidence-Based Medicine).

Introductory lecture – an hour on awareness raising

Any course you will teach will need to identify the key themes and concepts – to give a road map of where we are going and why. Initial concepts include the nature of EBM (sometimes called 'evidence-based practice'), the problem of information overload, the need to discriminate between good and poor quality evidence, and how EBM can help.

Important themes

Important themes include the attempt to keep up to date and the problem of how to select from the ever-increasing world literature. Over 20 000

"Evidence based medicine is the conscientious, explicit and judicious use of the best current evidence in making decisions about the care of individual patients"

Sackett et al 2000

"Change your thought and you change your world"

Norman Vincent Peale

"My students are dismayed when I say to them 'Half of what you are taught as medical students in 10 years has been shown to be wrong. And the trouble is, none of your teachers knows which half."

Dr Sydney Burwell, Dean of Harvard Medical School

"Doctors are inundated with new, often poorly evidence-based and sometimes conflicting clinical information. This is particularly serious for the generalist, with over 400 000 articles added to the biomedical literature each year"

Dave Davis

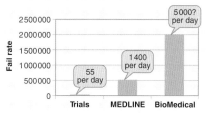

Fig. 30.1 The amount of medical research

randomized controlled trials (RCTs) are published each year (with a cumulative total of over 350 000) and approximately 50 new trials are published every day (Fig. 30.1). A general practitioner would have to read one RCT every half hour, night and day, to keep up to date just with the results of trials.

You might stop and ask your learners to reflect on how they currently learn and keep up to date. You might also ask them how much time is being spent on each process. Activities usually identified include: attending lectures and conferences; reading articles in journals; tutorials; using textbooks and clinical guidelines; clinical practice; small-group learning and study groups; using electronic resources, and speaking to colleagues and specialists. There is no right or wrong way to learn, a mixture of all of these methods will be beneficial in the overall process of gathering information.

It is helpful to think of learning needs, as a process of gathering information in two different ways: 'push' and 'pull'.

The 'push' is when we extract information from the array of resources that arrive in our post or email, on a variety of topics. This type of learning can be thought of as 'just in case learning'. When information is provided that is important to clinical practice and has already been appraised for certain validity criteria it can be very useful (see for example *Evidence Based Medicine* and *Clinical Evidence*, available in print versions as well as online; see Useful links at the end of this chapter).

Although we are not advocating any one style of learning over another, in medicine and all other healthcare areas, events are rapidly changing and we need to focus more on the 'pull' strategy: information to serve our current clinical problems. The 'pull' process, which can be thought of as a 'just in time' learning method, looks at how to formulate questions and 'pull' answers out of the literature as you need them. Effective strategies can lead to answers in less than two minutes!

Evaluate your own learning strategies and your learners
- Write down one recent patient problem.
- What was the critical question?
- Did you answer it? If so, how?

EBM is only one component of the many elements that go into teaching clinical practice. It supplements rather than replaces clinical expertise. It is a process of lifelong, self-directed learning in which caring for our patients creates clinically important information needs. Samples of introductory presentations are available free from the Oxford Centre for Evidence-Based Medicine website.

Asking answerable questions

Teaching the formulation of question is best done in small groups with approximately seven to eight students per tutor. If you are teaching this topic, think about recruiting some help (who is available in your department?) to guide the groups as they formulate their clinical questions. You should consider following or combining this session with searching skills.

"There is no such thing as a long piece of work, except one that you dare not start"

Charles Baudelaire

Your librarians may have skills, unbeknownst to you, that might help in this area.

Use the PICO principle to formulate the questions:

- **P**opulation/patient – what is the disease problem?
- **I**ntervention/indicator – what main treatment is being considered?
- **C**omparator/control – is this in relation to an alternative?
- **O**utcome – what are the main outcomes of interest to the patient?

Dissect the question into its component parts and then restructure it so that the components can be used to direct the search.

Scenarios are useful to teach question building

For the less experienced student, you might begin with short scenarios that lend themselves to splitting the question(s) easily. For the more experienced learners, let them loose on a scenario that incorporates all the types of questions that are possible. It is relevant to think of the type of question you want to ask, as it will affect where you look for the answer and what type of research you can expect to provide it.

While it sounds easy to teach question formulation, it is more difficult to get students to carry it out in their daily clinical duties.

How you are going to integrate asking questions into your own practice?

The challenge to the teacher is to identify questions that are both problem-based and orientated to the learners' needs; at the same time you will also be identifying gaps in your own knowledge which may need to be addressed. Think of how you and your students are going to keep track of the questions and come to a clinically useful answer.

One way is to use an educational prescription (Fig. 30.2), available for download from the Oxford Centre for Evidence-Based Medicine website. Another way is to provide clinical question 'logbooks', small pocket notebooks to store questions in. If you try and achieve two questions a week and ask your group to do the same, then time spent on answering them ought to be less than an hour. This means that in your small group, including yourself, you should be generating approximately 20 clinically useful answers each week.

Remember to recognise potential questions which are clinically useful to you and your learners, decide which of the questions to focus on, guide your learners in to developing useful questions, and assess their performance in building and asking answerable questions. Once clinical questions have been formulated (step 1) it is helpful to quickly follow up by letting students loose on searching for the answers.

Searching for the evidence

Resources that you will need include:

- if available, a computer laboratory with internet access
- one terminal for every two students

Typology for question building

Clinical findings: how to interpret findings from the history and examination.

Aetiology: the causes of diseases.

Diagnosis: what tests are going to aid you in the diagnosis?

Prognosis: the probable course of the disease over time and the possible outcomes.

Therapy: which treatment are you going to choose, based on beneficial outcomes, harms, cost and your patient's values?

Prevention: primary and secondary risk factors which may or may not lead to an intervention.

Cost-effectiveness: is one intervention more cost-effective than another?

Quality of life: what effect does the intervention have on the quality of your patient's life?

Phenomena: the qualitative or narrative aspects of the problem.

R̶x EDUCATIONAL PRESCRIPTION

Date and Place to be presented

THE PATIENT PROBLEM

The intervention:
(therapeutic, diagnostic, prognostic, causal)

Vs alternatives

The Target Outcome/s
(a change in the risk or likelihood of):

The Learner:

Presentations will cover:
1. HOW you found what you found, i.e. Search Strategies;
2. WHAT you found (the bottom line);
3. the VALIDITY and APPLICABILITY of what you found (the critical appraisal);
4. How what you found will ALTER your MANAGEMENT of such patients;
5. How WELL you think you DID in filling this Rx.

Fig. 30.2 Educational prescription (adapted with permission from the Centre for Evidence-Based Medicine)

- if available, data projection linked up to a computer with database access for students to view searches in action
- internet access or access to medical research databases.

We recommend the following two databases in searching for the evidence.

- *PubMed*, and
- *the Cochrane Library*

Use these two databases as a starting point because they are both free to access for users in many countries. Using PubMed allows all the concepts of proficient searching to be taught. It also has the very useful 'Clinical Queries' section: a question-focused interface with filters for identifying the more appropriate studies for questions of therapy, prognosis, diagnosis and aetiology. The Cochrane Library contains a number of databases, the Cochrane Database of Systematic Reviews, the Controlled Trials Register (CENTRAL) and the Database of Abstracts of Reviews of Effectiveness (DARE).

The success of problem-based learning depends on the ability to find the current best evidence effectively

Finding answers to questions can be highly rewarding when done well with speed or can be frustrating and time consuming when done poorly. A study of 103 GPs showed that they generated about ten questions over a two-and-half-day period. They tried to find the answers for about half of them. The most critical factor influencing which questions they followed up was how long they thought it would take to obtain an answer. If they thought the answer would be available in less than a couple of minutes, they were prepared to look for it. If they thought it would take longer, they would not bother. Only two questions in the whole study (0.2%) were followed up using a proper electronic literature search (Ely et al 1999).

A similar study in 64 hospital residents (Green et al 2000) revealed they asked an average of two questions per three patients. They pursued an answer for 80 questions (29%); their reasons for not pursuing answers were lack of time and because they forgot the question. When they did answer the question, textbooks were used 31% of the time, articles 21% and they asked their consultants 17% of the time.

How are you going to maintain searching skills?

In teaching searching skills think of the resources you have available to you. Librarians are currently changing the way they work; they often have knowledge in this area far beyond the skills of a busy clinician. They often run courses and workshops; if they aren't then consider approaching them to begin setting them up. On a personal level you should be proficient in searching; often you will be asked questions about searching strategies: 'Which database to use?' 'Why do I seem to get so many articles?'

Converting your question into a search strategy

It is often best to have a prepared scenario which generates a four-part question and leads on to demonstrating some of the key components of an effective search strategy. For example:

- In a five-year-old with a fever and a red bulging tympanic membrane should I prescribe antibiotics or watch and wait?
  (Clinically useful answer in the Cochrane database of systematic reviews in Glasziou et al 2004.)
- A 35-year-old lady came to clinic with a fresh dog-bite and she wanted to know whether she should have some prophylactic antibiotics.
  (Clinically useful answer in PubMed/Medline, in Cummings 1994.)

There are two main types of strategy for searching bibliographic databases: thesaurus searching (all articles are indexed under subject headings, so if you search for a specific heading you will pick up potentially relevant materials) and text-word searching (where you search for specific words or phrases in the studies' bibliographic record). Once the question has been broken down into its components (see Table 30.1), it can be combined using Boolean operators 'AND' and 'OR' (Fig. 30.3).

In combining terms into a search strategy, it can be useful to represent them as a Venn diagram (Fig. 30.4). Complex combinations can then be structured. Once this level of skill has been achieved, then it is time to let your students search on their own questions that they have generated.

Critically appraising the evidence for its validity and relevance

The initial steps in applying the evidence revolve around what to look out for in individual or combined trials to determine whether the results are valid and clinically useful. This process developed by epidemiologists and statisticians for assessing trials, is called 'critical appraisal'. Initially it is worth presenting in a lecture format some of the key concepts involved in appraisal, why it is important and some of the potential pitfalls. Flecainide

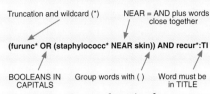

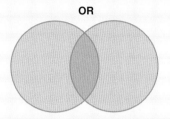

Fig. 30.3 Tips and tactics for searching

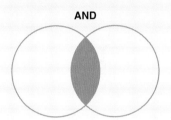

Fig. 30.4

Table 30.1 Applying the PICO principle

Question: In a 65-year-old man with heart failure does the addition of a beta-blocker compared with usual care improve survival?

Question part	Question term	Synonyms
Patient/problem	Adult, Heart failure	Left ventricular failure, congestive heart failure, NYHA classification
Intervention	Beta-blocker	Metoprolol, carvedilol,
Comparison	Usual care, standard therapy	
Outcome	Mortality	Death*, survival

use in the treatment of ventricular arrhythmias (Anderson et al 1981, Echt et al 1991) is an illustration of potential pitfalls.

If you are about to embark on teaching critical appraisal, consider how proficient you are yourself in appraisal of the following study types:

- therapy
- diagnosis
- systematic reviews
- harm/aetiology
- prognosis
- economic analysis optional.

If you do not feel confident, then refer back to the EBM book by Sackett and colleagues (2000) or consider attending a workshop on teaching and practising EBM (Oxford Centre for Evidence-Based Medicine).

Critical appraisal

Teaching the details of critical appraisal lends itself to small-group work. Small-group work allows generation of free discussion of these new concepts between the group leader and the participants, enabling them to gain knowledge from their peers. As with many intellectual skills, practice, discussion and feedback are helpful for faster and deeper learning.

Tutors can function in many different ways. They can identify errors in the group's interpretations of concepts and also act as a listener. The teacher's role is to set the ground rules for individual sessions. Pick out the educational needs and adapt the tutorial style accordingly (see chapter 7, Learning in small groups, and Elwyn et al 2001).

Working through critical appraisal

To help you, we suggest that you have some prepared critical appraisal worksheets to guide the process. You can design your own but there are many available which will help you. See for example:

- Oxford Centre for Evidence-Based Medicine (free downloads of critical appraisal worksheets)
- Centre for Health Evidence, University of Alberta
- Public Health Resource Unit
- Centre for Evidence-Based Medicine, Mount Sinai, Toronto
- Glasziou et al 2003
- Badenoch et al 1999.

Pitfalls and solutions

Small-group work can sometimes be relatively unprofitable when the individuals are not especially motivated. One useful trick here is to give the group a choice of content topics, e.g. by voting on which of several questions they wish to address. Since the appraisal process will be similar, this flexibility and choice improves engagement.

Participants may have differing levels of knowledge, resulting in time-consuming discussion about areas that some find boring. A way of

"Opportunity is missed by most people because it is dressed in overalls and looks like work"

Thomas A. Edison

dealing with this is to get the group to break into pairs for some periods, and allow more experienced students to help less experienced ones.

It is important to set clear objectives at the outset of a discussion. This helps to avoid heading off at tangents, with participants being left confused about what they are actually trying to learn. This can occur when the agenda is too large or varied.

It is useful to evaluate your performance by taking a few minutes at the end of the session to discuss whether participants felt their needs were met by this particular style of learning. This will not always be the case, and sometimes it will be seen that a more didactic approach is needed.

Crunching the numbers

You and the learners should become proficient with most of the outcome variables that are possible in trials. Results can be expressed in many ways and you should feel comfortable in demonstrating the calculations involved, such as those for:

- relative risk
- absolute risk reduction
- relative risk reduction
- number needed to treat (NNT)
- odds ratios
- sensitivity and specificity
- pre-test probabilities, likelihood ratios and post-test probabilities.

Do not expect your learners to calculate all of these variables all of the time, but they should be able to calculate NNTs and relative risks; however the more complex calculations may put them off. Introduce the use of a nomogram (Fig. 30.5) to aid diagnostic decision making.

Confidence intervals and *P* values

This is the branch of statistical analysis that will bring fear to some of your students. Remember that most people will only need to be users of statistics not 'doers'; interpretation is vital but calculation is unnecessary. So you might explain that all studies are subject to some random error, and that the best we can do is estimate the true risk based on the sample of subjects in a trial (called the point estimate). Statistics provide two estimates of the likelihood that a result was not due to random error:

- P values (hypothesis testing)
- confidence intervals (estimation).

Do not go into the statistical methods of calculating the answers. Provide discussion about the relevant methods and why an intervention can only be considered useful if the 95% confidence interval (CI) includes a clinically important treatment effect. Make a distinction between statistical significance and clinical importance:

- *Statistical significance* relates to the size of the effect and the 95% CIs in relation to the null hypothesis.

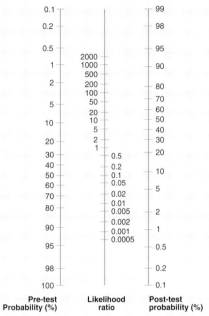

Fig. 30.5 Nomogram for converting pre-test probabilities into post-test probabilities for a diagnostic test result with a given likelihood ratio (reproduced with permission from the Oxford Centre for Evidence-Based Medicine)

"Statistics is a matter of common sense but it is a matter of ADVANCED common sense"

Stephen Senn

- *Clinical importance* relates to the size of the effect and to a minimum effect that would be considered to be sufficiently important to change practice.

Applying the evidence

The questions you should consider before you decide to apply the results of a study to your patient are:

- Is the treatment feasible in my setting?
- Is my patient similar to those of the study?
- What alternatives are available?
- Will the potential benefits outweigh the harms?
- What does the patient value?

Communication skills and risk

You can use the final step of reading a paper as a chance for your students to practise their communication skills. If you put a scenario to your learners before the outset of your critical appraisal and ask for their opinions based on their current knowledge, it can be enlightening to see how the evidence can alter management in the light of new information. Think of how you communicate risk: it isn't easy.

Two studies illustrate the point (Gigerenzer & Edwards 2003, Hoffrage & Gigerenzer, 1998). Doctors with an average of 14 years of professional experience were asked to imagine using the Haemoccult test to screen for colorectal cancer.

> *The prevalence of cancer was 0.3%, the sensitivity of the test was 50%, and the false-positive rate was 3%.*
> *The doctors were asked: "What is the probability that someone who tests positive actually has colorectal cancer?"*

The correct answer is about 5%. However, the doctors' answers ranged from 1% to 99%, with about half of them estimating the probability as 50% (the sensitivity) or 47% (sensitivity minus false-positive rate). If patients knew about this degree of variability and statistical innumeracy they would be justly alarmed.

Consider getting to grips with presenting information in terms of natural frequencies; information is often presented to us in confusing language, so it is no wonder that our own patients will often be confused.

Evaluating your own performance

The most important evaluations are the ones you and your learners design and carry out yourselves. The questions you might want to ask of yourself include:

- How many questions am I recording?
- Am I using different databases in my search strategies?

"Increasingly this is not good enough. There is a need for numbers, and many doctors don't feel easy with numbers. 'Can you,' asks Tze-Wey Loong, 'explain why a test with 95% sensitivity might identify only 1% of affected people in the general population?' My guess is that not one BMJ reader in a thousand could answer that question, but the numbers are in many ways the easy bit. The communication is the harder bit"

Richard Smith 2003, Editor of the BMJ

"I can live with doubt and uncertainty and not knowing. I think it is much more interesting to live not knowing than to have answers that might be wrong"

Richard Feynman

- Am I challenging my colleagues about everyday decisions?
- Am I answering my questions?
- Has my practice changed?

Think of how you might want to be evaluated. Small presentations such as in a journal club can be a valuable way of appraising students whilst increasing everyone's knowledge. Are you creating critically appraised topics (CATs)? These are structured appraisals incorporating all of the relevant points you would want to know from a study; a free downloadable version of a CAT-maker is available at the Oxford centre for Evidence-Based Medicine website. Are you setting clearly defined objectives in your small groups, and is this meeting the needs of your students? If your learners are creating important information, think of how you might want to store this resource. You might create a database that could be accessed by others in fields related to yours.

Integrating EBM into your curriculum

Consider finding a like-minded individual who will help you to design and carry out the introduction and maintenance of an EBM course. You can have a rapid introduction to EBM in one-day courses, and there are several good workbooks available to guide you in this process (Glasziou et al 2003). A one-day course would comprise an introductory lecture, and cover searching skills and critical appraisal in small groups.

It is possible to integrate EBM throughout the course of a year making your scenarios relevant to the different disciplines that a student will encounter. It is essential to demonstrate that you are practising EBM in your own clinical duties; leading by example is an excellent way to illustrate how evidence can be incorporated into your patient care. Be adventurous and try different strategies, mix and match lectures and small-group work; think about introducing a journal club for all those questions that still need answering. Join up with practitioners from different areas, and consider refreshing your skills at one of the many courses available (see for example, the Oxford Centre for Evidence-Based Medicine).

Summary

The traditional flow of continuing medical education (CME) is that research is formulated into guidelines or reviews (evidence-based we hope!), packaged into CME and presented in journals or at educational sessions, to be later retrieved and applied at the appropriate clinical moment. We suggest instead that the traditional flow should be reversed and the choice of topics on which to gather information should come directly from caring for our patients.

Use a variety of strategies to incorporate the five steps of EBM into your course. Essential to this process is the teacher's role as an effective practitioner of EBM.

"There is nothing more difficult to plan, more doubtful of success, nor more dangerous to manage than the creation of a new order of things. . . . Whenever his enemies have the ability to attack the innovator they do so with the passion of partisans, while the others defend him sluggishly, so that the innovator and his partner are vulnerable"

Niccolo Machiavelli, *The Prince*

"One must learn by doing the thing, for though you think you know it, you have no certainty until you try"

Sophocles, 400 BC

References

Anderson J L, Stewart J R, Perry B A et al 1981 Oral flecainide acetate for the treatment of ventricular arrhythmias. New England Journal of Medicine 305:473–477

Badenoch D, Straus S, Richardson W S et al 1999 Practising evidence based medicine. Evidence based medicine workbooks. BMJ Publishing Group, London

Centre for Evidence-Based Medicine, Mount Sinai, Toronto. www.cebm.utoronto.ca

Centre for Health Evidence, University of Alberta. www.cche.net/che/home.asp

Cochrane Library. www.cochrane.org

Cummings P 1994 Antibiotics to prevent infection in patients with dog bite wounds: a meta-analysis of randomized trials. Annals of Emergency Medicine 23(3):535–540

Echt D S, Liebson P R, Mitchell L B et al 1991 Mortality and morbidity in patients receiving ecainide, flecainide, or placebo. The Cardiac Arrhythmia Suppression Trial. New England Journal of Medicine 324:781–788

Elwyn G, Greenhalgh G, McFarlane F 2001 A guide to small group work in healthcare, management, education and research. Radcliffe Medical Press, Oxford

Ely J W, Osheroff J A, Ebell M H et al 1999 Analysis of questions asked by family doctors regarding patient care. British Medical Journal 319:358–361

Gigerenzer G, Edwards A 2003. Simple tools for understanding risks: from innumeracy to insight. BMJ 327:741–744

Glasziou P, Del Mar C, Salisbury, J 2003 Evidence based medicine workbook. BMJ Publishing Group, London

Glasziou P P, Del Mar C B, Sanders S L, Hayem M 2004 Antibiotics for acute otitis media in children (Cochrane review). Cochrane Library, issue 1. John Wiley, Chichester, UK

Green M L, Ciampi M A, Ellis P J 2000 Residents' medical information needs in clinic: are they being met? American Journal of Medicine 109:218–233

Hoffrage U, Gigerenzer G 1998 Using natural frequencies to improve diagnostic inferences. Academic Medicine 73:538–540

Oxford Centre for Evidence-Based Medicine. http://www.cebm.net/ ; downloads http://www.cebm.net/downloads.asp

Public Health Resource Unit. www.phru.nhs.uk/casp/appraisa.htm

PubMed. www.ncbi.nlm.nih.gov/entry/query.fcgi

Sackett D L, Straus S E, Richardson W S et al 2000 Evidence-based medicine: how to practice and teach EBM. Churchill Livingstone, New York

Useful links

Centre for Evidence-Based Medicine, Mount Sinai, Toronto. www.cebm.utoronto.ca

Centre for Health Evidence, University of Alberta. www.cche.net/che/home.asp

Clinical Evidence. http://www.clinicalevidence.com

The Cochrane Library. www.cochrane.org.

Evidence Based Medicine. http://www.ebm.bmjjournals.com

Oxford Centre for Evidence-Based Medicine. http://www.cebm.net/ ; downloads http://www.cebm.net/downloads.asp

Public Health Resource Unit. www.phru.nhs.uk/casp/appraisa.htm

Pub Med. www.ncbi.nlm.nih.gov/entry/query.fcgi

SECTION 6
ASSESSMENT

Chapter 31
Principles of assessment

M. Friedman Ben-David

Formative and summative assessment

Formative and summative assessment are two important concepts, which direct the design of an assessment system. The decision to employ summative, formative or a combination of both forms of assessment will guide the instrument selection, the manner by which assessment is implemented, the amount of manpower needed, the score interpretation and the use of assessment results.

In the formative process, we assess in order to intervene with intent to improve. In the summative process, we assess in order to make such decisions as good/bad, ready to move forward, repeat a programme.

In general, students' achievements are assessed for many purposes:

- assuring that an individual meets predetermined minimal qualifications
- identifying individuals who have achieved a level required for promotion to the next level or who need to repeat the programme.
- selecting the best candidates for a given programme
- allowing students to monitor their own learning
- providing information regarding student level of achievement
- generating performance profiles of students' strengths and weaknesses.

Traditionally, the first three of these are associated with summative assessment and the last three with formative assessment.

For selection and promotion purposes (graduation, licensure), summative assessment is the preferred approach. For feedback purposes to the learners, teachers or to the school, a formative assessment is the appropriate method.

However, a summative assessment system can contain a formative component by providing feedback to students on strengths and weaknesses. The combined approach must incorporate a programme for intervention and a subsequent opportunity for summative testing. One example of the combined approach is the 'early warning summative'. It is a 'trial' of the final examination, scored and returned but not recorded. The National Board of Medical Examiner (NBME) Shelf Boards are used for self-assessment purposes in preparation for the licensure examination in the United States.

"Formative assessment is usually contrasted with summative assessment in the following way: 'When the cook tastes the soup, that's formative evaluation. When the guests taste the soup, that's summative evaluation' "

Bob Stake 1991

"Formative assessment could become a powerful tool shaping students' performance"

Bloom & Hastings 1971

When students were asked about the purpose of assessment (Duffield et al 2002) in an ideal world, they ranked the following from high to low:

1. ensuring competence
2. providing feedback
3. evaluating the curriculum
4. guiding student learning
5. predicting performance as a doctor.

Of the five suggested purposes, only 1 and 5 are summative and 2, 3 and 4 are formative. Students in general would prefer assessment with a formative component, as this allows them to grow and learn especially where complex behaviours are measured.

Forms of assessment most suitable for formative methods are portfolios (Friedman et al 2001; see also chapter 37, Portfolios, projects and dissertations), objective structured clinical examinations (OSCE) (van der Vleuten & Swanson 1990; see also chapter 35, Performance assessment), modified essay questions (MEQs) (Knox 1980) and multiple choice questions (MCQs) (Scriven 1991; see also chapter 34, Written assessment).

The more sophisticated the assessment strategies, the more appropriate they become for feedback and learning (Friedman 2000). Thus those designing summative evaluation should strive to include formative information. This will turn the assessment exercise into the educational concept of a 'teachable moment'. One should continuously ask the following question when designing a test: 'What type of learning experiences can be incorporated in this examination, either immediately prior to the examinations, during, or after the examination?' As assessment becomes a learning experience, students and medical trainees will appreciate the assessment experience and will value the additional learning opportunities (Abraham 1998).

The progress test

Learning objectives or outcome-based frameworks require a series of levels that progressively approach the defined outcomes. Assessment must focus on the definition and evaluation of student progress to ensure that trainees are 'on track' in achieving the outcome objectives.

A progress test is an assessment tool, administered on multiple occasions, in order to measure progress relative to previous individual test performance. Incremental gains of knowledge and abilities through the curriculum phases are the units of measurement.

Three main factors may influence students' progress (Brown et al 1995):

- the logical structure of concepts within each discipline
- the sequencing and nature of teaching and activity both within and outside the school
- the changing motivation and intellectual growth of the student.

Consequently learning progress is an outcome of multiple factors, some directly related to formal courses and some to informal learning where students' progress is stimulated by their own individual experiences.

"Assessment of student learning or learning through assessment"

Friedman 2000

"If the feedback information which proceeds backwards from the performance is able to change the general method and pattern of the performance, we have a process, which may very well be called learning"

Weiner, cited in Ende 1983

"Curriculum schemes and assessment programs are based on the assumption of a common model of progression in what students learn"

Brown et al 1955

The measurement of progress is not limited only to incremental gains in knowledge but rather to any form of development of skills or competence. Table 31.1 is an example of student progress in undergraduate medical education with regard to a number of abilities. The elements of progress shown are not inclusive. They are polarised to better define and measure students' growth towards the defined outcomes. In later phases of the curriculum, abilities can be combined in order to approach a more authentic integrated performance.

Once the end-points of learning objectives have been defined (van der Vleuten et al 1996), a progress test could be constructed that takes into account all the core learning objectives required at the time of graduation. When students take different forms of the progress test on multiple occasions throughout the curriculum, they are expected to show gains in their attainment of the school's learning objectives, matched to their level. Students' progress will reflect knowledge and competencies gained in formal courses as well as through informal experiences.

Measuring progress in acquiring core knowledge and competencies may be a problem if the examinations are designed to measure multiple integrated abilities, such as factual knowledge, problem solving, analysis and synthesis of information. Students may advance in one ability and not in another. Therefore, progress tests that are designed to measure growth from the onset of learning until graduation should measure discrete abilities.

A major concern in undergraduate medical education is ensuring that students are mastering the core knowledge. Tests such as modified essay questions (MEQs), or constructed-response questions (CRQs), which are based on multiple elements of a few clinical scenarios, are examples of time-consuming forms of examination which may not allow adequate sampling of core knowledge. Multiple-choice questions (MCQs) provide

> From the student perspective, core curriculum is what is contained in lectures. From the perspective of faculty it is the knowledge required upon graduation.

Table 31.1 Medical students' levels of progression (Friedman 2000)

Initial level	Advanced level
Discrete concepts	Integration
Simple	Increased complexity
Directed	Self-directed
Structured environment	Unstructured environment
Limited responsibility	Increased responsibility
Independent work	Teamwork
Foundations of knowledge	Reflection in action
Public knowledge	Personal knowledge
Certainty	Increased uncertainty
Recognising error	Management of error

a good method of core knowledge sampling, some schools prefer not to use this mode of examination because of its cueing nature, particularly in problem-based programmes (Muijtjens et al 1998). True/false or short-answer type questions eliminate the cueing problem and thus offer an alternative for measuring progress in acquiring core knowledge. Whatever type of questions are used, the effect of guessing should be considered (Friedman et al 1987)

The progress test also addresses the concern that knowledge of basic sciences is not reinforced in the later years of medical school curricula. This issue is resolved by having the same test that includes sampling of all core knowledge for the whole undergraduate curriculum, administered at the same time to all students from all years. Junior students will attempt all questions but will answer correctly only the questions covered already by their formal learning. However, they may also answer correctly higher-level questions for which they have gained knowledge through their informal learning. As the students move through their learning phases, their core knowledge, including their grasp of basic sciences, can be measured in the later years.

A large data pool of questions provides an adequate supply for a yearly repeated administration of one test that measures the core knowledge for the entire curriculum. Thus, each year, a sample of about 250 questions is drawn from a pool of questions generated by a blueprint of the exam. The blueprint ensures construction of parallel forms of the tests according to phase, subject and school learning objectives (Arnold & Willoughby 1990, Verhoeven et al 1999). The progress test could be administered more than once during a year or phase of the curriculum (van der Vleuten et al 1996); in this case more questions would be needed for the repeated parallel forms of the test. The databank of questions may contain anything from 3000 to more than 10 000 questions, which are written and reviewed by special test committees (Arnold & Willoughby 1990) to ensure core knowledge is measured.

Usually, students are not required to study for the test. Immediate feedback is given to students by means of profiles. The score profiles indicate students' performance relative to their classmates, on the overall test, according to subject matter, compared with a previous test administration or matched against a standard of achievement for their current level of studies.

Schools may design the progress test as a summative or formative test for each phase of the curriculum. When progress tests are summative, feedback information is still given to students, thus providing ongoing feedback on progress throughout the curriculum.

In summary the progress test:

- samples core knowledge
- may be administered in parallel test forms once or several times a year
- measures student progress relative to the individual's previous performance
- does not require students to study for it

Students are expected to maintain knowledge acquired during previous formal learning and indicate incremental gains of new knowledge.

Student progress is documented according to the relative gain of knowledge between yearly examinations or between repeated administrations in the same year.

- facilitates reinforcement of already gained knowledge
- allows students to monitor their learning
- allows immediate feedback through score profiles.

Mastery testing

The purpose of mastery testing is to indicate whether an individual has mastered a given subject, in other words, whether they have attained a 'mastery' level of achievement. Mastery testing requires that 100% of the items are answered correctly. In non-mastery testing, in contrast, a cut-off point of 65%, for example, might be set: attainment of 65% of the tested material is considered sufficient.

The concept of mastery testing stems from criterion-referenced tests, first proposed by (Glaser & Nitko 1971). In criterion-referenced tests, individual performance is judged by the degree to which an acceptable standard is attained in the test material ('assessment to a standard'). This is different from norm-referenced testing in which an individual score is interpreted relative to the scores obtained by others on the same test. Commonly, the purpose of norm-referenced testing is to discriminate between low- and high-performing students. Consequently, norm-referenced tests are used mainly for selection purposes. The tests are designed to include a range of item difficulty which usually results in a normal distribution of scores. Norm-referenced tests show up differences between individuals and score variability is built into the test.

In contrast, mastery tests may contain only easy, but essential core items. In an ideal situation all students may attain a score of 100%, resulting in zero variability among scores with no individual differences. However, due to measurement error and other confounding factors, it is reasonable to set the mastery level score at 85%.

Results are usually categorised as 'mastery' or 'non-mastery'. Students who did not attain the mastery level may return to take tests as many times as needed to reach mastery. At the end of the instructional unit all students are expected to achieve the same score.

Reliability and validity of mastery tests

As mastery testing minimises individual differences and thus reduces variability, the classical test methods for establishing the reliability and validity of tests are not applicable. Therefore, in the construction of criterion-referenced tests one must ask:

- How many items must be used for adequate sampling of the content domain?
- What proportion of items must be answered correctly for a reliable determination of mastery?

The test–retest method is one way of establishing the reliability of a mastery testing. Students taking the test may be retested within a reasonable time to ensure reproducibility of the test scores. Students studying at a higher level may take a lower-level test to ensure validity of the test

"Criterion-referenced testing uses as its interpretive frame of reference a specified content domain, rather than a specified population of persons"

Anastasi 1976

The purpose of mastery testing is not to identify low- or high-ability students, but rather requires that all students attain the content domain sampled by the test.

Individual differences are manifested in learning time, rather than in the final score.

Mastery testing requires allocation of time and resources for multiple test administration for students who do not achieve the mastery level score.

"Programs that employ Mastery Testing systems are oriented towards competency-based education"

Alverno College Faculty 1985

content. If core materials are assessed, one would also expect more senior students to demonstrate mastery of the test content.

Global rating scales

Global rating scales are measurement tools for quantifying behaviours. Raters use the scale either by directly observing students or by recalling student performance. Global rating scales are distinguished from other rating forms in that raters judge a global domain of ability for example:

- clinical skills
- communication skills
- problem solving etc (ACGME 2000).

When simple recording of discrete behaviours is needed, for example evaluation of taking a blood pressure, a checklist will be a more appropriate method. Specific behaviours are listed, and the rater makes a binary decision, 'yes' if the behaviour was demonstrated, and 'no' if the behaviour was not demonstrated.

Checklists are commonly employed in methods such as the objective structured clinical examination (OSCE). For some checklists, where little clinical judgement is required, non-clinicians, usually standardised patients, are employed as raters. Global ratings fall into two main categories:

- behaviourally anchored scales
- Likert scales.

Behaviourally anchored scales

Smith & Kendall introduced the concept of the 'behaviourally anchored' scale in 1963. The scale is constructed by describing examples of behaviour, called 'anchors', from the domain under study, and a group of experts rank the behaviours on a scale from low to high. Numerical values are assigned to each anchor to provide a score.

Behaviour descriptions can also be developed, using the critical-incident technique (Rhoton 1989). In this technique, a series of interviews are carried out with students or faculty, investigating, for example, a communication domain. Students are asked to identify incidents where communication was exceptionally good/effective and incidents where it was bad/ineffective.

The behaviours are then analysed and aggregated into several aspects of the domain. For each aspect, behaviourally anchored descriptors are developed.

The number of points on the scale is determined by the number of anchors and by the ability of the rater to discriminate among the points on the scale (Spector 1992). In some cases (see, for example, Table 31.2) the scale is grouped into three main anchors, with three scale points assigned to each anchor; this allows the raters flexibility in choosing a point on the scale for each anchor.

Table 31.2 is an example of an anchored scale for one aspect of skills in communication with patients, that is, sensitivity to the patient's concerns.

Global rating scales allow assessment of behaviours which are not amenable to measurement by written tests.

Global ratings include interpretation and judgement, because of the broad nature of the behavioural domains.

Table 31.2 Behaviourally anchored scale: communication skills with patients

Low				Sensitivity to patient's concerns				High
1	2	3	4	5	6	7	8	9
lack of sensitivity to patient's problem, does not follow up on patient's concern			concentrates mostly on the medical problem with some questions related to patient's concern			is skilful in integrating questions regarding the medical problem and patient's concern		

In performance assessment, when rating takes place in a real or simulated environment, the case scenarios are chosen or developed to elicit the behaviours it is desired to measure.

The reliability of a global rating scale must be established before it is used for formative and summative assessment.

Other aspects of communication with patients might concern empathy or sensitivity to the patient's understanding, for example.

Likert scales
Another global rating technique was developed by Likert (1932). Raters mark behaviours on a continuum, for example from 'excellent' to 'poor'. A numerical value is assigned to the categories. Likert scales are commonly divided into *agreement scales* (agree–disagree), evaluation scales (excellent–poor) and frequency scales (never–always). The scale points in these three categories are arranged on a continuum from low to high (Table 31.3). The number of points may vary based on the construct measured (Spector 1992).

Overcoming the drawbacks of global rating scales
Although global rating scales are easy to use and develop, a high degree of error is evident. The different forms of error commonly result in a low reliability of global rating scales. One frequent error is the 'halo effect'. In this case, raters are influenced by one or more factors related to the examinee, and thus disregard the diverse meanings of the items and consistently rate the examinee at the same scale point, along the items

Table 31.3 Frequency Likert scale: communication with patient

	Seldom		Frequently		Always	
	1	2	3	4	5	6
1. Sensitivity to patient concern						
2. Empathy						
3. Sensitivity to patient understanding						
4. Orientation to socio-economic issues						

domain and across domains. Another common error is the 'central tendency', in which raters tend to avoid extreme positions and choose the middle range to mark performance. Raters may also tend to make severe or lenient judgements due to their own subjective expectation relative to performance on a specific domain.

There are ways to overcome problems of low reliability, both intrarater where one rater is inconsistent in making judgement for the same individual, or interrater, where two or more raters do not agree. In the case of low interrater reliability, an extensive programme for training raters to use the rating form is required. Such programmes will improve intrarater, as well as interrater reliability. It is also necessary to employ a significantly high number of raters to achieve an aggregate reliable score. In structured assessment programmes such as an OSCE, where standardised patients undergo extensive training for using a global rating scale and all examinees are observed under the same conditions, ten standardised patient raters are sufficient to produce an aggregate reliable score (Ziv et al 1998). However, when observations are carried out in real-life situations which are not structured and examinees are exposed to raters under different conditions, a higher number of raters is required to produce a reliable score. Extensive training programmes may reduce the number of raters needed.

Generalisability analysis (Brennan 1983) is employed to estimate the number of raters needed to achieve an acceptable reliability that may range from .75 to .90 in value. Written comments on global rating scales forms may provide useful feedback to students and may also contribute to pass/fail decisions.

Global rating scales can be combined with checklists. When the global judgemental score is given independently of the checklist items, it may add valuable information about the relative weights of the checklist items (Keynan et al 1987) and can also be used to set standards for performance (Dauphinee et al 1997). Checklists are useful for detailed feedback on process items, whereas global ratings generate feedback on more integrated complex behaviours.

Self-assessment

Medical professional associations consider self-reflection, self-regulation and self-monitoring to be vital aspects of the lifelong performance of physicians. Lifelong learning requires that individuals are able not only to work independently, but also to assess their own performance and progress (Falchikov & Boud 1989). Consequently, undergraduate medical education is expected to incorporate student self-assessment exercises to build their abilities to self-regulate their behaviour and self-monitor their studies.

The process of self-assessment may include:

- students' review of own performance
- students' explanation of the process used
- description of breakthroughs in their development

"Self-assessment may be regarded as a skill and, as such, needs to be developed"

Falchikov & Boud 1989

- evaluation of their own performance, employing criteria
- identification of strengths and weaknesses.

(Alverno College Faculty 1985)

Every form of assessment can be used as a self-assessment exercise, as long as students are provided with 'gold standard' criteria for comparing their own performance against an external reliable measure.

Faculty or experts may provide a form of gold standard for student self-assessment (Sclabassi & Woelfel 1984). Peer assessment is another form of standard with which students can compare their self-assessment (Calhoun et al 1990). A set of criteria, developed for a performance domain and known to students in advance, is another form of gold standard against which self-assessment can be compared. However, standards for comparisons may vary on a continuum of objective/subjective judgement. For example, standards for MCQs are objective: the students' responses to the question are either right or wrong. However, standards for essay questions are subjective, since interpretation of student response may vary among examiners. Therefore, when designing self-assessment exercises, attention must be given to the method of feedback in the form of an external gold standard. In relative forms of gold standards, examples of poor work and excellent work can be provided to students, for instance, along with the associated criteria. Such exercises may also enhance student ability to self-reflect as they analyse the work examples against the associated criteria and against their own work. Logbooks (Paice et al 1997) and portfolios (Friedman et al 2001; see chapter 37) are assessment methods which require a high level of self-reflection on one's own performance.

The development of self-assessment skills may require that students progress from measuring their performance using absolute or simple relative standards to using highly complex relative standards. The broader the performance domain, the more challenging is the self-assessment exercise.

There have been attempts to investigate the extent to which students are capable of self-marking their own assessment work compared with marking by faculty. When such a method is employed, the issue of student 'outliers', who systematically underestimate or overestimate their work, becomes a problem that interferes with the accuracy of self-marking (Frye et al 1991). Issues of self-confidence, class standing and other personality variables may affect student underestimation and overestimation when self-marking. More research is needed to identify student 'outliers' and further examine how under- or overestimation behaviours affect their learning strategies, and their clinical decision-making.

Table 31.4 summarises approaches to self-assessment with different assessment methods. It is important to note that, as in any form of feedback, immediate opportunity to compare one's work with a gold standard is central to the success of self-assessment programmes. With the facilities offered by computer software, self-assessment programmes can incorporate a self-assessment exercise with immediate feedback from tutors, other work samples, peer-evaluation, predetermined criteria, correct responses, and so on.

When an assessment method is chosen as a self-assessment exercise, faculty must be informed about how to discuss self-assessment results relative to that modality.

Table 31.4 Self-assessment approaches

Assessment method	Suggested 'gold standard'	Nature of standard
Written examinations		
Multiple-choice questions (MCQs)	Faculty judgement	Objective
True/false	Faculty judgement	Objective
Essays		
Modified-essay questions (MEQs)	Faculty judgement	Objective
Constructed-response questions (CRQs)	Faculty judgement	Objective
Performance examinations		
Checklists	Standardised patients/ faculty/peers	Objective/Subjective
Global ratings	Standardised patients/ faculty/peers	Subjective
Video	Performance criteria/faculty	Subjective
Student logbook	Performance criteria/faculty	Objective/Subjective
Portfolio	Performance criteria/faculty	Subjective

Summary

This chapter takes a broad overview of several key aspects and current trends in assessment:

- formative and summative assessment
- progress testing
- mastery testing
- global rating scales
- self-assessment.

A well-referenced description of the role and principles of each is provided, which prepares the reader for the more detailed practical descriptions in the subsequent chapters in this section.

References

Abraham S 1998 Gynaecological examination: a teaching package integrating assessment with learning. Medical Education, 32:76–81

ACGME Outcomes Project 2000 Toolbox on assessment methods. Accreditation Council for Graduate Medical Education and American Board of Medical Specialties, September. Online. Available: http://www.acgme.org/Outcome/assess/Toolbox.pdf

Alverno College Faculty 1985 Assessment at Alverno College. Alverno College, Milwaukee WI

Anastasi A 1976 Psychological testing (4th edn) Macmillan Publishing, New York

Arnold L, Willoughby T L 1990 The quarterly profile examinations. Academic Medicine, 65:515–516

Bloom B S, Hastings G J 1971 Handbook on formative and summative evaluation of students' learning. McGraw-Hill, New York

Brennan R L 1983 Elements of generalisability theory. American College Testing, Iowa

Brown M, Blondel E, Simon S, Black P 1995 Progression in measuring. Research Papers in Education 10:143–170

Calhoun J G, Ten Haken J D, Woolliscroff J D 1990 Medical students' development of self-assessment and peer-assessment skills: a longitudinal study. Teaching and Learning in Medicine 2:25–29

Dauphinee W D, Blackmore D E, Smee S M, et al 1997 Optimizing the input of physician examiners in setting standards for a large scale OSCE. In: Advances in Medical Education. pp 656–658

Duffield K E, Spencer J A 2002 A survey of medical students' views about the purposes and fairness of assessment, Medical Education 36:879–886

Ende J 1983 Feedback in medical education. JAMA 250:777–781

Falchikov N, Boud D 1989 Student self-assessment in higher education: a meta-analysis. Review of Educational Research S9:345–430

Friedman M, Hopwood L E, Moulder J E, Cox J D 1987 The potential use of the discouraging random guessing (DRG) approach in multiple choice exams in medical education. Medical Teacher 9:33–41

Friedman Ben-David M 2000 The role of assessment in expanding professional horizons. Medical Teacher 22:472–477

Friedman Ben-David M, Davis M H et al 2001 AMEE Medical Education Guide no. 24 Portfolios as a method of student assessment. Medical Teacher 23:535–551

Frye A W, Richards B F, Bradley E W, Philip J R. 1991 The consistency of students' self-assessment in short essay subject matter examinations. Medical Education 23:310–316

Glaser R, Nitko A J 1971 Measurement in learning and instruction. In: Thorndike R L (ed.) Educational measurement, 2nd edn. American Council on Education, Washington DC

Keynan A, Friedman M, Benbassat J 1987 Reliability of global rating scales in the assessment of clinical competence of medical students. Medical Education 21:477–481

Knox J D E 1980 How to use modified essay questions. Medical Teacher 2:20–24

Likert R A 1932 A technique for the measurement of attitudes. Archives of Psychology 140:1–55

Muijtjens A M M, Hoogenboom R J I, Verwijnen G M, van der Vleuten C P M 1998 Relative or absolute standards in assessing medical knowledge using progress tests. Advances in Health Sciences Education 3:81–87

Paice E, Moss F, West G, Grant J 1997 Association of use of a logbook and experience as a pre-registration house officer: interview survey. BMJ 314:213–215

Rhoton M F 1989 A new method to evaluate clinical performance and critical incidents in anaesthesia: quantification of daily comments by teachers. Medical Education 23:280–289

Sclabassi S E, Woelfel S K 1984 Development of self-assessment in medical students. Medical Education 84:226–231

Scriven M 1991 Evaluation thesaurus (4th edn). Sage Publications, Newbury Park CA

Smith P C, Kendall L M 1963 Retranslation of expectations: an approach to the construction of unambiguous anchors for rating scales. Journal of Applied Psychology 47:149–155

Spector P E 1992 Summated rating scale construction. Sage Publications, Newbury Park CA

van der Vleuten C P M, Swanson D B 1990 Assessment of clinical skills with standardized patients: state of the art. Teaching and Learning in Medicine 22:58–76

van der Vleuten C P M, Verwijnen G M, Wijnen W H F 1996 Fifteen years of experience with progress testing in a problem-based learning curriculum. Medical Teacher 18:103–110

Verhoeven B H, Verwijnen G M, Scherpbier J A et al 1999 Quality assurance in test construction: the approach of a multidisciplinary central test committee. Education for Health 12:49–60

Ziv A, Curtis M, Burdick W P et al 1998 An holistic and behaviorally anchored measure of interpersonal skills; issues of rater consistency. Proceedings of The 8th International Ottawa Conference on Medical Education and Assessment

Chapter 32
Standard setting

J. Norcini

Introduction

In the context of this chapter, a standard is a single score on a test that serves as the boundary between qualitatively different performances. For example, the most common standard is 'pass–fail', where a single score is chosen as the cut-off. Examinees who achieve that score or better pass, while those below it fail. Passing implies sufficient knowledge or skill given the purpose of the test, while failing implies insufficient knowledge or skill.

Unlike many medical tests, educational assessments only rarely have a gold standard against which to establish their validity. The nature of a 'competent' physician or an 'unsatisfactory' medical student varies over assessment, time, location, and a series of other factors. Consequently, standards on educational tests are an expression of judgement in the context of a particular assessment, its purpose, and the wider social/professional environment.

Because standards are based on judgement, methods for selecting them are not intended to discover an underlying truth. Instead, they are a means for gathering a variety of perspectives, blending them together, and expressing them as a single score on a particular assessment. As a consequence, the methods do not differ in the correctness of the standards they yield, but in their credibility.

This chapter is based on previous work (Norcini 2003, Norcini & Guille 2002, Norcini & Shea 1997). It describes:

- the types of standards
- the characteristics that lead to their credibility
- the more popular methods for setting standards
- variations of the methods for use with clinical examinations.

Types of standards

There are two types of standards:

- relative
- absolute

Relative standards are expressed in terms of the comparative performance of the examinees. For instance, a relative standard may be that the 120 examinees with the highest scores are admitted to medical school.

This type of standard is appropriate for assessments intended to select a certain number or percentage of examinees, such as tests for admissions or placement.

Absolute standards are expressed in terms of the performance of examinees against the test material. For instance, a passing score may be that any examinee who correctly answers 75% or more of the questions knows enough anatomy to pass. This type of standard is appropriate for assessments intended to determine whether examinees have the necessary knowledge or skills for a particular purpose, such as course completion or graduation from medical school.

Credibility of standards

The credibility of standards depends on:

- the standard setters
- the method they use
- the outcome of their efforts.

Standard setters

The standard setters must understand the purpose of the test, know the content, and be familiar with the examinees. In a low-stakes setting like a course, a single faculty member is credible, but standards will vary over time and he or she has a conflict of interest in being both the teacher and assessor. In a high-stakes setting like licensure, a significant number of standard setters need to be involved because this increases the reproducibility of standards and reduces the effects of 'hawks' and 'doves'. Ideally, the group would be free of conflicts of interest, include a mix of educators and practitioners, and be balanced with regard to gender, race, geography, and the like.

Method

The specific method is not as important as whether it produces standards fit for the purpose of the test, relies on informed expert judgement, demonstrates due diligence, is supported by a body of research, and is easy to explain and implement.

Fit for purpose. The method must produce standards that are consistent with the purpose of the assessment. Methods that turn out relative standards are to be used when the purpose is to select a specific number of examinees. Methods that turn out absolute standards are to be used when the purpose is to judge competence.

Based on informed judgement. Methods for setting standards can be based entirely on empirical results (e.g., consequences, performance on criteria), entirely on expert judgement, or on a blend of the two. With the exception of a few admissions testing situations (where outcome data, like successful completion of a course, are available and relative standards are being used), there are only rarely instances in which it is possible to base a standard entirely on empirical results in medical education.

In contrast, most of the methods allow a standard to be based solely on the judgement of experts, without reference to performance data (e.g., the difficulty of the questions, the pass rate, etc.). Moreover, standard setters sometimes become uncomfortable when data are presented, thinking that it 'biases' their judgements.

In fact, methods for setting standards are not intended to discover an underlying truth but to create a credible standard out of the judgements of experts. Such credibility derives from decisions that are based on all of the available information. Consequently, methods that permit and encourage expert judgement in the presence of performance data are preferable.

Demonstrates due diligence. Methods that require the standard setters to expend thoughtful effort will demonstrate due diligence and this lends credibility to the final result. In contrast, methods that require quick, global judgements are less credible and methods requiring several days of effort are unnecessary.

Supported by research. Methods supported by a research literature will produce more credible results. Ideally, studies should show that standards are reasonable compared to those produced by other methods, reproducible over groups of judges, insensitive to potentially biasing effects, and sensitive to differences in test difficulty and content.

Easily explained and implemented. Credibility is enhanced if the method is easy to explain and implement. This decreases the amount of training required for the judges, increases the likelihood of their compliance, and assures examinees that they are being treated fairly.

Realistic outcomes

A standard that produces unreasonable outcomes (far too many or too few examinees pass) will not be viewed as credible regardless of the care with which it was derived. Therefore, it is important to collect data that support the fact that the stakeholders believe the standard is correct and that it has reasonable relationships with other markers of competence.

For example, it would be supportive of the standard if the faculty generally believed that an appropriate number of students passed the summative assessment at the end of medical school. Moreover, it would be useful to gather evidence that the students who passed also performed well in the next phase of their training.

Methods for setting standards

There is a host of methods for setting standards and many have variations. Reviews and descriptions are available elsewhere (Berk 1986, Cusimano 1996, Jaeger 1989), but according to Livingston & Zeiky (1982) they fall into four categories:

- relative methods
- absolute methods based on judgements about individual examinees
- absolute methods based on judgements about test questions
- compromise methods.

If the test is very long and security is not a major issue, have the standard setters meet and judge 30–40 items. Then ask them to do the remainder at home.

A reliable standard will result even when subsets of standard setters make judgements about subsets of the items on a test, as long as there are enough doctors involved.

If the standard setters have not taken the assessment, they should take it before the meeting because it prevents overconfidence and unrealistically high standards.

Give the standard setters the correct answers during the meeting unless they are overconfident. It prevents embarrassment.

All of the methods require that several standard setters be selected and that they meet as a group. As the name implies, relative methods produce relative standards and thus judgements are made about what proportion of the examinees should pass. The two groups of methods for setting absolute standards differ in the type of judgements that are being collected. In one group, the standard setters consider whether individual examinees should pass and these judgements are aggregated to derive the cut-off. In the other group, the standard setters consider individual test questions and these judgements are combined to calculate the cutting score. The compromise methods require judgements both about what proportion of the examinees should pass and what score they need to achieve to do so. The final result is a compromise between these two types of judgements.

Before the meeting

Prior to the meeting, the method for setting standards needs to be selected, depending on the purpose of the test, the stakes, and the resources available. Once this is done, the standard setters should be chosen to be broadly representative of the relevant perspectives. They should all review the assessment in detail so that they are familiar with the content and scoring. This is particularly important for the methods that do not require a review of the test as part of the standard setting process.

During the meeting

At the beginning of the meeting the methods should be explained to the standard setters. They should then engage in a discussion of the purpose and content of the test and the abilities of the examinees. These discussions are critical because they focus the standard setters on the task and guide them as they begin to make judgements.

Once this discussion is completed, the standard setters should practise the method, where practical with data that are not part of the test. Throughout the practice period and the remainder of the meeting, the standard setters should be given feedback about the consequences of their judgements (e.g., what percentage of examinees they would pass).

It is important that all standard setters attend the entire meeting and that there are not interruptions. Absences, even for a short time, will generate missing data and could influence the standard more broadly by altering the discussion.

Relative methods

In the *fixed-percentage* method, following the preliminaries, each standard setter announces what percentage (or number) of examinees is qualified to pass. Their judgements are recorded for all to see and they then engage in a discussion, often led off by those with the highest and lowest estimates. All are free to change and when the discussions are over the estimates are averaged. The standard is that score which passes the average percentage (or number) of examinees.

In the *reference group* method, the process is exactly the same except that the standard setters have a particular group of examinees in mind (e.g., graduates of a certain set of schools or examinees with specific educational experiences). The selection of this reference group is based on the fact that the standard setters are most familiar with them and able to make good judgements about them. The cutting score established for this reference group is applied without modification to all other examinees.

These methods are quick and easy to use, they only have to be repeated occasionally, the standard setters are comfortable making the required judgements, and they apply equally well to all different test formats. However, the standards will vary over time with the ability of the examinees and they are independent of how much examinees know and the content of the test.

Absolute methods based on judgements about individual examinees
In the *contrasting groups* method, a random sample of examinees is drawn before the meeting. The entire test paper of each member of this randomly selected group is taken to the meeting and given, one at a time, to the standard setters. They decide as a group whether each performance is passing or failing. To calculate the standard, the scores of the passers and failers are graphed separately but on the same piece of paper. The cutting score can then be derived in a variety of ways. For example, the point where the curve of the passers overlaps least with the curve of failers could be taken as the standard. Figure 32.1 provides an illustration.

Standard setters are usually comfortable making the judgements required by this method and it has the advantage of informing them with the actual test performance of examinees. Further, by shifting where the standard is set, it is possible to maximise or minimise false-positive and false-negative decisions. However, it is difficult for the standard setters to produce a balanced judgement when the test is relatively long. In addition, a large number of examinees need to be judged to produce precise results.

Absolute methods based on judgements about test questions
The two most popular methods in this category have been proposed by Angoff and Ebel. Both methods require that the standard setters specify the characteristics of a borderline group of examinees. The borderline group excludes examinees that would clearly pass or fail and is composed of those about whom the standard setters are uncertain.

In Angoff's method, the standard setters estimate the proportion of the borderline group that would respond correctly to an item. These are discussed with all being free to change their estimates and the process is repeated for all items on the test. To calculate the standard, the estimates for each item are averaged and the averages are summed. Table 32.1 provides an example.

In Ebel's method, the standard setters build a classification table for the items in the test. For example, they might decide to classify items by difficulty (easy, medium, and hard) and frequency with which encountered in practice (common and uncommon). The standard setters then assign each item to one of the categories. After all items are assigned, they estimate the proportion of items in a category that borderline

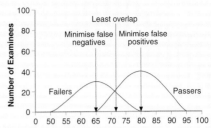

Fig. 32.1 This is an example of an application of the contrasting groups method to a 100-item test. A sample of students is drawn at random and the standard setters review the first student's answers to the entire test. After making a decision as a group about whether the performance merits a pass or a fail, the standard setters make similar decisions about the remaining students one by one. After judgements have been made about all the students, the scores of the failing group and passing group are graphed separately. The cut score is usually set at the point of least overlap between the two distributions, 72 in this example. If there is a need to minimize false negatives the cut score is set at 65 and if there is a need to minimize false positives it is set at 80.

The contrasting groups method is especially useful when there is a need to directly manipulate the number of false-positive or false-negative decisions.

Studies of Angoff's method demonstrate that when it is properly applied, the results are reliable and consistent over time, level of expertise does not affect the judgements, and the standards are sensitive to content differences.

Ebel's method is especially useful when there are natural categories of responses like 'indicated' or 'contraindicated' options.

Table 32.1 Angoff's method. This is an example of an application of Angoff's method to an 8-item test. The meeting of the five standard setters begins with a discussion of the characteristics of a borderline group of students. When the standard setters reach consensus, they turn to a consideration of the first item. The standard setters each estimate aloud what proportion of the hypothetical borderline group would respond correctly to the question. Their estimates are written on a board for all to see and a discussion ensues, led by the standard setters with the highest and lowest estimates. All standard setters are free to change their estimates. The standard setters proceed in this manner through all of the items on the test. The cut score is taken as the sum of the standard setters' mean estimates for each question.

	Standard setter					Mean
	1	2	3	4	5	
Question						
1	.90	.85	.80	.75	.85	.83
2	.60	.55	.40	.35	.50	.48
3	.70	.60	.65	.50	.55	.60
4	.85	.75	.80	.65	.70	.75
5	.95	.90	.85	.75	.80	.85
6	.50	.50	.45	.40	.50	.47
7	.65	.55	.45	.45	.60	.54
8	.85	.70	.80	.65	.75	.75
Standard (cut score)						5.27

examinees will answer correctly; see Table 32.2. As with Angoff's method a discussion ensues and estimates can be changed. To determine the standard, the estimates for each category are averaged, multiplied by the number of items in the category, and summed.

Both of these methods are widely used in high-stakes testing situations. There is a considerable body of research supporting them, especially Angoff's method, and they are relatively easy to apply. In addition, they force the standard setters to review every item on the test and thus result in more informed judgements. However, the standard setters sometimes have difficulty envisioning the performance of a borderline group and so feel that they are simply making up numbers. These methods can also be time consuming for long tests.

Compromise methods

The Hofstee method is the most popular exemplar of this class of methods. The standard setters are asked to produce four judgements: the maximum and minimum acceptable pass rates and maximum and minimum acceptable cut-off scores. These judgements are discussed and changed, as with the other methods, and the final results for the four estimates are obtained by averaging across standard setters. The percentage of examinees who

Table 32.2 This is an example of an application of Ebel's method to a 100-item test. The standard setters begin with a discussion of how the test questions should be classified. In this example, they choose two dimensions: frequency and difficulty. As a group, they go through all of the questions on the test, one by one and place them into one of the categories (e.g., easy and common). After this task is complete, the standard setters discuss the characteristics of a borderline group of students. When the group reaches consensus on these characteristics, they turn to a consideration of the first category of questions. The standard setters each estimate aloud what proportion of the hypothetical borderline group would respond correctly to the questions in the category. Their estimates are written on a board for all to see and a discussion ensues, led by the standard setters with the highest and lowest estimates. All standard setters are free to change their estimates. When done, the group proceeds through the rest of the categories. To derive the cut score, the average proportion correct is multiplied by the number of questions in each category to produce expected scores. These expected scores are summed to calculate the standard.

Category	Average proportion correct	No. of questions	Expected score
Common			
Easy	.95	20	19
Medium	.80	40	32
Hard	.70	10	7
Uncommon			
Easy	.70	15	10.5
Medium	.50	10	5
Hard	.30	5	1.5
Standard (cut score)			75

would pass for every possible value of the cut score on the test is graphed and a rectangle is superimposed as defined by the four judgements of the standard setters. A diagonal is drawn through the box and the standard is the point where it intersects the examinee performance curve. Figure 32.2 provides an illustration.

This method is efficient and the standard setters feel capable of making the judgements necessary for it. In some instances, however, the curve for examinee performance does not fall within the area circumscribed by the rectangle and in this case the minimum or maximum acceptable pass rate is selected by default to provide a standard. Because it includes elements of a relative standard, this method is not ideal for regular use in a high-stakes setting. However, it is suitable occasionally, or for use in a low-stakes application.

After the meeting

Outliers

Common to all of the methods is the possibility that a standard setter with extreme views might significantly influence the results. Livingston &

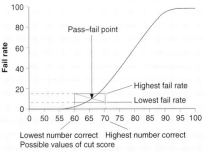

Fig. 32.2 This is an example of an application of the Hofstee method to a 100-item test (see 1 below). The standard setters are asked to answer four questions: What are the minimum and maximum acceptable fail rates and what are the minimum and maximum acceptable cut-off scores? After a discussion where these estimates can be changed, means over all standard setters are calculated. These are graphed as a rectangle and a diagonal is drawn through it. The performance of the students is graphed (see 2 below). The standard is the point where the performance curve intersects the diagonal.

1. The scores in this case are the numbers of items answerd correctly
2. Showing what the fail rate would be at each possible value for the cut-off.

Zeiky (1982) review methods for dealing with this problem, such as removing outlying judgements from the calculations or using the median instead of the mean. The removal of data should be a last resort, however, since it undermines the credibility of the process and the selection of standard setters.

Reliability

It is important to determine whether the results would be the same if the method was repeated with more or different standard setters. This is reliability or reproducibility, and there are a variety of ways of calculating it but generalisability theory offers a good alternative (Brennan & Lockwood 1980, Kane & Wilson 1984). If the results of this analysis are unacceptable given the purpose of the assessment, standard setters can be added in a second application of the method. The data from this second application should be combined with those of the first unless there were significant problems associated with it.

Outcomes

As mentioned above, a standard setting process will not be credible if it produces an unreasonable outcome. In an assessment programme that continues over time, it is important to ensure that the stakeholders view the results as reasonable and that these results are related to the other indicators of proficiency.

Variations for clinical examinations

Although the methods described above were developed for multiple choice examinations, they can be applied directly to clinical examinations, such as OSCEs, without modification. The fixed percentage, reference group, and Hofstee methods require no additional effort. However, direct application of the other methods can become cumbersome. For example, applying the Angoff or Ebel approaches to an OSCE may necessitate some type of judgement about all of the items on all of the checklists. Similarly, applying the contrasting groups method to an OSCE would require the standard setters to apprehend and then judge the performance of each examinee across all of the checklists on all of the stations.

In a variation intended to make the Angoff and Ebel methods more efficient, standard setters are asked to provide judgements at the level of the station rather than at the level of individual items on the checklist. For instance, in Angoff's method the standard setters would be asked to treat the entire OSCE station checklist as a single item and estimate the score of the borderline examinees on it. These scores would be averaged for each station and summed to determine the standard.

In a variation that makes the contrasting groups method more efficient for an OSCE, the standard setters consider the performances of a sample of examinees on each case. They sort them into 'acceptable' and 'unacceptable' groups, identify the score separating them, and then sum these scores across all of the stations to arrive at the standard for the test.

Finally, a technique proposed by Dauphinee et al (1997) combines elements of both the Angoff and contrasting groups methods. When physicians are used to observing and scoring OSCE stations, they can be asked to rate each examinee in such a way that borderline performances are identified. The scores of the examinees with these borderline performances are averaged and then combined over all the stations in the assessment.

Summary

A standard is a single score on a test that serves as the boundary between qualitatively different performances. These standards are an expression of judgement in the context of a particular assessment, its purpose, and the wider social/professional environment. Consequently, methods for selecting them are a means for gathering a variety of perspectives, blending them together, and expressing them as a single score. This chapter described the two types of standards, the characteristics that lead to their credibility, the more popular methods for setting standards, and some efficient variations for use with clinical examinations.

References

Berk R A 1986 A consumer's guide to setting performance standards on criterion-referenced tests. Review of Educational Research 56:137–172

Brennan R L, Lockwood R E 1980 A comparison of the Nedelsky and Angoff cutting score procedures using generalizability theory. Applied Psychological Measurement 4:219–240

Cusimano M D 1996 Standard setting in medical education. Academic Medicine 71:s112–s120

Dauphinee W D, Blackmore D E, Smee S et al 1997 Using the judgments of physician examiners in setting standards for a national multi-center high stakes OSCE. Advances in Health Sciences Education 2:201–211

Jaeger R M 1989 Certification of student competence. In: Linn R L (ed.) Educational measurement. American Council on Education and Macmillan Publishing Company, New York

Kane M. 1994 Validating the performance standards associated with passing scores. Review of Educational Research 64:425–461

Kane M, Wilson J 1984 Errors of measurement and standard setting in mastery testing. Applied psychological measurement 8(1):107–115

Livingston S A, Zeiky M J 1982 Passing scores: a manual for setting standards of performance on educational and occupational tests. Educational Testing Service, Princeton NJ

Norcini J J 2003 Setting standards on educational tests. Medical Education 37:464–469

Norcini J J, Guille R A 2002 Combining tests and setting standards. In: Norman G, van der Vleuten C, Newble D (eds.) International Handbook of Research in Medical Education. Kluwer Academic, Dordrecht, The Netherlands. pp 811–834

Norcini J J, Shea J A 1997 The credibility and comparability of standards. Applied Measurement in Education 10:39–59

Chapter 33
Choosing assessment instruments

S. McAleer

Introduction

When it comes down to deciding on the best instrument for assessment the choices on offer are not as depressing as those suggested by Woody Allen. Nevertheless getting it right or wrong can have long-term effects for the students involved in the process. Therefore in selecting appropriate assessment instruments it is essential to understand the key principles involved. Assessment is a measure of performance which can be used as a feedback mechanism for three important aspects of the learning situation. It can provide:

- a measure of the level of student performance
- an indication of the effectiveness of the teaching situation
- a measure of the appropriateness of the content input.

There are some important questions which must be asked before making a choice of assessment method:

- What should be assessed?
- Why assess?

When an assessment instrument is being considered you must also ask:

- Is it valid?
- Is it reliable?
- Is it feasible?

In answering these questions the basic principles of assessment will be brought into play. What is assessed and which methods are used will play a significant part in what is learnt. Decisions on what students should learn and the reasons for making those decisions must be established first. Afterwards the type of assessment can be determined. For example, if you want your students to read a textbook then tell them there will be a series of multiple-choice questions (MCQs) on each chapter in their end-of-term examination. If you want your students to show competence in minor surgical techniques then inform them that there will be a practical examination in these skills.

At this stage it is probably useful to make the distinction between assessment method and assessment instrument. For example, the method of assessment selected may be self-assessment and the instruments used

"More than at any other time in history, mankind faces a crossroads. One path leads to despair and utter hopelessness. The other, to total extinction. Let us pray we have the wisdom to choose correctly"

Woody Allen, *Side effects* (1980)

Also think about the effect the assessment may have on the students. Will it be a motivation for learning? Will it create a healthy educational environment?

"Examinations are formidable even to the best prepared, for the greatest fool may ask more than the wisest man can answer"

Charles Caleb Colton, 1780–1832

could be MCQs or perhaps an objective structured clinical examination (OSCE). Table 33.1 illustrates the difference by comparing assessment to travel and instruments to types of conveyance. Of course, different assessment instruments may be used within a particular method.

There is currently a wide range of assessment instruments available and in order to make an informed choice it is necessary to be familiar with what is on offer:

Table 33.1 Difference between methods and instruments

Method of travel	Conveyance	Method of assessment	Instrument
By land	Train/bus/car	Performance	Checklist/ simulators
By sea	Ferry/speedboat/liner	Written	Essay/MCQs
By air	Helicopter/glider/jet		

- essays
- patient management problems
- modified-essay questions
- checklists
- objective structured clinical examinations
- projects
- constructed-response questions
- multiple-choice questions
- critical reading papers
- rating scales
- extended matching items
- tutor reports
- portfolios
- short case assessments
- long case assessments.

What should be assessed?

Harden (1979) suggested that many teachers failed to address this question with sufficient thought. This claim is still worthy of consideration as it stresses the importance of educational objectives defined by Mager (1984) as the performance to be exhibited by a learner before being considered competent – 'An educational objective is therefore an intended result of instruction, rather than the process itself.'

Useful objectives relate to:

- the task the student is to perform
- the conditions under which the performance should be exhibited
- the level of performance that will be considered acceptable.

Clear objectives are important in the planning of authentic assessment. These objectives should not only be worth measuring but they

Try to use more than one assessment instrument, and more than one assessor especially if you are looking at skills and attitudes. Gather as much data on the candidate as is feasible.

"the most useful objective is the one that allows us to make the largest number of decisions relevant to its achievement and measurement"

Mager 1984

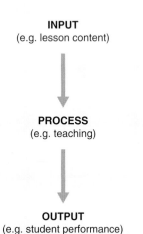

In determining good learning outcomes it is important to ensure that they can be:
- observed
- measured
- carried out by the learners.

INPUT
(e.g. lesson content)

↓

PROCESS
(e.g. teaching)

↓

OUTPUT
(e.g. student performance)

Fig. 33.1 The assessor must focus on the output

"The first step in making choices of measurement instruments is to determine the purpose and desired content of evaluation, as it is important to choose the measurement methods that are congruent with the evaluation questions"

Andrew Wojtczak 2002

should also be measurable. The more specific the objective, the more useful it is likely to be in indicating the assessable behaviours expected of students. Specific objectives are also extremely useful as a springboard for developing a suitable assessment programme. Morgan & Irby (1978) emphasise the importance of the precise wording of objectives so that student, teacher and assessor are all exactly clear about what must be performed to show competence. For example, rather than saying that a medical technologist should '*know* the characteristic appearance of different types of blood cell', the objective should state that 'the medical technologist will *identify* and *interpret* blood cells on a blood smear.'

Writing objectives that are well defined and precise can be difficult and can be influenced by the subject being taught. Objectives are always output measures and in determining what they are, the assessment writer has to start at the end of the process illustrated in Figure 33.1. The teacher usually thinks about the content first and then develops the assessment instruments second. Focusing on the output measures, although educationally sound, goes against the natural instincts of many teachers.

Output measures should contain:

- a knowledge component
- a skill component
- an attitudinal component.

The knowledge component domain relates to the learners' ability to remember and understand. The skill component encompasses those psychomotor tasks which are deemed prerequisite for professional competence. The attitudinal component includes the key personal qualities thought necessary of a professional. Before choosing an assessment instrument it is vital to define clearly what exactly is to be assessed. What may be appropriate for testing knowledge is unlikely to be useful for assessing psychomotor skills. A number of taxonomies are available which can help by providing lists of the competencies available and in setting an appropriate level of performance: for example, Bloom (1956), Harrow (1972) and Krathwohl et al (1964).

Why assess?

Assessment is an important part of the curriculum for the following reasons:

- It is an integral part of the learning process in which students are informed of any weaknesses and of how to improve the quality of their performance.
- It illustrates progress and ensures a proper standard has been achieved before the student moves to a higher level of training.
- It provides certification relating to a standard of performance, e.g. the award of a degree.

- It indicates to students the areas of a course which are considered important.
- It acts as a promotion technique.
- It acts as a means of selection for a career or as an entrance requirement for a course.
- It motivates students in their studies.
- It measures the effectiveness of training and identifies curriculum weaknesses.

Validity

Whatever assessment instrument is used it must be valid for the task it is to do. In other words the answer to the question 'Am I measuring what I am supposed to be measuring?' must be positive. A particular examination might be valid for one purpose but invalid for another. For example, a series of MCQs which test factual recall may be a valid measure of whether a student has read a textbook on diabetes but invalid as the indicator of whether that same student can actually manage a patient suffering from diabetes.

The measure of validity is not a straightforward process as a variety of types of validity are described and 'degrees of validity' are recognised. Building up a dossier to support a claim of validity can involve looking at five major types:

- content validity
- concurrent validity
- predictive validity
- construct validity
- face validity.

It is important to be familiar with all of these but the emphasis attributed to each is dependent on the reasons for assessing.

Content validity

This refers to the extent to which a test or examination actually measures the intended content area. For an examination to have content validity it must have 'item validity' and 'sampling validity'. These terms are best explained in the following example. If a test is designed to measure knowledge of the human anatomy then good item validity is present if all the questions deal with facts pertaining to the human body. However, poor sampling validity will be apparent if all the questions focus on the lower limbs.

The issue of content should be seen in relation to:

- the subject matter you are teaching
- the students who are being taught.

How to establish content validity

- Define the subject matter being assessed.
- Identify the cognitive/behavioural/attitudinal process involved.

"Either he's dead, or my watch has stopped"

Groucho Marx 1895–1977

The terminology surrounding validity can be confusing, with many 'new' varieties emerging. Keep in mind the basic definition 'the extent to which an assessment measures what it is supposed to measure'.

Examine your assessment closely, note the specific outcomes and determine how well each outcome is covered by the test items.

- Establish the outcomes expected.
- Draw up a specifications grid (see Table 33.2).

Table 33.2 Table of specifications for an MCQ in physiological psychology

Content	Knowl-edge	Compre-hension	Appli-cation	Higher processing	Total
Neurones/ gross anatomy	6	4	2	1	13 (26%)
Motor mechanisms	4	3	2	1	10 (20%)
Sensory systems	3	2	2	1	8 (16%)
Alerting mechanisms	3	2	2	1	8 (16%)
Motivation/ emotion	2	2	1	1	6 (12%)
Memory/ learning	2	2	1	–	5 (10%)
Total	20 (40%)	15 (30%)	10 (20%)	5 (10%)	50 (100%)

"An expert is one who knows more and more about less and less"

Nicholas Murray Butler 1862–1947

The term criterion validity is sometimes used to incorporate concurrent and predictive validity.

This type of grid should:

- identify the content areas (n = 6)
- specify learning outcomes (n = 4)
- determine the number of items for each content area and learning objective
- ensure that the number of items in each cell is in proportion to the time spent in teaching and learning.

Content validity is based on expert judgement and the assessor should compare what is taught with what is measured by the examination. If you are testing for achievement you must ensure content validity.

Concurrent validity

This refers to the degree to which scores on a test correlate with the scores on an established test administered at the same time. The procedure is to:

- Administer the new test.
- Administer the established test.
- Correlate the two sets of scores.
- The greater the positive correlation, the greater the validity.

Predictive validity

Predictive validity relates to the certainty with which a test can predict future performance. It is particularly important if you are using your assessment for selection purposes. No test will have perfect predictability so it is wise to base any decision on more than one predictor. The procedure is to:

- Administer your test.
- Collect measures of the new behaviour.
- Correlate the two results.
- The magnitude of the correlation coefficient will indicate the predictive validity.

Construct validity

Construct validity is the extent to which a test measures a hypothetical construct (e.g. empathy, intelligence) or a trait that explains behaviour but is not easily observed. For example, if a theory of schizophrenia hypothesised that high scorers on a test will take longer to problem solve than low scorers, then if high scorers do indeed take longer it would provide evidence for construct validity. It can be difficult to determine and all forms of validity should be used as evidence for its presence.

Face validity

Face validity is concerned with appearance; i.e. does the exam *seem* to measure what it is supposed to measure? If candidates feel that the assessment is fair and relevant then they will be better motivated. The teaching and learning environment will also benefit. Face validity is determined by feedback received from all those involved in the assessment.

Factors influencing validity

There are a variety of factors which may influence the validity of an assessment instrument. Check for the following:

- vague or misleading instructions to candidates
- inappropriate vocabulary or overcomplicated wording
- too few test items causing poor sampling validity
- problems of time – insufficient time for answers turns the test into one based on speed
- items inappropriate for the outcomes being measured
- item difficulty – items that are too easy or too difficult will fail to discriminate.

Reliability

It is important to be able to trust any assessment instrument used. Reliability is the degree to which a test consistently measures whatever it is supposed to measure. The more reliable the examination, the greater the confidence that the result would be the same if the examination were re-administered. For example, if a student scored 60% in an MCQ examination and in two subsequent sittings shortly afterwards scored 30% and 90% then you would assume the test lacked reliability. As with validity a number of different kinds of reliability are described, as outlined below.

"Face validity pertains to whether the test 'looks valid' to the examinees who take it, the administrative personnel who decide on its use, and other technically untrained observers"

Anastasi 1988

"Concerns about the valid interpretation of assessment results should begin before the selection or development of a task or assessment instrument. A well-designed scoring rubric cannot correct for a poorly designed assessment instrument"

Moskal & Leydens 2000

"Problems of the dependability of scores and grades occur when papers are marked by many assessors"

Satterly 1994

Test–retest reliability

Test–retest reliability measures the consistency of an examination over time. It is calculated by correlating the scores on a test with scores produced by a repeat administration to the same group. A high positive correlation indicates good reliability. One problem is deciding on the appropriate time period between the two administrations. If it is too short then the students are likely to remember their previous answers. If there is too lengthy a gap then students may have benefited from further learning. This type of reliability is important for tests used as predictors.

Equivalent forms reliability

This type of reliability refers to the consistency of scores across two different formats of the same test. The tests are identical in terms of number of questions, structure and the level of difficulty. The only difference is in the wording of the specific items but both tests measure the same objectives. To calculate reliability the scores on format 1 of the test are correlated with the scores from format 2. Not surprisingly a major difficulty is constructing two versions of the same examination that are essentially equivalent. The main use for this form of examination is in studies which require a pre-test and a post-test to be given.

Split-half reliability

The internal consistency of an examination is measured by this method. With split-half reliability the examination is divided into two parts, e.g. all the odd numbered questions and all the even numbered questions. The scores for both halves are correlated and the degree of correlation reflects the internal consistency of the instrument. Only one administration of the test is necessary and the method is particularly suitable for tests with many items. The more questions in an examination, the greater the likelihood of high reliability. There are various statistical techniques for discovering the internal consistency of a test. The KR20 and Cronbach's alpha are two of the most common.

Scorer/rater reliability

If you are using an instrument where the scoring involves a certain amount of subjectivity it is important to check for both interrater reliability and intrarater reliability. The first type refers to the reliability of two or more independent markers to give the same marks to each student. The second kind relates to the scoring of assessors: will a marker give the same score to a student if the work is remarked at a later date? The reliability for both versions is calculated by correlational statistics.

Factors influencing reliability

- Test length. The more items included in an examination, the greater the reliability.
- Objectivity in scoring. Lack of objectivity, for example, will reduce the reliability of long essay questions.

One of the most common measures of reliability associated with assessment is Cronbach's alpha coefficient which determines the internal consistency of a test.

Make sure examiners and students are absolutely clear about the marking criteria used.

- Environmental effects. Performance may be poor in candidates who are required to sit an examination at the end of a long day.
- Processing errors. Mistakes may be made in calculating candidates' marks.
- Classification errors. A marker may interpret what may really be a candidate's anxiety as rudeness.
- Generalisation errors. The examiner may generalise from a specific answer.
- Bias errors. Some examiners may place too great an emphasis on a particular trait. Others may be prejudiced against certain students. The previous overall impression of a student can sometimes influence the mark given to a student. Certain examiners may be 'easy' markers while others may be 'hard' markers.

Feasibility

When selecting an assessment instrument it is paramount to check that it will be feasible to use it. This will involve calculating the cost of the assessment, both in terms of resources and time. The following questions should be asked:

- How long will it take to construct the instrument?
- How much time will be involved with the marking process?
- Will it be relatively easy to interpret the scores and produce the results?
- Is it practical in terms of organisation?
- Can quality feedback result from the instrument?
- Will the instrument indicate to the students the important elements within the course?
- Will the assessment have a beneficial effect in terms of student motivation, good study habits and positive career aspirations?

Summary

In selecting an assessment instrument it is necessary to know exactly what it is that is to be measured. This should reflect the course outcomes, i.e. what it is you want your students to be able to do. Different learning outcomes necessitate the use of different instruments. It is inappropriate to assess a performance skill with an MCQ.

It is essential to use an instrument that is valid, reliable and feasible. An instrument may be perfectly reliable but totally invalid. For example, an MCQ examination may show high reliability but is it really a valid measure of whether students are competent in resuscitation skills? Finally, no assessment instrument is of any value if it is unfeasible to use it.

If a full variety of instruments are used then there will be more confidence that the results obtained are a true reflection of the students' performance.

"I am free of all prejudice. I hate everyone equally"

W. C. Fields 1880–1946

Always look at the way you assess and ask 'How will this benefit my students?'

"If I ran a school, I'd give the average grade to the ones who gave me all the right answers, for being good parrots. I'd give the top grades to those who made a lot of mistakes and told me about them, and then told me what they learned from them"

R. Buckminster Fuller

References

Anastasi A 1988 Psychological testing. Macmillan, New York

Bloom B S (ed) 1956 Taxonomy of educational objectives. Handbook I: Cognitive domain. David Mckay, New York

Harden R M 1979 How to assess students: an overview. Medical Teacher 1(2):65–70

Harrow A J A 1972 A taxonomy of the psychomotor domain. David Mckay, New York

Krathwohl D R, Bloom B S, Masia B B 1964 Taxonomy of educational objectives. Handbook II: Affective domain. David Mckay, New York

Mager R F 1984 Preparing instructional objectives. Pitman Learning, California

Morgan M K, Irby D M (eds) 1978 Evaluating clinical competence in the health professions. C V Mosby, St Louis

Moskal B M, Leydens J A 2000 Scoring rubric development: validity and reliability. Practical Assessment, Research and Evaluation 7(10). Online. Available: http://pareonline.net/getvn.asp?v=7&n=10

Satterly D 1994 Quality in external assessment. In: Harlen W (ed.) Enhancing quality in assessment. Paul Chapman Publishing, London

Schuwirth L W T, van der Vleuten C P M 2003 ABC of learning and teaching in medicine. Written assessment. BMJ 326:643

Further reading

Cummings R 1988 How should we assess and report student generic attributes? In: Black B, Stanley N (eds) Teaching and learning in changing times. Proceedings of the 7th Annual Teaching Learning Forum, University of Western Australia, February 1998. UWA, Perth, Australia. Online. Available http://lsn.curtin.edu.au/tlf/tlf1998/cummings.html

Jolly B, Grant J 1997, The good assessment guide. OUCEM Publications Milton Keynes

Thomson B, Daniel L G 1996 Seminal readings on reliability and validity: a 'hit parade' bibliography. Educational and Psychological Measurement 56(5):741–745

Chapter 34
Written assessments

L. W. T. Schuwirth, C. P. M. van der Vleuten

Introduction

Written assessment formats are probably the most well-known and most widely used assessment methods in medical education. Their popularity is mainly due to their logistical advantages and their cost-effectiveness. In comparison with many other methods (computer-based, oral, patient-based, etc) they are quite easy and cheap to run. Also, they can produce reliable scores. But they are not a panacea: to test medical competence comprehensively a variety of written and nonwritten methods is needed. The purpose of this chapter is to provide some background information about strengths and weaknesses of written assessment methods. First, some general issues concerning written assessments will be discussed. Subsequently, individual formats will be presented with their advantages and disadvantages. Finally, some tips concerning their use and some item construction rules are given.

Question format

Often a distinction is made between open-ended and closed question formats. 'Closed questions' refers to all formats in which the answers are provided in the form of options, and 'open-ended' refers to all question types in which the candidate has to construct the answer spontaneously. Often multiple-choice items are deemed unfit for the testing of higher-order cognitive skills (e.g., medical problem solving) because of the so-called cueing effect. This effect implies that the correct answer can be produced by recognition of the correct option rather than by spontaneous generation. Although this is intuitively plausible the vast amount of research in this area does not, in fact, sustain this notion. On the contrary, the format of the question seems to be far less important than the stimulus in determining what cognitive skills are being tested.

Response format versus stimulus

In more technical terms, the distinction between open-ended and closed question formats pertains to the response format (how the response is recorded). From the literature in which response formats are compared, one can definitely conclude that the response format (open-ended or closed) is not so important, but that the stimulus (what you ask) is essential.

A variety of written and non-written methods of assessment are required to test medical competence comprehensively.

Response formats
Closed questions – require candidates to select answers from a list of options.
Open-ended questions – require candidates to generate answers spontaneously.

"The positive cueing effect is considered as a disadvantage of the MCQ, and has been documented consistently. However, MCQs apparently also cue in the opposite direction: they lead the examinee to choose the wrong answer"

Schuwirth et al 1996

Consider for example these two questions regarding the response format:

You are a general practitioner and you have made a house call on a 46-year-old patient. She appears to have a perforated appendix and she shows signs of a local peritonitis.
Which is the best next step in the management?

and

You are a general practitioner and you have made a house call on a 46-year-old patient. She appears to have a perforated appendix and she shows signs of a local peritonitis.
Which of the following is the most appropriate next step in the management?
a   give pain medication and re-assess her situation in 24 hours
b   give pain medication and let her drive to the hospital in her own car
c   give no pain medication and let her drive to the hospital in her own car
d   give pain medication and call an ambulance
e   give no pain medication and call an ambulance

In these two questions there is very little difference in what is asked, whereas the way the response is recorded differs.

Now consider these two questions regarding stimulus format:

What is the most prevalent symptom of meningitis?

and

Make a swot analysis of the government's new regulations to reduce the waiting lists in the health care system.

In these questions the response format is similar, but the content of the question is completely different. In the second question the expected thought processes are completely different from those evoked by the first.

For the rest of this chapter we will therefore use the distinction between response formats and stimulus formats.

Quality control of items

No matter which assessment format is used, the quality of the examination is always directly related to the quality of the individual items. Therefore it is of no use discussing strengths, weaknesses and uses of various item types if we cannot assume that optimal care has been taken to ensure their quality. One aspect of quality of an item is its ability to discriminate clearly between those candidates who have sufficient knowledge and those who do not. So they are a 'diagnostic for medical competence'. This implies that when a student who does not master the subject matter answers a question correctly, this can be regarded as a false-positive result, and the opposite would signify a false-negative result. In quality control procedures, prior to test administration the diag-

Stimulus formats
The content of a question will determine the thought processes required to answer it.

nosis and elimination of sources of false-positive and false-negative results is essential. In addition, determining the relevance of the items, the congruence between curricular goals and test content, and the use of item analysis and student criticisms are other important factors in quality control of assessment, but in this chapter we will focus on quality aspects of the individual items.

Response formats

Short-answer open-ended questions

Description

This is an open-ended question type which requires the candidate to generate a short answer of often no more than one or two words.
For example:

> *Which muscle origin is affected in the condition "tennis elbow"?*

When to use and when not to use

Open-ended questions generally take some time to answer. Therefore, fewer items can be asked per hour of testing time. There is a relationship between the reliability of test scores and the number of items, so open-ended questions will lead to less reliable scores. Also, they need to be marked by a content expert which makes them logistically less efficient and more costly.

For these reasons short-answer open-ended questions should only be used if closed formats would not do.

A question such as:

> *Which kidney is positioned superior to the other one?*

is not very sensible. Theoretically, there are only two possible answers, so the content prescribes a two-option multiple choice.

On the other hand a question like:

> *In elderly people with vague complaints of fatigue, thirst and poor healing of wounds which diagnosis should be thought of spontaneously?*

would be ludicrous in a multiple-choice format.

In general, the advice concerning the use of short-answer open-ended questions is not to use them unless the content of the question requires it.

Tips for item construction

Make sure the question is phrased unambiguously. Tests of medical competence are not tests of reading ability. The ability to read complicated sentences can be required from an academic but when it is not the purpose of the test it is a source of error. Use short sentences and avoid double negatives. If in doubt as to whether to use more words for clarity or fewer words for brevity it is best to opt for more clarity.

Make sure a well-defined answer key is written. Correct and incorrect answers must be clarified and possible alternative answers identified

For short-answer, open-ended questions it should be clear beforehand what would be correct answers and what would be incorrect answers.

(perhaps by a panel of examiners) beforehand. This is especially necessary if more than one person is to correct the test papers.

Make sure that it is clear to the candidates what kind of answer is expected. A disadvantage of open-ended questions may be that it is not fully clear to the candidates what kind of answer is expected. This may be due to confusion about the required level of detail. For example in the answer to a question on chest infection, is the expected answer: pneumonia, bacterial pneumonia or even pneumococcal pneumonia?

There may be lack of clarity about what type of answer is expected:

What is the main difference between the left and right lung?

Is the expected answer: mirror image, the number of lobes, the angle of the main bronchus, the surface, the contribution to gas exchange?

Indicate a maximum length of the answer. Students often apply a 'blunderbuss' approach, which means that they will write down as much as they can in the hope that part of their response will be the correct answer. By limiting the length of the answer this can be prevented.

Use multiple correctors effectively. If more than one teacher is involved in correcting the test papers it is better to 'nest' them within questions than within students. This means that it is better that one corrector scores the same item(s) for all students and another corrector scores another set of items for all students, than for one corrector to score the whole test for one group of students and another the whole test for another group of students. In the latter case a student can be advantaged by a mild corrector or be disadvantaged by a harsh one; in the former the same group of examiners will be used to produce the scores for all students, which leads to a better reliability with the same effort.

Essay questions

Description

Essay questions are open-ended types of questions that require a longer answer. Ideally, they are used to ask the candidate to set up a reasoning process, to evaluate a given situation or specifically to apply learnt concepts to a new situation. An example is:

John and Jim, both 15 years old, are going for a swim in the early spring. The water is still very cold. John has the idea of seeing who can stay under water the longest. They both decide to give it a go. Before entering the water John takes one deep breath of air, whereas Jim exhales deeply about 10 times and dives into the cold water. When John cannot hold his breath any more he surfaces. Much to his shock he sees Jim on the bottom of the swimming pool. He manages to get Jim on the side, and a bystander starts resuscitation.

Explain at the pathophysiological level what has happened to Jim, why he became unconscious, and explain why this has not happened to John.

Of course it is important that the situation of John and Jim is new to the students, and that it has not already been explained during the lectures or practicals. A question such as:

Explain the Bohr effect and how it influences the O_2 saturation of the blood.

is therefore less suitable as an essay type of question. Although the knowledge asked may be relevant, the question asks for reproduction of factual knowledge, which is more efficiently done with other formats.

When to use and when not to use

It is essential to use essay questions only for specific purposes. The main reason for this is the lower reliability and the need for hand-scoring.

Essay questions are therefore best used when the answer requires spontaneous generation of information and when more than a short text is required. Examples are:

- Evaluating a certain action or situation, for example:

  Make a swot analysis of the government's new regulations to reduce waiting lists in the healthcare system.

- Application of learnt concepts on a new situation or problem, for example:

  During your course you have learnt the essentials of the biofeedback mechanism of ACTH. Apply this mechanism to the control of diuresis.

- Generating solutions, hypotheses, research questions.
- Predicting or estimating.
- Comparing, looking for similarities or discussing differences.

Tips for item construction

For essay questions, essentially the same item construction suggestions apply as for short-answer open-ended questions:

- The question must be phrased extremely clearly; the candidate must not be left in the dark as to what is expected.
- The answer key must be well written, including alternative correct answers and plausible but incorrect answers. This must not be simply left to the corrector.
- The maximum length of the answer must be stipulated, to ensure a concise response and avoid the 'blunderbuss' approach.

A special type of essay question is the modified essay question. This question consists of a case followed by a number of questions. Often these questions follow the case chronologically. This can lead to the problem of interdependency of the questions. So, if candidates answer the first question incorrectly they are likely to answer all subsequent parts of the question incorrectly also. This is a serious psychometric problem which can only be avoided by an administrative procedure in which the candidates hand in the answers before they are allowed to

It can be difficult to score answers submitted as an essay without being influenced by the student's literary style.

proceed to the next question. Currently, the key-feature approach case-based assessment, which will be discussed below, is more popular.

True–false questions

Description

True–false questions are statements to which the candidate has to indicate whether the given answer is true or false. For example:

> *Stem:* *For the treatment of a Legionella pneumophila pneumonia a certain antimicrobial agent is most indicated. This is:*
>
> *Item:* *erythromycin* *True/False*

The first part, the stem, is information that is given to the candidate. It is always correct, so the candidates do not have to include it in their considerations. The item is the part for which the candidate has to indicate whether it is true or false.

When to use and when not to use

True–false questions have the possibility of covering a broad domain in a relatively short period of time, which leads to broad sampling. They are often used mainly for testing of factual knowledge, and it seems as if this is indeed what they are most suited for. Nevertheless, they have some inherent disadvantages. First, they are quite difficult to construct flawlessly. Very careful item construction is needed to ensure that the answer is defensibly true or false. This often leads to quite artificial construction. For example:

> *Stem:* *Certain disorders occur more often together than is to be expected on the basis of pure coincidence. This is the case for:*
>
> *Item:* *diabetes and atherosclerosis* *True/False*

A second disadvantage is that when candidates answer a false-keyed item correctly one can only conclude that they knew that the statement is untrue, and not whether they would have known what would have been true. For example in the question:

> *Stem:* *For the treatment of an acute attack of gout in elderly patients certain drugs can be indicated. Such a drug is:*
>
> *Item:* *allopurinol* *False*

If a candidate answers 'false' one cannot conclude that they would have known which drugs are indicated.

Tips for item construction

Use stems when necessary. It is useful to put all information that is not part of the question in the stem. That way it is perfectly clear to the candidate what should and should not be considered. Also most item construction flaws are avoided.

Avoid semiquantitative terminology. Words such as 'often', 'seldom', etc. are difficult to define. Different people assign different meanings to those words, so whether the answer is 'true' or 'false' is then a matter of opinion and not of fact. In such cases one has to revert to statements indicating exact percentages such as:

Stem: *In a certain percentage of patients with an acute pancreatitis the disease is self-limiting*
Item: *This percentage lies closer to 80 than to 50%*

Avoid terms that are too open or too absolute. Words such as 'can', 'is possible', on the one hand, or 'never', 'always', on the other lead test-wise students to the correct answer. The most probable answer to statements which are too open is 'true' and the most probable answer to statements which are too absolute is 'false'.
The same applies to equality, synonymy, etc.
Make sure the question is phrased so that the answer is defensibly correct.

Stem: *The cause of atherosclerosis is*
Item: *hypercholesterolaemia*

In this case one could argue that there are many causes or that there is a chain of aetiological factors that cause atherosclerosis. In such a case, for example, it would be better to ask for risk factors than causes.
Avoid double negatives. Although double negatives are to be avoided in all types of questions, it is especially important in true–false questions, as the answer-key 'false' can be seen as a negative also. Unfortunately, this cannot be avoided in all cases.

Stem: *For patients with hypertension certain drugs are contraindicated. Such a drug is:*
Item: *corticosteroids*   *False*

The double negative 'contraindicated' and 'False' (answer key) cannot be simply removed by using the combination 'indicated' and 'True', because then the question would not be correct.

Multiple-choice questions

Description
This is certainly the most well-known item format. It is often also referred to as single-best option multiple-choice or A-type. It consists of a stem, a question (called the lead-in) and a number of options. The candidate has to indicate which of the options is correct.

Stem: *During resuscitation of an adult, compressions of the thorax have to be performed to produce circulation. For this one hand has to be placed on the sternum and the other has to be placed on this hand in order to give correct compressions.*
Lead-in: *Which of the following options indicates the most correct position of both hands?*
Option: *a   the junction between manubrium and sternum*
b   the superior half of the sternum
c   the middle of the sternum

d   the inferior half of the sternum
e   the xiphoid process of the sternum

When to use and when not to use

Multiple-choice items can be considered the most flexible question type. They are reasonably simple to produce and to administer. They are not time-consuming in answering and scoring, and they are logistically efficient. This does not mean however that they can test all aspects of medical competence. They are therefore best used if broad sampling of the domain is required and if large numbers of candidates are to be tested. They yield reliable testing scores per hour of testing time. The two main reasons for not using them are:

• when spontaneous generation of the answer is essential (this is explained in the paragraph on short-answer open-ended questions)
• when the number of realistic options is too large.

In all other cases multiple-choice questions are a good alternative to open-ended questions.

Tips for item construction

The general tips mentioned in the preceding paragraphs all pertain to multiple-choice questions also (clear sentences, defensibly correct answer key, etc.), but there are some tips that apply uniquely to multiple-choice questions:

Use equal alternatives.

Sydney is:
a   the capital of Australia
b   a dirty city
c   situated at the Pacific Ocean
d   the first city of Australia

In this case the options all relate to different aspects and in order to produce the correct answer the candidate has to compare apples to oranges. A better and more focused alternative would be:

Which of the following is the capital of Australia?
a   Sydney
b   Melbourne
c   Adelaide
d   Perth
e   Canberra

Use options of equal length. Often the longest option is the correct one, because often more words are needed to make an option correct than to make it incorrect. Students know this and will be guided by this hint.

Avoid fillers. Sometimes it is difficult to find sufficient realistic options. Unfortunately, it is often prescribed to have four or five options where only three realistic ones can be found. This leads to the production of nonsense options (fillers). There is much to be said against this.

- Candidates will recognise the fillers and discard them immediately.
- You will underestimate the guessing chance.
- It will take a lot of item-writing time to find the extra option before you decide for the filler (this time would better be used for another question).
- Authors may use combination options ('all of the above' or 'none of the above') instead, which is ill-advised.

Use simple multiple-choice formats only.

The major symptoms associated with cardiovascular disease:
1   *are chest pain, dyspnoea, palpitations*
2   *appear to worsen during exertion*
3   *are fatigue, dizziness and syncope*
4   *appear during rest*

a   *(1), (2) and (3) are correct*
b   *(1) and (3) are correct*
c   *2) and (4) are correct*
d   *only (4) is correct*
e   *all are correct*

In this case the question is unnecessarily complicated. Not only can it lead to mistakes by candidates in selecting between all the combinations, which has nothing to do with medical competence, but the combinations could also give important clues as to which answer is correct simply by logic. The rule for these formats is simple: do not use them.

Try to construct the question in a way so that theoretically the answer could also be given without seeing the answer options. This ensures that there is a clear and well-defined lead-in and that all the alternatives are aimed at the same aspect. So after a stem or case description, the lead-in *Which of the following is true?* is too open, but the lead-in *Which of the following is the most probable diagnosis?* is well defined and could theoretically be answered as if it were an open-ended question.

Multiple true–false questions

Description
In this question format more than one option can be ticked by the candidate. There are two versions. In one candidates are told how many options they should select or this is left open. The former is used when there is no clear distinction between correct and incorrect, for example:

Select the two most probable diagnoses

The latter version is used if there is a clear distinction, for example:

Select the drugs that are indicated in this case

Scoring of such items can be done in various ways. The standard approach is to treat all options as true–false items and then regard a ticked option as 'true' and the others as 'false'. The score on the item is the total of correctly ticked and nonticked options divided by the total number of options. An alternative scoring system is to indicate a minimum of correct answers for a score of 1 and to score all other responses as 0.

When to use and when not to use
The main reason for using this format is when a selection of correct options from a limited number of options is indeed required, and when short-answer open-ended questions cannot be used.

Tips for item construction
There are no specific tips concerning this question type other than those applying to multiple-choice and short-answer open-ended questions.

Stimulus formats

Extended-matching questions

Description
Extended-matching items consist of a theme description, a series of options (up to 26), a lead-in and a series of short cases or vignettes.

Theme: diagnosis
Options:

a hyperthyroidism	*d hyperparathyroidism*	*g....etc....*
b hypothyroidism	*e phaeochromocytoma*	
c prolactinoma	*f Addison's disease*	

Lead-in:
For each of the following cases select the most likely diagnosis
Vignettes:
A 45-year-old man consults you because of periods of extensive sweating. One or two times per day he has short periods during which he starts sweating heavily. His wife tells him that his face is all red. He feels very warm during this period. He has had this now for over 3 weeks. At first he thought the complaints would subside spontaneously but now he is not sure any more. Pulmonary and cardiac examination reveal no abnormalities. His blood pressure is 130/80, pulse 76 regular.

When to use and when not to use
Because the questions ask for decisions and the stimuli are cases, extended-matching items focus more on decision making or problem solving. The large number of alternatives reduces the effect of cueing. Because the items are relatively short and can be answered quickly, extended-matching questions cover a large knowledge base per hour of testing time. They are best used in all situations where large groups of candidates have to be tested in a logistical and feasible way.

Tips for item construction
First determine the theme. This is important because it helps you to focus all the alternatives on the same element. To minimise the influence of cueing it is important that all the options could theoretically apply to all vignettes.

The options should be short. The shorter and clearer the options the less likely it is that any hints as to the correct answer may be given. It is good to avoid using verbs in the options.

The lead-in should be clear and well-defined. A lead-in such as 'for each of the following vignettes select the most appropriate option' is too open and often indicates that the options are not homogeneous or the vignettes are not appropriately related to the options.

Key-feature approach questions

Description

A final format is the key-feature approach. It consists of a short clearly described case or problem and a limited number of questions that aim at essential decisions. Key-feature approach tests can therefore consist of many different short cases enabling a broad sampling of the domain. They often produce a reliable examination per hour of testing time and are demonstrated to be valid for the assessment of medical decision making or problem solving. Although often certain response formats are prescribed, the most versatile way to use them is to select the response format according to the content of the question (this is explained in the paragraphs above)

Tips for item construction

Apart from all the tips concerning the other question types, some tips are specifically pertinent to key-feature tests.

Make sure all the important information is presented in the case. This does not only mean relevant medical information, but also contextual information (where you see the patient, what is your function, etc.). After you have written the questions it is good to re-address the case to check whether all the necessary information is provided.

Make sure the question is directly linked to the case. It should be impossible to answer the question correctly if the case is not read. Ideally, all the information in the case must be used to produce the answer, and the correct answer is based on a careful balancing of the all the information.

The question must ask for essential decisions. An incorrect decision must automatically lead to an incorrect management of the case. In certain instances the diagnosis may not be the key feature, for example if different diagnosis would still lead to the same management of the case. Another way to check this is to see whether the answer key would change if certain elements of the case (such as location of the symptoms, age of the patient, etc.) were to be changed.

Summary

It must be stressed again that there is no one single best question format; for a good and comprehensive assessment of medical competence a variety of instruments is needed. This chapter has provided a brief overview of various written question formats with some of their strengths and weaknesses and some hints for their use. The reference and further reading lists suggest more detailed literature.

In constructing EMI questions:
- Determine the theme first.
- Keep the individual options short.
- The lead-in should be clear and well-defined.

"it has proven to be ill-advised to make up cases without consulting others"

Schuwirth et al 1999

For key-feature approach questions:
- Make sure all the important information is presented in the case.
- Make sure the question is directly linked to the case.
- The question must ask for essential decisions.

"Exam questions which relate to patient situations we will have to deal with as junior doctors seem more relevant than those testing simple factual knowledge"

Medical student

"A final piece of advice would be the suggestion...to look for the possibility of co-operation with other departments or faculties since the production of high quality test material can be tedious and expensive"

(Schuwirth et al 1999)

References

Schuwirth L W T, van der Vleuten C P M, Donkers H H L M. 1996 A closer look at cueing effects in multiple-choice questions. Medical Education 30:44–49

Schuwirth L W T, Blackmore D B, Mom E M A et al 1999 How to write short cases for assessing problem-solving skills. Medical Teacher 21:144–150

Further reading

Bordage G. 1987 An alternative approach to PMPs: the 'key-features' concept. In: Hart I R, Harden R, editors. Further developments in assessing clinical competence, Proceedings of the Second Ottawa Conference. Montreal. Can-Heal Publications pp 59–75

Cantillon P, Hutchinson L, Wood D 2003 editors. ABC of learning and teaching in medicine. BMJ publishing Group, London

Case S M, Swanson D B. 1993 Extended-matching items: a practical alternative to free-response questions. Teaching and Learning in Medicine 5:107–115

Case S M, Swanson D B. 1998 Constructing written test questions for the basic and clinical sciences. National Board of Medical Examiners, Philadelphia

Norman G R, Swanson D B, Case S M 1996 Conceptual and methodology issues in studies comparing assessment formats, issues in comparing item formats. Teaching and Learning in Medicine 8:208–216

Schuwirth L W T, Van der Vleuten C P M, Donkers H H L M 1992 Open-ended questions versus multiple choice questions. In: Harden R, Hart I R, Mulholland H (eds) Approaches to the assessment of clinical competence, Proceedings of the Fifth Ottawa Conference. Page Brothers, Norwich, Great Britain. p 486–491

Swanson D B, Norcini J J, Grosso L J. 1987 Assessment of clinical competence: written and computer-based simulations. Assessment and Evaluation in Higher Education 12:220–246

Chapter 35
Performance assessment

M. Marks, S. Humphrey-Murto

Introduction

Performance-based assessment is not a new concept. All readers will probably have had a performance-based assessment at some time. Your earliest assessment of this type probably occurred as a child when you were assessed for the next level of a sporting or musical activity. Or perhaps your first experience was when you were assessed for your ability to drive a car. In each of these incidences you had to *demonstrate* to an examiner and *be observed* doing the task being certified. It would never occur to anyone to consider examining for these skills using only a written examination.

Miller (1990) proposed a framework for clinical assessment which progresses through four levels:

- knows
- knows how
- shows how
- does.

This same framework can be applied to the assessment of any skill set. Let us consider the skills of driving and obeying the rules of the road. A pen and paper test can assess whether an individual *knows* the actual rules, for example, a red light means stop. One may be able to describe the process of applying gradual pressure to the brake pedal to stop a vehicle when a red light appears – *knows how*. However, during a road test one has to actually demonstrate the ability to smoothly bring a vehicle to a stop at the red light – *shows how*. The police monitor compliance with the rules of the road, checking that a driver actually stops at a red light – *does*. As every new driver realises, knowing what to do and actually doing it during the road test is definitely not the same thing.

As with driving a car, a clinician's performance must be measured using performance-based testing. To practise competently, clinicians require proficiency in a number of different skills. The idea of implementing a performance-based examination to assess this vast array of skills may seem an insurmountable task. Thus, for many years medical student evaluation focused on the assessment of knowledge using written tests that are easily administered, cover broad content and have proven reliability.

"The fundamental concept of performance-based testing is that a candidate must 'show how' and/or be observed 'doing' the behaviour to be assessed"

Dauphinee 1995

"No single assessment method can provide all the data required for judgment of anything so complex as the delivery of professional services by a successful physician"

Miller 1990

"Performance based testing is required for national certification by:
- *Medical Council of Canada*
- *General Medical Council of the United Kingdom*
- *Educational Commission for Foreign Medical Graduates in the United States*
- *National Board of Medical Examiners in the United States (planned for 2005)"*

Adamo 2003

A PubMed search retrieves 133 papers with OSCE in the title.

"The OSCE is now used in over 50 countries world-wide. There is a national OSCE in Canada, taken by all medical school graduates before they are granted a licence to practice"

Hart 2001

Oral examinations

The traditional oral examination continues to be a 'rite of passage' for physicians in some countries. Oral examinations provide a means of assessing student knowledge and sometimes performance within a clinical context. After assessing a real patient, usually unobserved, the student is asked a series of questions about the patient. If the student is not observed, this examination does not meet the criterion of 'shows how' to actually make it a performance-based examination. Furthermore, different examinees seeing different patients, limited sampling, and low reliability are some of the major limitations to this type of examination (Petrusa 2002). Due to these limitations, oral examinations are no longer used as certification assessments by many specialty boards in the United States and Canada.

In-training assessments

Assessment of skills in the settings in which they are learned is very appealing and certainly appears to have greater face validity than any exam model. However, problems with in-training evaluations are multiple: lack of standardisation, limited observation of performance and limited sampling of skills are all issues of concern (see chapter 36, Work-based assessment). While these evaluations are important for formative assessment, they may not have adequate reliability and validity to be useful as a high-stakes summative evaluation.

Introducing an objective structured clinical exam

The next best thing to using real patients to assess students is to use standardised patients in simulated clinical encounters. Lay persons can be trained to assume the role of a patient, providing a consistent history, communication style and physical findings (see chapter 8, Teaching in the clinical skills centre). Harden & Gleeson (1979) introduced the idea of the objective structured clinical examination (OSCE). In this examination students moved in turn through 5-minute 'stations' in which they were presented with a specific clinical scenario and had to demonstrate specific clinical examination skills. A key feature of the OSCE was that each student performed the same series of tasks and was graded using a standardised scoring scheme. The OSCE was one of the first performance-based examinations to be used in assessing physician competence and is now considered the prototype of performance-based assessment.

Over time, the OSCE has been adapted to assess multiple skills: physical examination skills; interpretation of radiographs, EKGs and laboratory results as they relate to a patient encounter; communication skills; technical skills and teaching skills. The use of genital, rectal and breast models, heart sound simulators and more complex cardiovascular simulators have expanded the skills that can be tested. Surgical skills, such as the excision of a sebaceous cyst and incision and drainage of an abscess, have been included in surgical performance-based assessments (Friedlich et al 2002). Depending on the complexity of the skill being assessed the length of the stations can vary from 5 to 30 minutes. Thus, the format and content of multistation performance-based assessments can be varied to meet the needs of diverse groups.

There is little disagreement that an OSCE style examination provides a more valid assessment of clinical skills than a written or oral examination. With training of those involved in conducting and presenting the examination, the reliability of OSCEs, in terms of standardised patient portrayal, interrater agreement, exam reliability and standardisation across multiple testing sites, has been shown to be acceptable.

Reliability can be further increased with larger numbers of stations and examinees (Petrusa 2002). Some would suggest that a minimum of about 20 stations is needed to obtain the minimum reliability (Shumway & Harden 2003). However, in a high stakes examination in Canada, with large numbers of candidates, the number of stations has been reduced from 20 to 12 without significant reduction in test reliability (D Blackmore, personal communication, 2004).

The feasibility of OSCE-type performance-based assessments must be considered. A 25-station OSCE over 8 hours may provide excellent reliability and validity, but is not realistic for most universities. In our experience 10–12 stations seems to be a reasonable compromise for a local medical school examination. The length of our stations is 8 minutes with 2 minutes for feedback and 1 minute to move to the next station.

In Dundee, multiple (25–35) 4- or 5-minute stations are the norm. Thus most exams provide a total testing time per candidate of 100–120 minutes. Some high-stakes examinations may be slightly longer in length.

Making it happen: implementing a performance-based examination

Once the decision has been made to use a performance–based assessment, time and effort will be required to plan, develop and implement a multistation examination. If this is the first OSCE-type examination in your centre a site visit or communication with individuals who have done similar examinations may be invaluable. The following section will outline the required steps to organise the exam. The examples given are from OSCEs; however the same principles can be applied to any performance-based test. Table 35.1 provides an OSCE planning checklist that may be valuable to those planning their first OSCE. Each of the components of the checklist will be considered below.

Examination content – what do you want to assess?

Examination blueprint
Before developing stations for your exam, you need to know what skills you should assess. That is, your examination should reflect the training objectives of the education programme. One way to ensure this is by developing a blueprint or template for the examination. Ideally it should be developed by a group of individuals familiar with the training objectives. For a general undergraduate medical OSCE, a useful approach is to consider the skills students should have mastered for their level of training,

The OSCE is all about measuring outcomes.

The OSCE allows very specific feedback, not only to the candidates, but also to those who taught them and those who set the examination.

"If there are a set of explicit learning objectives for the course, these can be used along with imagination to develop a series of stations that can test them in as close to real-life situations as possible"

Hart 2001

Table 35.1 Exam-planning checklist

Exam content
- Blueprint
- Recruit case authors
- Finalise case content

Standard setting
- Decide on a pass mark

Standardised patients
- Recruitment
- Training

Logistics
- Location of the exam
- Number of tracks required
- Staff
- Equipment and models

Examiners
- Recruitment
- Training

Budget
- Administrative staff
- Examiners
- Standardised patients
- Food
- Equipment
- Site
- Parking

Post-exam review
- Feedback on cases and process from
  - students
  - examiners
  - administrative staff
- Review pass marks
- Recommend changes to stations

such as history taking, physical examination skills, patient management, counselling, communication skills and procedural skills.

Specific domains of practice should then be outlined, such as internal medicine, surgery, psychiatry, obstetrics, paediatrics, family medicine and emergency medicine. Decide on the number of stations required for each skill and content area and plan accordingly. Each station will cover at least one skill and one domain of practice (Table 35.2).

How to develop cases/scenarios

Content experts, with some knowledge of the trainees to be tested and their required skill level, should write the cases. Case authors should be provided with a specific skill and domain of practice to be assessed and asked to base their case on an actual patient they have encountered. In addition to adding to the authenticity of the examination, using actual cases leaves less room for error and omissions in developing cases for the exam. The authors are asked to provide the following components for each case:

Table 35.2 Sample template for an exam blueprint

	History	Physical examination	Coun- selling	Procedural skills	Manage- ment	Investi- gations
Internal medicine	1				1	1
Surgery		1		1		
Paediatrics	1					
Psychiatry	1					
Obstetrics and gynaecology			1			
Family medicine		1				1

1. *Define the purpose of the station*
   State the skill and domain to be tested. For example:
   Skill – physical examination. Domain – internal medicine/cardiology.

   The purpose of this station is to assess the ability of candidates to complete a physical examination of a patient with congestive heart failure.

2. *Candidate instructions*
   Candidate instructions must be clear and concise. Always ask a colleague to interpret the instructions you provide to ensure they are indeed clear. Make sure the task can be completed in the allocated time.

   Complete a focused physical examination in a patient with suspected congestive heart failure. You have eight minutes to complete this station.

3. *Scoring checklist*
   The checklist should be complete and include the main components of the skill being assessed. However, exhaustive checklists are not necessary. Table 35.3 provides a sample checklist for assessment of a physical examination. If deemed appropriate, checklist items can be weighted to reflect the importance of one item over another.

4. *Standardised patient instructions*
   These instructions must be detailed enough to guarantee standardisation across candidates and across more than one standardised patient playing the same role. Indicate the gender and age of the standardised patient and the type of clothing that should be worn. Provide all relevant data including the presenting complaint and history of present illness, past medical history, medication, family history and social history. The history of the

Table 35.3 Sample of examiner checklist for assessment of a physical examination

Candidate's Instructions: Mrs/Mr C. presents with a sore swollen ankle for 6 weeks. He/she cannot recall any trauma. **Please examine his/her right ankle.**

	Done/asked satisfactorily √
1. Introduces self to patient	
2. Explains to the patient what will be done	
3. Demonstrates concern for patient i.e. is not excessively rough	
4. Inspection for any of swelling, erythema, deformity	
5. Compares to the other side	
6. Inspection: • Standing • From anterior • And posterior	
7. Inspection of gait	
8. Palpation • Anterior joint line (tibiotalar) • Medial malleolus • Lateral malleolus • Achilles tendon	
9. **ROM** • Checks active and passive ROM • Tibiotalar (true ankle joint) plantar dorsiflexion • Midtarsal (grasps the forefoot, stabilises the heel and internally/externally rotates • Subtalar (grasps the heel and internally/ externally rotates)	

Score: _____ / 17

present illness will require details such as when did the chest pain begin, location, quality, severity, alleviating/aggravating factors and so forth. It is also necessary to standardise how much information the standardised patient will give to open-ended questions. Finally, any specific questions to be asked by the standardised patient must be outlined, including instructions as to when in the scenario the questions are to be asked.

5. *Instructions for station set-up*

List all equipment required for the station. A simple list of necessary equipment may be all that is needed for a physical examination skills station. However, a detailed outline of how equipment is to be presented to each candidate is necessary for stations where models, technical equipment and simulators are being used. All candidates should be presented with the same equipment, in the same manner, throughout the exam.

Ideally, cases should be reviewed and finalised by a committee of case authors. The reality is often that one or two individuals do most of the writing. For new authors, an example of a previous case can be helpful; most who have not had previous experience with performance-based examinations using clinical simulations fail to appreciate the amount of detail required to guarantee standardisation.

Once the case is written, ask a colleague to go through the station. This will highlight any difficulties with the candidate instructions and identify required revisions in the checklist items. It will also ensure the length of the station is appropriate and whether the information provided for the standardised patient is sufficient. Five to ten minutes spent with a colleague asking, 'What would you do based on these candidate instructions?' may save hours of frustration for candidates, standardised patients and examiners later.

Weighting of checklists and rating scales

Most checklists require the examiner to indicate whether an item has been performed satisfactorily. One method of highlighting items felt to be more important is to include weighting. For example most items would be worth 1 mark, but giving oxygen to a hypoxic patient may be worth 5 marks. It would therefore contribute more to the final mark.

Likert rating scales are very useful for skills such as communication where a binary rating may not reflect the range of skill being demonstrated by a variety of candidates. Table 35.4 provides an example of a communication checklist. Calculating the final mark will require a decision on the weighting of the communication checklist. In our institution it is included on all history taking and counselling stations and is worth 20% of the mark. In other examinations, the communication skills checklist can account for up to 50% of the mark for a station.

Recruitment and training of standardised patients

Standardised patients are trained to portray a specific clinical scenario in a reliable and consistent fashion. They may be volunteers or paid employees. While volunteers may frequently be recruited for a small OSCE exam, access to a programme that recruits and trains standardised patients can be extremely valuable for larger scale examinations. Many institutions also have trainers who review the case with the standardised patients and help them practise their role until standardisation has been achieved. Ideally, a physician will also observe the standardised patients demonstrating their scenario before the examination. Training for these

"Skills are actions (and reactions) which a person performs in a competent way in order to achieve a goal.

One may have no skill, some skill or complete skill. Acceptable mastery must be set appropriate to the level of the student's training: not yes/no, but analogue along a spectrum"

Hart 2001

Table 35.4 Sample communication skills checklist	1 Poor	2 Fair	3 Good	4 Very good	5 Excellent
1. Interpersonal skills:					
– Listens carefully					
– Treats patient as an equal					
2. Interviewing skills:					
– Uses words patient can understand					
– Organised					
– Does not interrupt, allows patient to explain					
3. Patient education:					
– Provides clear, complete information					
– Encourages patient to ask questions					
– Answers questions clearly					
– Confirms patient's understanding/opinion					
4. Response to emotional issues:					
– Recognises, accepts and discusses emotional issues					
– Controls own emotional state					

Score: ____/20

individuals can vary from 30 minutes to 15 hours depending on the complexity of the case.

Paying standardised patients does allow the institution to demand regular attendance and a higher standard of performance. The rate of remuneration is around $10 to $15 per hour in the US (Adamo 2003). Do not forget that during the examination standardised patients may require periodic rests, especially in physically demanding stations.

Examiner recruitment and training

Examiners can be faculty clinicians or senior trainees, depending on the examination. Standardised patients or trained observers have been used to complete checklists and global rating scales (Martin et al 1996).

Using physician examiners may have several advantages: there is increased validity in having a member of the profession examine candidates; physicians can be used for standard setting using the modified borderline group method, and can also provide immediate feedback during practice exams. Disadvantages include difficulty with recruitment in some institutions and the costs incurred if examiners are paid.

Examiner training usually consists of a short introduction to the purpose of the examination and a basic review of checklist completion, the global rating scale and providing feedback. Physicians are provided with their station assignment. More extensive training that is case-specific may be beneficial, but not realistic, in many centres. If trained observers, such as standardised patients, are used more training is required. Examiner recruitment should be done weeks or months in advance of the examination. The orientation is best completed just preceding the examination to ensure attendance by all examiners.

Standard setting: pass or fail?

There is no consensus regarding which method should be used for standard setting, or deciding on a pass/fail mark, in any examination, including the OSCE. Most authors would agree that standard setting should be criterion-referenced to ensure candidates have a minimum acceptable level of competency. Usually a percentage score in the examination is agreed upon by a group of examiners as reflecting the minimal level of competence required (see chapter 32, Standard setting).

If clinician examiners are used in an OSCE, then the modified borderline group method may be used to set a pass mark. At the end of each encounter the examiner is asked to complete a global rating scale independently of the checklist. The examiner is asked, 'Did the candidate meet the needs of the patient?' The rating scale includes 'Unsatisfactory' (inferior, poor, borderline) or 'Satisfactory' (borderline, good, excellent).

Checklist scores for all candidates rated as borderline (Unsatisfactory and Satisfactory) are summed, and the mean becomes the cut score to pass that station. Thus the pass/fail score is the average of the borderline performances that several examiners have identified. We have used this method with as few as 60 candidates and it appears to provide defensible results. The risk with small numbers of candidates is that very few will be identified as borderline and the pass mark will be less reliably established. Cusimano (1996) has reviewed in detail the topic of standard setting in performance-based examinations.

Running the exam: logistics

Examinations may be run in test centres or outpatient clinics during evenings and weekends. In the latter situation, basic equipment such as examining tables and blood pressure cuffs are available and in a teaching hospital the space is usually free of charge. It is crucial that detailed instructions for station set-up be provided for each station to ensure

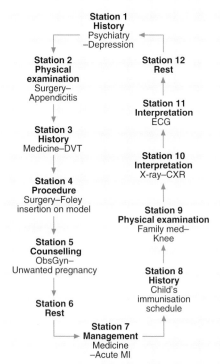

Fig. 35.1 Example of a 10-station OSCE accommodating 12 students

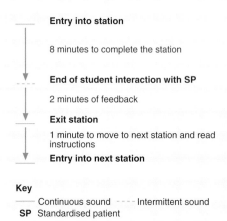

Key

—— Continuous sound   - - - - Intermittent sound
SP Standardised patient

Fig. 35.2 Signalling station changes

standardisation across sites. A map of the facility being used, including location of specific stations, is also helpful for planning. Arrows on the walls or floor can assist candidates and staff with the rotation from station to station.

Space requirements

The number of candidates and available rooms will determine how many tracks (each track contains the full examination) and administrations (how many times the tracks will have to be run) you will require. For example, we have 65 students but only three tracks, each with 10 stations. We therefore administer the examination simultaneously in three tracks (30 students), and run it twice (60 students). The extra five students are accommodated in 'rest stations' within the tracks. Figure 35.1 shows how 12 students may be accommodated in a 10-station track. To ensure exam security, students in the first administration of the exam must be sequestered until the second set of students has begun.

In addition to the examination rooms for each station, orientation rooms are required for the examinees and examiners. Other rooms may be required to register staff and provide food.

Signalling station changes

During the student orientation students receive instruction on how to progress from one station to the next, and that a buzzer or bell will signal entry into a station and another indicates time to exit from the station. During practice exams we provide an intermittent buzzer to signal the beginning of a 2-minute time for feedback from the examiner. When the end-of-station buzzer sounds, candidates have one minute to move to the next station and read the candidate instructions posted on the door. The next buzzer signals entry into the next station (Fig. 35.2).

Exam day

On the day of the examination staff will be required to register the candidates, direct them to stations, time the exam, indicate station changes using buzzers or bells and assist with set-up and dismantling of the stations. Each station must have the station number and candidate instructions posted on the door. The standardised patients, examiners and candidates must be matched to the appropriate stations. Examiners and standardised patients should be in the examination rooms 30 minutes before the start of the exam to review checklists and rating scales. A final dry run of the station is advisable to help the standardised patient get into the role for the exam.

Collecting results

If printed checklists are used they must be distributed in each station and gathered at the end of the examination. Handheld computers have the potential to replace these sheets and provide immediate automated feedback to each candidate as well as provide group data to the organisers. Schmidts (2000) found that examiners required only 15 minutes of training to use these devices that have the potential to significantly improve efficiency in grading and marking of examinations with multiple stations.

Budget and dedicated staff

Running an OSCE can be resource intensive. While some institutions have separate examination centres, teaching hospitals often provide clinic space free of charge for an evening to run a multiple-station examination. Required equipment is also often available within the hospital clinic rooms.

Standardised patients may have to be paid. If your institution has a standardised patient centre for teaching purposes the same individuals can often be used during examinations. In such situations funding may be available through the university to support a standardised patient programme. Having a full-time administrator for the programme and a trainer for the standardised patients is almost essential as busy clinician educators are unlikely to be able to assume these roles.

Data entry and analysis of multiple checklists for multiple stations will require administrative support.

Examination review

Once the OSCE has been successfully completed take time to reflect on the process and make recommendations for improvements to the next exam. Often logistics can be improved. Candidate and examiner feedback should be collected on questionnaires at the completion of the examination and reviewed by the physician in charge. Stations may be modified depending on the comments received. Review the scores for each station and the pass/fail rates; identify stations that were too difficult or too easy and consider modification. With practice, the process of running these examinations will become more routine and refined.

Ten OSCE pearls

When an OSCE is run for the first time, what can go wrong, will go wrong. Here are some examples of lessons learned through our experiences in administering OSCEs

- Make all stations the same length. All candidates must rotate at the same time so one station cannot be a few minutes longer than the others.
- Stations that are coupled or linked require forethought. For example, in an OSCE of 5-minute stations, station 8 is a patient encounter and station 9 provides a radiograph based on the patient encounter. No candidate can therefore start the OSCE on station 9. A staggered start is required. One candidate starts station 8 at 5 minutes before the start of the main exam. At the start of the main exam a second candidate can then start in station 8 when the first has moved on to station 9. The staggered start candidate will complete the OSCE 5 minutes before the others.

- Have spare standardised patients and examiners available for the exam as life is unpredictable.
- Have back-up equipment, such as alternative view boxes for X-rays, extra batteries for equipment, extra checklists, etc.
- Have staff available during the examination to maintain exam security and help candidates 'find' the next station. Nervous candidates often require guidance for the first few rotations.
- If there is a missing candidate, move a sign labelled 'missing candidate' to each empty room as the exam proceeds. This avoids confusion as other candidates may skip stations, moving into the next room vacated by the preceding candidate.
- Remind candidates to remain in the room until the buzzer sounds, even if they have completed the station. This avoids loitering outside the rooms. Likewise, tell standardised patients to always remain 'in role' as candidates will often pause, only to resume and acquire additional checklist items.
- Maintain exam security. If you are administering the examination twice to accommodate all candidates, make sure the first group is kept away from the second group who are waiting for the start of their examination.
- The timer is in a position to do the most damage. Choose this individual carefully. Make sure the bells or buzzers can be heard from all locations with the doors closed.
- If the rotation has been compromised and confusion reigns, stop the exam, sort out the problem and then resume the examination. If a candidate has managed to miss a station, let the exam carry on and allow them time to do the station at the end.

Summary

Performance-based testing has become an expectation for the assessment of physician competency. As described by Miller (1990), physicians must *show* or *demonstrate* their skills, as well as provide evidence of having a sound base of medical knowledge. An OSCE-style examination provides a valid, reliable and feasible means of assessing the range of skills physicians require to practise competently; it has become the prototype performance based examination to assess the skills required of physicians.

The logistics of developing and running a large scale OSCE are significant. Adequate planning and support for the examination are essential to ensure the following tasks are completed appropriately:

- setting an examination blueprint
- developing cases with checklists and rating scales
- recruiting and training examiners
- recruiting and training standardised patients
- planning space and equipment needs
- identifying budgetary requirements
- preparing for last-minute emergencies.

"The great end in life is not knowledge but action"

Thomas Huxley

References

Adamo G 2003 Simulated and standardized patients in OSCEs: achievements and challenges 1992–2003. Medical Teacher 25(3):262–270

Cusimano M D 1996 Standard setting in medical education. Academic Medicine 71(10):S112–120

Dauphinee W D 1995 Assessing clinical performance: Where do we stand and what might we expect. Journal of the American Medical Association 274(9):741–743

Friedlich M, Wood T, Regehr G et al 2002 Structured assessment of minor surgical skills (SAMSS) for clinical clerks. Academic Medicine 77(10):S39–S41

Harden R M, Gleeson F A 1979 Assessment of clinical competence using an objective structured clinical examination (OSCE). Medical Education 13:41–54

Hart I 2001 Object clinical examinations: In Dent J, Harden RM (eds) A practical guide for medical teachers, 1st edn, Churchill Livingstone, Edinburgh, pp 357–368

Martin J A, Reznick R K, Rothman A et al 1996 Who should rate candidates in an objective structured clinical examination? Academic Medicine 71(2):170–174

Miller G E 1990 The assessment of clinical skills/competence/performance. Academic Medicine 65(7):S63–S67

Petrusa E R 2002 Clinical performance assessments. In: Norman G R, van der Vleuten C P M, Newble D I, (eds) International Handbook of Research in Medical Education. Kluwer, Dordrecht, p 673–709

Schmidts M B 2000 OSCE logistics – handheld computers replace checklists and provide automated feedback. Medical Education 34(11):957–958

Shumway J M, Harden R M 2003 The assessment of learning outcomes for the competent and reflective physician. Medical Teacher 25(6): 569–584

Useful links

NCBI (National Center for Biotechnology information http://www.ncbi.nlm.nihi.gov.PubMed

Chapter 36
Work-based assessment

M. H. Davis, G. G. Ponnamperuma

Introduction

Miller (1990) took forward thinking about assessment in the healthcare professions by identifying four levels of assessment: *knows, knows how, shows how,* and *does.* Miller's work focused attention on a largely unassessed level: what the doctor does in real-life settings. Rethans et al (1991) emphasised that scores awarded to general practitioners by simulated patients in an examination setting were significantly higher than the scores awarded for the same tasks in a real-life setting. This and other studies have drawn attention to the need to assess what healthcare professionals do in practice. Traditional examinations cannot assess what the candidate 'does' in real-life settings (Davis & Harden 2003) and a battery of new assessment tools is needed to assess performance: work-based assessment.

Judgement of performance

Norcini (2003) classified judgements about performance into three broad categories.

- outcomes of care
- process of care
- practice volume.

Outcomes of care

Outcomes of care refer to the patient outcomes as a measure of performance. Historically these outcomes were confined to mortality and morbidity. The outcomes, however, have been expanded to include various other patient end-points such as patient satisfaction, functional status of the patient and cost-effectiveness of care.

Advantages   The main advantage of utilising patient outcomes to judge performance is that they reflect the quality of care that the doctor provides and enable the public, patients and other doctors to identify the level of performance of the doctor concerned.

Disadvantages   Not every patient outcome can be attributed to the doctor's performance. The doctor usually works in a healthcare team and may not necessarily be the team leader. She/he might not be responsible for selecting the other team members. Hence, the doctor may no longer be solely responsible for the patient outcome. Several other factors, such as the patient's condition, the patient's compliance, the number of patients in the practice or the type of unit in which the patient is treated, may contribute to the patient outcome.

Process of care

Process of care bases the judgement of performance on the procedures or investigations, such as screening for cancer, diabetes and ischaemic heart disease, that have been carried out by the doctors on their patients.

Advantages   The main advantage of this method is that the judgement is less dependent upon the patient's health status. The doctor is more in control of the process of care. Since some procedures such as immunisation have to be carried out on the whole population, these methods enable standardisation and comparison of performance among doctors.

Disadvantages   The major disadvantage is that performance of a procedure does not indicate how well or otherwise the procedure has been carried out.

Practice volume

This suggests that the judgement should be based on the number of patients that the doctor has attended to. The rationale for this stems from the research evidence that quality of care is associated with higher practice volume.

Advantages   The doctor may become more experienced by handling a larger number of patients. It is assumed that the quality of care may improve when there are more opportunities to learn (i.e. more patients).

Disadvantages   Counting patient throughput has its limitations. More patients than the doctor can handle may be detrimental to the quality of patient care provided.

Tools for assessing performance in the workplace

Work-based assessment can be considered under four categories (Norcini 2003).

- clinical records
- administrative data
- diaries or logbooks
- observation of practice.

Clinical records

Clinical records are the notes written by the doctor on the patient's overall health condition and management. These may include records of history and examination findings, investigations, and management.

Advantages   The main advantage is that clinical records reflect the quality of care over time. Clinical records may be one of the best sources for studying the doctor's performance in relation to patient care.

Disadvantages   The disadvantages relate to patient confidentiality and the cost-effectiveness of the process. Records may also be lost,

"A doctor's portfolio might contain data on outcomes, process, or volume, collected through clinical record audit, diaries, or assessments by patients and peers"

Norcini 2003

incomplete or inaccurate. Moving to a fully computerised, virtual health-care environment may overcome some of these problems.

Administrative data

Administrative data held in central databases may relate to patient numbers, prescribing information, procedures performed or investigations ordered.

Advantages   These records are accessible and inexpensive. They are helpful in estimating aspects of an individual doctor's care such as cost-effectiveness.

Disadvantages   Qualitative information may be lacking in these records.

Diaries or logbooks

Diaries kept by trainees may provide useful insights into trainee achievements and other qualitative information. Logbooks can indicate the accomplishment of a list of tasks.

Advantages   If maintained properly, diaries and logbooks will provide a comprehensive account of what the trainee has done. The logbook demonstrates the scope of the trainee's activities, while the diary may additionally demonstrate progression of learning.

Disadvantages   Data may be incomplete, as considerable intrinsic motivation is required to keep diaries and logbooks up-to-date. The logbook may lack qualitative information. Verifying the accuracy of diaries is taxing. Setting standards or uniform criteria for summative assessment is difficult, particularly if the diaries are not structured.

Observation of practice

Observation of performance may be direct, or indirect such as the use of video consultations for formative (Campbell & Murray 1996a) and summative (Campbell & Murray 1996b) assessment by the Royal College of General Practitioners in the UK.

Who observes performance?

The trainee performance may be observed by either trainees/students themselves, i.e. self-assessment, or by others, such as patients, peers, tutors, and members of the healthcare team.

Self-assessment of performance

Self-assessment implies reflection on one's own performance with a view to improving it. An example of a self-reflection instrument is the Jefferson scale of physician empathy (Hojat et al 2002). Self-assessment may be affected by gender and personality traits such as self-confidence. The trainees may find it difficult to compare their own performance with that of the expected standard. These drawbacks mostly limit the role of self-assessment to formative assessment.

Patient observation

Today's patient-centred healthcare systems place high value on patient satisfaction. Patient surveys have the potential to add an important dimension to the development of the healthcare professional. Patient observation may be documented in a 'patient satisfaction questionnaire'. The items included in such a questionnaire may relate to the consultation, doctor accessibility, availability of appointments, and other facilities. Such patient surveys not only provide information valuable for formative assessment, but may also be used for summative assessment if the data collection process meets the requirements of reliability and validity (Swing & Bashook 2000). Doubts relating to the reliability of assessment by untrained observers, however, have precluded the widespread use of patient satisfaction questionnaires in high-stakes assessment.

Peer observation

Evaluation forms have been designed for use by peers; for example, Ramsey and colleagues (1996) developed a hospital-based peer-rating form to assess the performance of practising physicians. The peer evaluation questionnaires designed by Hall and by Thomas and their colleagues (Hall et al 1999, Thomas et al 1999) have been effective in formative assessment. Although peers can be a strong source of feedback on attributes such as integrity, teamwork, communication skills and leadership, a conflict of interest may arise if peer trainees are also being assessed by one another. This will lead to a desire to mark colleagues down (i.e. lower than oneself) or to a situation where 'you scratch my back, and I scratch yours' thrives.

Tutor observation

Assessments such as CEX (clinical evaluation exercise) (Kroboth et al 1992) and mini-CEX (mini clinical evaluation exercise) (Norcini et al 2003) are based on tutor observation. For content-related competencies such as clinical skills, the tutors or other senior members of the profession are the most appropriate to evaluate a trainee's performance.

Observation by other members of the healthcare team

Comments and ratings by the other members of the healthcare team such as nurses, physiotherapists, and social workers are increasingly being used with the aim of achieving 360-degree assessment (Swing & Bashook 2000). Healthcare team members may observe aspects of trainee behaviour which other types of assessment fail to capture, for example attitude towards juniors. The major disadvantages in this type of assessment relate to the difficulty of training the observers, leading to concerns regarding the reliability of information, and the unnecessary tension that such an assessment may give rise to in the workplace.

How are the observations recorded?

What has been observed may be recorded using:

- unstructured reports, e.g. references
- checklists
- rating scales
- structured reports.

Unstructured reports

A written report is useful for obtaining an individual opinion regarding a trainee or student. The report can pull together qualitative and quantitative information from areas which are difficult to test by conventional methods. The disadvantages of this method include subjectivity and low reliability because of its unstructured nature.

Checklists

Checklists contain a list of items or statements about the trainee's behaviour or performance in an identified situation. The person checking the items directly observes the trainee during a procedure, task or performance of a skill. The checklist can accommodate sequential or nonsequential items.

They:

- provide a convenient method of recording trainee performance, which is not time consuming
- are objective
- can be standardised as the observers mark all the trainees using the same checklist
- are ideally suited for tasks that can be broken down into several steps by task analysis and where the performance of these steps is an 'all or none' process that needs no grading, e.g. asking the patient's name.

Checklists, however, do not give information about how well a task has been performed, and so are limited to assessing procedures that do not require estimation of the quality of performance.

Rating scales

Rating scales can be global measures of overall performance or several rating scales may measure different aspects of performance. If suitably 'anchored' with behavioural descriptors or rubrics, rating scales can provide objective information which also indicates the standard of performance.

Rating scales are particularly useful for assessing areas that are difficult to test by conventional methods, such as personal attributes, attitudes, generic competencies and professional attributes such as reliability, trustworthiness and time keeping.

Advantages of rating scales

- Rating scales can be validated to suit a particular group of candidates.
- They are flexible and can be used in different settings, e.g. ward, community, etc.
- They have high validity, if they are designed to assess important learning outcomes of the course.
- They are standardised. The same rating scales are used to assess all the trainees.
- They can be used to show whether or not the trainee has reached the required standard, i.e. the required standard can be indicated on the rating scale.

"In contrast with the unstructured descriptions of behaviour gathered in anecdotal records, rating scales provide a systematic procedure for reporting observers' judgements"

Gronlund & Linn 1990

"The specific learning outcomes specify the characteristics to be observed and the rating scale provides a convenient method of recording our judgements"

Gronlund & Linn 1990

- Such assessments provide ratings of trainee behaviour under usual practice circumstances. Thus, they have high authenticity.
- They can be used to quantify the trainees' ability in a given area by calculation of the average of the trainee ratings.
- Rating scales can be used to provide feedback to both the trainer and trainee, particularly if the scale is anchored on observable, clearly defined behavioural descriptors.
- The progress of the trainee over time can be profiled. This will assist early identification of poor performers in order to initiate remedial action.
- This method of assessment is unobtrusive.
- The cost is minimal.
- Rating scales can assess sustained performance over a period of time, in contrast to the snapshot obtained from an examination; rating scales measure actual and ongoing performance.

Disadvantages of rating scales

Disadvantages include:

- rating problems in applying the scale
- subjectivity
- low reliability
- potential for adverse influence on the relationship between tutor and student.

Problems applying the scale Guilford in *Psychometric methods* (1974) lists six common errors made by raters when using rating scales:

- Error of leniency. Difficulties may arise if the rater likes the candidate. Some raters may give the candidate a higher rating than is appropriate, while others may overcompensate and give a lower rating.
- Error of central tendency. Many raters tend to ignore the extremes of the scales and concentrate on the rating points near the centre of the scale.
- 'Halo' effect. The appearance of the student may influence the rater's judgement.
- Logical error. Where competencies appear to be logically related, e.g. empathy and verbal communication, the raters tend to give similar ratings.
- Proximity errors. Raters tend to give similar ratings to traits which are placed close together especially if they are not disparate traits, e.g. reflective ability and professionalism.
- Contrast error. If raters think that they are exceptionally good at certain skills, they tend to rate candidates lower than most other raters.

Subjectivity   If there is only one rater, even when well-designed rating scales are employed, there is a possibility that the assessment may be subjective and open to the influences of 'hawks' and 'doves'.

Low reliability   The reliability of the tutor ratings may be low when only one tutor's view is represented and when the contact time between student and tutor has been short.

Raters should be made aware of this potential problem and trained to separate their rating of candidate's performance from their feelings about the candidate.

Instruct raters to make full use of the scale, and anchor points on the scale using descriptors.

The provision of clear descriptors distinguishing the competencies will help to avoid this tendency.

Place similar traits some distance apart on the rating form.

Point out this tendency during rater training sessions.

Adverse influence on relationship between tutor and student A potential risk is that the observation of the student necessary for continuous assessment may affect the relationship between the student and the tutor. Emphasis placed on a consistently high level of performance during the observation period, in order to obtain the highest point on the scale, may be unrealistic and students may be discouraged.

Improving the quality of rating scales

Several measures can be employed to improve the quality of rating scales.

Provide feedback to raters on the quality of ratings The quality of rating scales can be variable and depends on the effort the individual expends in ensuring high standards and in following best practice when completing the rating scale. It is important to maintain pressure on raters to ensure that the rating scales are taken seriously and that adequate attention is paid to their completion. Those who are consistently harsher or more lenient than others in their ratings should be informed of their stance.

Provide training in the use of the rating scales Training in the use of rating scales improves reliability. Training should be directed at ensuring that raters understand the scale, are given practice in their use, understand the common errors listed above and can defend their views, particularly to their superiors. When a consensus view is needed, there may be a tendency for the views of the head of department to dominate. Raters need to be trained to defend their views on students and for heads of department to accept consensus opinions.

Use several raters Increasing the number of raters may accommodate the views of several tutors and other members of the healthcare team working with the student. The use of several raters who reach a consensus when rating a candidate on a given scale is likely to improve both objectivity and reliability.

Recognise the limitations Use of a rating scale is not a good way of testing knowledge.

Anchor the rating scales Where rating scales are employed it is important to 'anchor' the scales: that is, to define points on the scale concretely, in order to reduce the effect of 'doves' and 'hawks' and to improve reliability.

Compensate for a central tendency Raters may be unwilling to rate students at either end of the scale. This may effectively reduce a five-point scale to one of three points, which may be insufficiently discriminating. This problem can be overcome as follows:

- The scale is anchored with clearly defined descriptors.
- Seven or more points are used in the scale, so that raters still have the choice of a number of points. In practice it is wise to limit the number of points to less than ten, as beyond this anchoring is difficult and the range of choice becomes confusing.
- The number of points on the scale is varied so that raters cannot run down a central point on all scales.

Use several raters' opinions to minimise the positive and negative influences of attributes that are not being assessed.

- Even numbers of points are used so that raters must choose one or other side of the midline, assuming the midline is the indicator of acceptable performance.

Ensure adequate contact time between rater and student   In practice, where the clinical attachment is under four weeks the use of rating scales is not likely to be worthwhile.

Structured reports

Structured tutor reports include a number of rating scales anchored by descriptors to record the trainee performance in a holistic and coherent way. There is a danger that report forms may appear complex, deterring the rater from using them. They must therefore be designed to facilitate ease of use. However, the design and testing of the report forms are time-consuming and it may be useful to pilot the reports in restricted situations before full implementation.

Designing a structured report form begins with identifying the outcomes and competencies to be assessed. These will probably include aspects of clinical skills (including attitudes and professionalism), relationship with patients, attendance, interest and motivation, reliability, and dress code/appearance.

Rating scales are then developed for each competency with clearly defined descriptors. The following are examples from tutor report forms used in phase 3 of the undergraduate medical programme at the University of Dundee.

Clinical skills

1 Unable to demonstrate basic procedures appropriate to stage in course.
2 Minimal level of basic skill. Needs work on procedures. Little progress.
3 Satisfactory basic skill appropriate to stage in course. Steady improvement.
4 Demonstrates superior mastery of basic skills. Performs in advance of clerkship level.
—Not observed or applicable.

Relationships with patients

1 Causes concern by being discourteous and/or not empathetic with patients. Puts personal convenience above patients' needs.
2 Fair rapport. Occasionally discourteous if patient is hostile.
3 Generally good rapport with patients but may be erratic.
4 Widely recognised as being courteous and empathetic. Gives patient's needs priority even with hostile/unpleasant patients.
— Not observed or applicable.

Attendance

1 Zero attendance.
2 Sporadic attendance.
3 Occasional unexplained absence. Does not always produce supportive documentation.

4 Attends all sessions. If absent makes request known in advance or produces support documentation, e.g. medical certificate.

— Not observed or applicable.

Interest and motivation

1 Poor self-motivation. Has to be prompted to participate in activities. Sometimes refuses to participate. Shows little interest.
2 Frequently needs prompting to participate. May lack confidence. Demonstrates variable level of interest.
3 Always participates. Asks spontaneous questions.
4 Highly self-motivated. Mature approach to activities. Makes specific requests.

— Not observed or applicable.

Reliability

1 Poor reliability. Work not well done or incomplete. Often absent/late for duties.
2 Occasionally forgetful.
3 Usually reliable. Work always done. Always present and prompt for clinical responsibilities.
4 Always reliable. Takes initiative for routine matters.

— Not observed or applicable.

Dress code/appearance

1 Appearance may cause offence to patients.
2 Dress/appearance may be inappropriate, unkempt or immodest.
3 Generally conforms to standard but may be untidy.
4 Appearance appropriate. Conforms with professional image.

— Not observed or applicable.

The development of accurate descriptors is a skilled process requiring knowledge of student behaviour at different ability levels in the range of competencies being assessed. Facility with language and an accurate description of the behaviours being described are also required. The descriptors should paint a picture of real and recognisable behaviour. The ability of the tutors to identify the described behaviour is the key to the success of the structured tutor report. The descriptors minimise the effects of the presence of hawks and doves among raters and increase interrater reliability.

The number of contact hours between student and tutor should be noted somewhere on the report. There should be space in the report for a written comment on the student and completion of this area should be enforced.

Reports that are discussed with the trainee at the end of the attachment/rotation or, better still, at an intermediate point during the period of training, are useful for providing feedback to the trainee.

It is also important to include in the report a written comment area where tutors can list the major strengths and weaknesses of the student and identify what specific feedback points have been given to the student.

Summary

In postgraduate medical education, the context of learning is shifting from the classroom to the workplace. This shift is reflected in a growing interest in work-based assessment. The ability to assess the actual performance of trainees, based on predetermined competencies and meta-competencies may also be a contributory factor to the popularity of work-based assessment.

Patient outcomes, process of care or practice volume or both, can be the basis of judging performance, using tools such as clinical records, administrative data, diaries/logbooks and direct or indirect observation of performance.

Observation may be by the trainee his- or herself, by patients, peers, tutors or/and other members of the healthcare team, and may be recorded in unstructured reports, checklists, rating scales or structured reports. All the above recording methods have their advantages and disadvantages, and a combination of methods is required to provide a holistic view of the trainee's performance. The 'record of in-training assessment' or RITA, an example of work-based evaluation in postgraduate medical education in the UK, assesses the trainee in a range of competencies using a variety of tools, including logbooks; reports from supervisors, training programme directors and other colleagues; results from formal examinations; certificates of courses attended; and other material collected by the trainee.

References

Campbell L M, Murray T S 1996a The effects of the introduction of a system of mandatory formative assessment for general practice trainees. Medical Education 30(1):60–64

Campbell L M, Murray T S 1996b Summative assessment of vocational trainees: results of a three-year study. British Journal of General Practice 46:411–414

Davis M H, Harden R M 2003 Competency-based assessment: making it a reality. Medical Teacher 25(6):565–568

Kroboth F J, Hanusa B H, Parker S et al 1992 The inter-rater reliability and internal consistency of a clinical evaluation exercise. Journal of General Internal Medicine 7:174–179

Gronlund N E, Linn R L 1990 Measurement and evaluation in teaching, 6th edn. Macmillan, New York

Guilford J P 1974 Psychometric methods, 2nd edn. McGraw-Hill, New York

Hall W, Violato C, Lewkonia R et al 1999 Assessment of physician performance in Alberta: the physician achievement review. Canadian Medical Association Journal 161:52–56

Hojat M, Gonnella J S, Nasca T J et al 2002 Physician empathy: definition, components, measurement, and relationship to gender and specialty. American Journal of Psychiatry 159:1563–1569

Miller G E 1990 The assessment of clinical skills/competence/performance. Academic Medicine 65(9):s63–s67

Norcini J J 2003 Work based assessment. British Medical Journal 326:753–755

Norcini J J, Blank L L, Duffy F D, Fortna G S 2003 The mini-CEX: a method for assessing clinical skills. Annals of Internal Medicine 138(6):476–483

Ramsey P, Carline J D, Blank L L, Wenrich M D 1996 Feasibility of hospital-based use of peer ratings to evaluate the performance of practising physicians. Academic Medicine 71:364–370

Rethans J J, Sturmans F, Drop R et al 1991 Does competence of general practitioners predict their performance? Comparison between examination setting and actual practice. British Medical Journal 303:1377–1380

Swing S, Bashook P G. 2000 Toolbox of assessment methods version 1.1 ACGME Outcome Project ACGME (Accreditation Council for Graduate Medical Education), ABMS (American Board of Medical Specialties). Online. Available: http://www.acgme.org/Outcome/assess/Toolbox.pdf [Accessed 10 April 2004]

Thomas P, Gebo K, Hellmann D 1999 A pilot study of peer review in residency training. Journal of General Internal Medicine 14:551–554

Further reading

Rethans J J, Norcini J J, Baron-Maldonado M et al 2002 The relationship between competence and performance: implications for assessing practice performance. Medical Education 36:901–909

Chapter 37
Portfolios, projects and dissertations

M. H. Davis, G. G. Ponnamperuma

What are portfolios?

A portfolio is a collection of student work, which provides evidence of the achievement of knowledge, skills, attitudes, understanding and professional growth through a process of self-reflection over a period of time. Portfolios have been used for several decades to assess students, for example, in the fine arts where material such as artwork produced by students is as important as written material.

Portfolios and logbooks

The crucial difference between a logbook and a portfolio is student reflection. Reflection is the purposive, deliberate revisiting of an experience, to explore and extract the learning offered by the experience. Reflection can promote learning, personal and professional development and improvement of practice.

Uses of portfolios

Interest in the use of portfolios for assessment in the healthcare professions has developed as part of the move away from testing and 'snapshot' examinations, towards a broader use of assessment. This assessment culture includes:

- closer links between assessment and learning
- the use of assessment to improve learning outcomes through the provision of feedback
- attempts to assess students in areas such as attitudes, personal attributes and professionalism that are difficult to assess by traditional methods.

   The use of portfolios provides an opportunity to assess:

- *Student coursework and its documentation*, such as material written by the student, videos, photos, CD ROMs, etc.
- *Student attitudes*. These may be assessed through rating scales completed by tutors, peers, students themselves, patients, other healthcare professionals, or through material that the students have selected for inclusion in their portfolio. What students include in their portfolio highlights what they value and consider to be important.

"Assessment is undergoing a paradigm shift, from psychometrics to a broader model of educational assessment, from a testing and examination culture to an assessment culture"

Gipps 1994

- *Student learning and progression of learning during the course.* Through the use of reflective student commentaries on their learning experiences during the course and annotations of submitted work, teachers can explore and discuss student learning.
- *Student performance* in the wards, outpatient departments, and general practice healthcare centres and with patients in the community, through the use of rating scales or reports.

Portfolio contents

Undergraduate portfolios

Portfolios used for assessment purposes in undergraduate medical education may include:

- case reports
- a checklist of practical procedures undertaken
- videotapes of consultations
- research project reports
- published work
- evidence of other achievements: for example, work undertaken on behalf of the student body for the organisation of meetings or conferences
- reflective material, that is student reflection on what he/she has learned.

Postgraduate portfolios

Portfolios used formatively in postgraduate general practice training by Snadden & Thomas (1998) include:

- critical-incident reports of trainees' experiences with patients
- reflections on their difficulties and successes during the training period.

Continuing education portfolios

Portfolios used for revalidation purposes by Scottish general practitioners (Snadden & Bruce 2002) include relevant personal and practice information, and evidence of fulfilment of each of the outcomes identified by the General Medical Council (GMC) in *Good medical practice* (GMC 2001). General practitioners may collect this evidence in the form of signed statements, analysis of practice data, peer observation data, patient satisfaction surveys, written accounts, logbooks, investigation data, a reflective diary, practice accreditation certificates, minutes of meetings attended and patient/peer feedback.

The GMC has identified a portfolio approach to revalidation for all UK doctors from 2005. Suggested portfolio contents include:

- a description of the individual doctor's medical practice
- evidence of participating in a quality-assured appraisal scheme
- evidence of compliance with the local clinical governance requirements
- certification of freedom from significant unresolved concerns about fitness-to-practise
- indications of competence in the principles set out in *Good medical practice* (GMC 2001)

"The evidence in portfolios is limited only by the degree of the designer's creativity"

Friedman Ben-David et al 2001

"Summary of portfolio contents:
- *Products of students' learning experiences*
- *Cumulative – work completed over a period of weeks or months*
- *Material selected from the on-going work*
- *A reflective component"*

Stecher 1998

Teaching portfolios should be self-portraits of teachers, providing vivid representations of themselves.

"Four models of portfolio structure:
- *Shopping trolley – everything that the student has undertaken during the course.*
- *Toast rack – a number of 'slots' to be filled for each module/unit/placement.*
- *Cake mix – integrates portfolio material to provide evidence of achievement of the learning outcomes.*
- *Spinal column – students collect evidence (nerve roots) to demonstrate the mastery of a series of competency statements (vertebrae). Each piece of evidence is used only once against a certain competency statement"*

Webb et al 2002

The five-step portfolio assessment process:
1. Collection of evidence of learning
2. Reflection on learning
3. Evaluation of evidence
4. Defence of the portfolio
5. Assessment decision.

Teaching portfolios

Many teachers in the healthcare professions now assemble a teaching portfolio for job-seeking and career development purposes. Teaching portfolios:

- are reflective compendia of self-selected artefacts
- are representations of teaching credentials and competencies
- offer holistic views of teachers
- provide documentation for strengthening interviews.

Portfolio structure

If the portfolio is to be used for assessment purposes, a framework is necessary to ensure that the portfolio contains appropriate evidence of student achievement of the learning outcomes that are to be assessed. Tensions, however, exist between structure and selection; a too stream-lined and structured portfolio may become 'sterile and counterproductive' (Stockhausen 1996). The framework should be sufficiently flexible to allow inclusion of material selected by the individual student.

Portfolio assessment

There are five steps in the portfolio assessment process.

1. Collection of evidence of learning The students may be given guidance in general terms about what contents to include, but they should where possible select the individual items for inclusion in the portfolio.

2. Reflection on learning The student:
- reflects on the learning experience
- identifies how the learning experience contributes to the learning outcomes
- identifies what has been learned
- identifies what further learning is required
- undertakes the further learning
- describes the further learning achieved.

3. Evaluation of evidence Examiners decide whether the student has reached the required standard in each of the outcomes. They identify the student's strengths and weaknesses in terms of the outcomes, based on the evidence in the portfolio.

4. Defence of evidence Examiners question the student regarding portfolio contents to probe and confirm or refute the evidence of the student's strengths and weaknesses.

5. Assessment decision This is a consensus approach involving all the examiners, with an assessment decision, based on predetermined criteria.

Advantages of portfolio assessment

The advantages of portfolio assessment include:

- *The ability to assess difficult-to-test areas*. There has been increasing interest in the use of portfolio assessment to assess curriculum outcomes that are not easily measured by conventional tests. These outcomes include taking responsibility for continuing professional development, professionalism, attitudes and student progress towards the learning outcomes.

- *The ability to test a range of curriculum outcomes within one assessment framework.* By structuring the portfolio content to include material relating to all the curriculum outcomes, previously ignored areas such as critical thinking or health promotion and disease prevention can be assessed. Thus, the importance of all the curriculum outcomes can be emphasised.
- *More effective student learning.* Portfolios promote active, deep, peer-supported, self-directed, adult learning through self-reflection and self-assessment. The portfolio also accommodates diverse student learning styles and facilitates the integration of learning and assessment: assessment supports learning.
- *Learning partnerships between students and teachers are encouraged* through discussion of learning needs and provision of feedback.
- *Continuous assessment.* Opportunities for continuous assessment are provided through regular submission of material that is then marked by the student's educational supervisor or tutor.
- *Assessment of student performance in authentic, real-life settings,* usually through the use of rating scales.
- *Incorporation of multiple assessment methods*: these may be qualitative and quantitative, formative and summative and objective and subjective.
- *The ability to identify poor performers early* through scrutiny of marked portfolio material.
- *Assessment of extent of learning.* Both the breadth and depth of student learning can be assessed through the portfolio.
- *Demonstration of self-expression and creativity.* Opportunities for self-expression and creativity are provided through selection of material and its presentation.
- *Provision of feedback.* Opportunities for feedback to the student are provided during discussion of the portfolio with the tutor/teacher, and when marked portfolio components are returned to the student. Snadden & Thomas (1998) emphasise the portfolio's usefulness for exploring attitudes and values to stimulate feedback.

"The potential of portfolios to drive student learning in an educationally desirable direction may be one of the reasons for the current wave of enthusiasm for portfolios in the healthcare professions"

Davis et al 2004

Disadvantages of portfolio assessment

The main disadvantages associated with portfolio assessment concern the following issues:

- *Reliability, especially interrater reliability* (Pitts et al 2002; Roberts et al 2002). Reliability may be improved by measures such as the validation of the rating scales used to assess performance, and examiner training to ensure that the examiners share an understanding of the outcomes being assessed and the standard required in each outcome.

- *Student attitudes towards portfolios* (Davis et al 2001). Students are notoriously conservative regarding examinations and they may find it difficult to accept an innovative approach, at least initially. The cultural environment within which the portfolio is implemented may also affect student attitudes. In an authoritarian teacher-centred environment or when portfolios are used for summative assessment, students may be reluctant to disclose their weaknesses to the examiners. Considerable student induction may be required for the success of portfolio assessment.
- *Practicability/feasibility* (Friedman Ben-David et al 2001). The organisation of a portfolio assessment process includes data collection by the institution as well as by the students; meeting deadlines for submission of material; collection of portfolios and their distribution among the examiners; training the tutors who mark the portfolio components, and organising student orientation programmes. In addition, the portfolio reading and marking process is time consuming and taxing for the examiners.

Assessment criteria

Examples of some of the assessment criteria employed to give feedback to the students regarding their portfolios are presented in Table 37.1.

Implementing portfolio-based learning and assessment

Careful planning is necessary if the introduction of portfolio-based learning and assessment is to be a success. The following list is provided by Friedman Ben-David and colleagues (2001) to guide the successful implementation of portfolio assessment.

1. Define the purpose of the portfolio. Is it for formative or summative purposes? What is the relationship between the portfolio and other assessments?
2. Determine the outcomes to be assessed. The exit learning outcomes of the course are the framework on which the portfolio is built.
3. Identify the contents of the portfolio. The contents should provide evidence of achievement of the learning outcomes. The contents and the outcomes provide the blueprint for assessment.
4. Develop a marking system. A marking system that can be employed for all the portfolio components will aid the assessment process.
5. Plan the examination process. What is needed in terms of time, numbers of academic and support staff, space and administration?
6. Develop guidelines for assessment decisions, such as pass, fail and distinction/honours, if these are to be awarded.
7. Orientate the students. Student induction programmes, written guidelines and tips from students who have previously undertaken

Examiners should be warned about the time needed to read portfolios.

Guidance for students in portfolio building is essential, to prevent valuable information on student progress being submerged in the irrelevant and redundant detail that students tend to include in their portfolios.

Portfolios are important records of student achievements. A public display of portfolios provides useful information for various stakeholders in medical education, for example, members of faculty, other students and employing authorities.

Table 37.1 Criteria used in portfolio assessment

Points awarded	Grade	Descriptor
Record keeping		
This scale is designed to assess presentation of portfolio content		
1	Fails to meet the standard	Chaotic, no emphasis, accessing items generally difficult
2	Borderline	Disorganised/muddled at times. Some difficulty accessing material. Little attempt at emphasis
3	Meets the standard	Clear layout, organised material, easily accessed. Key points emphasised
4	Exceptional	Shows flair in layout and organisation. Portfolio 'shines'
Discussion of the portfolio		
Students are asked to identify the important features of an individual patient		
1	Fails to meet the standard	Failure to identify salient features
2	Borderline	Identifies clinical features only in relation to presenting complaint
3	Meets the standard	Correctly identifies key features and links them to patient's ideas, concerns and contexts
4	Exceptional	High level of empathy with patient's situation. Student appropriately identifies key features and links them to patient's ideas, concerns and contexts
Patient management		
This scale is designed to assess the patient management outcome		
1	Fails to meet the standard	No suggestions
2	Borderline	Is able to provide one option but is unable to supply reasons regarding its acceptability or suitability
3	Meets the standard	Provides at least one acceptable management option with reasons
4	Exceptional	Is able to provide a range of different management options with reasons for acceptability or lack of it
Task-based learning		
This scale is designed to assess the student's ability to link theory to practice		
1	Fails to meet the standard	Inability to link relevant theory to the cases discussed
2	Borderline	Sometimes uses inappropriate linkage of theory to the case
3	Meets the standard	Demonstrates ability to link theoretical aspects of the course appropriately to the cases discussed
4	Exceptional	The case is instrumental in driving theory acquisition

Continued

Table 37.1   Criteria used in portfolio assessment—Cont'd

Points awarded	Grade	Descriptor
Further learning		
This scale is designed to assess utilisation of educational resources		
1	Fails to meet the standard	Doesn't know what educational resources are available. Doesn't ask others
2	Borderline	Unsure of educational resource availability. Leans heavily on referral to colleagues/other healthcare professionals
3	Meets the standard	Makes a reasonable attempt to answer patient problems by accessing other healthcare professionals plus more than one educational resource
4	Exceptional	Uses a wide range of learning resources including other healthcare professionals and knows how to access them without support
Scientific behaviour/critical thinking		
Is the student able to reflect on what has been learned from seeing the patient?		
1	Fails to meet the standard	Only addresses the issues of what, when and where
2	Borderline	Analytical skills becoming evident but poorly constructed
3	Meets the standard	Demonstrates the ability to analyse the case critically. Adequately assesses the whys and hows
4	Exceptional	Demonstrates the ability to analyse the case critically and apply the analysis to his or her own potential future situation

portfolio assessment help to inform the students about the portfolio assessment process and reduce their anxiety.

8. Select and train examiners. Staff development workshops are essential.
9. Establish reliability and validity evidence. Pilot studies are helpful in providing such evidence.
10. Design evaluation procedures. Student and staff feedback is essential to fine tune the process.

Conclusion

Portfolios can be used to:

- teach/learn and assess attitudes and professionalism that are otherwise difficult to assess
- teach/learn and assess a range of outcomes
- assess all four levels of Miller's pyramid (knows, knows how, shows how and does), if results from exams such as multiple-choice tests

and competence-based measures such as OSCEs (objective structured clinical examinations) are included in the portfolio
- provide feedback to both the learner and the teacher/examiner
- provide a holistic picture of the individual student's fitness to practise.

Projects and dissertations

What are projects and dissertations?
A dissertation is a piece of written work based on personal research. The research may be either a literature review or a piece of original work or both. The research is usually supervised and the level of supervision needs to be identified before the research starts. Discussion between the student and the supervisor is required to identify the appropriate level of supervision.

The term 'project' is usually applied to a smaller piece of research that may be carried out either individually or by groups of students. Medical students may be asked to carry out projects as part of the undergraduate programme, often over a period of several weeks.

Some examples of different types of project are given below, with examples of topics that might be studied:

- Questionnaire surveys:
  — of staff: violence and abuse in teaching hospitals
  — of students: student attitudes to assessment in the undergraduate curriculum
  — of patients: a survey of patients in a city general practice who are prescribed H_2 antagonists
  — other groups: a look at stress in the parents of autistic children, and the provision and adequacy of services provided to such families
- Interview surveys:
  — of staff: which drugs do GPs carry in their emergency bags and are they in date?
  — of patients: what women want from antenatal care; the opinions of pregnant women in two areas of Scotland with regard to provision of antenatal care
  — of other groups: a comparative view of school carers' and patients' perceptions of feeding difficulties occurring in children with neurological problems
- Literature reviews
  — investigations into medicinal uses of maggots
- Practical research
  — laboratory: does the activity of glutathione-S transferase modulate the expression of multiple self-healing squamous epitheliomata?
  — clinical: the effects of local anaesthetic on intravenous cannulation
- Audit projects
  — assessing the quality of dialysis using the quality of dialysis scoring system

"Most tutors will at some stage have faced a pile of written projects which are derivative, tedious, full of unreferenced, photocopied, unacknowledged material, which represent a vast amount of student work but do not represent a vast amount of student learning"

Brown & Knight 1994

If the student is allowed to select the area of research, it is likely to be personally relevant and motivation may be increased.

- Case note surveys
  — the outcome of diabetic pregnancies in an identified geographic region.

The outcomes of the research may be presented by the individual student or by the group as a report, a poster, a videotape, an audiotape, a short computer program, an oral presentation or as written material.

Advantages of projects and dissertations

Projects and dissertations can be used to assess a range of curriculum outcomes. They can provide evidence of creativity through the way that the students present their results. They promote knowledge of the literature in the area of the research topic and an understanding of the importance of carrying out literature searches.

Through project work students can acquire a range of competencies:

- knowledge of a specific topic
- improved communication skills through interview surveys
- competence in practical procedures such as laboratory techniques or investigative procedures
- heightened awareness of ethical stances through access to patients and their records
- accuracy in dealing with data
- ability to handle and retrieve information
- improved critical thinking
- problem-solving skills
- writing skills
- time management.

Because the research is carried out over a period of time, projects and dissertations provide the opportunity to assess continuous work. They overcome the problems inherent in the 'big-bang' examination when short-term illness or an 'off-day' may adversely influence performance.

The research work may produce publishable material for inclusion in the student's portfolio.

Disadvantages of projects and dissertations

Identification of a piece of research that is capable of completion within the available time is critical to the success of this type of assessment. Experienced supervisors are necessary who can recognise over-ambitious projects.

The research needs to be realistically costed in terms of staff time, resources and finance, and adequate funds to cover the cost of the work must be identified. The agreed level of supervision must be provided and a series of short-term goals are useful for monitoring progress.

Fraud and plagiarism are potential problems with this type of assessment. The requirement of a signed statement stating that the work is original is one way of validating this work.

Structure of a dissertation or project report

Although there is no specific format for writing a project report or dis-

Projects prepared by students can be used to teach subsequent cohorts of students, capitalising on the saying that 'to teach is to learn twice'.

sertation there are some general guidelines that may be of help. The subject matter of the study will determine to a large extent how it is presented on the page. It is important that the student and supervisor draw up a plan and discuss the intended format. The following is a frequently adopted structure.

- Title page – provides a clear and informative title.
- Contents page – should list all the main sections and subsections and their page numbers.
- Abstract – explains what the project is about, how it has been carried out, a summary of the results and the implications of the work.
- Introduction – this may explain the general topic area and justification for the study. Background information may be included. This chapter should answer the question 'Why am I writing this dissertation?'
- Literature review – this is a key part of the project and should involve a comprehensive, focused and critical review of the published work in the research area. It should move from the general to the specific. This section should end with the research questions or hypotheses. The literature review should answer the question 'What has already been found out about this research area?'
- Methods – this chapter should focus on the design of the study and the procedures carried out. It should clearly describe the subjects and any sampling methods used and provide good reasons for selecting the study method. If there are different possible ways of carrying out the project, this section should state what they are and why the chosen method was selected. This chapter should answer the question 'What did I do?'
- Results – a clear and logical display of findings is necessary. Tables and figures must be labelled and accompanied by relevant descriptive text. Sufficient detail should be available so that inferences can be drawn. This chapter should answer the question 'What did I find out?'
- Discussion – this chapter should look at the findings and discuss their significance in relation to what has already been published. Move from the specific to the general. This is the opportunity to explain how the research questions are answered and how they are linked to previous studies. The discussion should be rich in analysis and may be broken into logical segments using subheadings. It should answer the question 'How do my findings relate/add to what is already published?'
- Conclusions/recommendations – it is quite common, but not essential, to have a final chapter on the way ahead or plans for future studies. This is usually not as lengthy as the discussion. It should answer the question 'What is the way ahead?'
- References – this should contain full references for all works cited in the text.
- Appendices – additional relevant data should be included in the appendices.

How to assess projects and dissertations

Preparing a dissertation requires the ability to handle large quantities of information and to criticise, analyse and evaluate the information.

Deadlines need to be met. The work needs to be presented in a coherent, lucid and compelling way. The significance of the conclusions needs to be appreciated and made explicit.

Criteria for assessment of the project or dissertation should be based on the competencies being assessed and need to be identified before the work begins. Rating scales are useful for this purpose, particularly where a number of people are involved in assessing the projects/dissertations. Peer assessment of project work, for example, voting on the best poster presentation, adds excitement to the process and is motivating for students and supervisors alike.

Summary

A portfolio is an innovative method of assessing student achievement of learning outcomes that are less suitably assessed by traditional examinations. Students not only choose the material that they wish to include in their portfolio but also reflect on their work to identify what has been learned and what is yet to be learned.

The completion of a project or a dissertation usually takes several weeks of part-time study during a senior year of the undergraduate medical course. Whether a survey, practical work or an audit project is chosen, close supervision and guidance from a tutor are required. Innovative methods of assessment can be employed to add extra interest to this approach.

References

Brown S, Knight P 1994 Assessing learners in higher education. Kogan Page, London

Davis M H, Friedman Ben-David M, Harden R M et al 2001 Portfolio assessment in medical students' final examinations. Medical Teacher 23:357–366

Davis M H, Ponnamperuma G G, Pippard J, Ker J 2004 Student perceptions of a portfolio assessment process. Medical Teacher. (Submitted)

Friedman Ben-David M, Davis M H, Harden R M et al 2001 AMEE Guide No.24: Portfolios as a method of student assessment. Medical Teacher 23(6):535–551

GMC 2001 Good medical practice, 3rd edn. Online. Available: http://www.gmc-uk.org/standards/GMP.pdf

Gipps C 1994 Beyond testing. Falmer, London

Pitts J, Colin C, Thomas P, Smith F 2002 Enhancing reliability in portfolio assessment: discussions between assessors. Medical Teacher 24(2):197–201

Roberts C, Newble D, O'Rourke A J 2002 Portfolio-based assessments in medical education: are they valid and reliable for summative purposes? Medical Education 36(10):899–900

Snadden D S, Thomas M L 1998 Portfolio learning in general practice vocational training – does it work? Medical Education 32:401–406

Snadden D, Bruce D 2002 East of Scotland GPASC (General Practice Administration System for Scotland) Annual report 2002/2003. Tayside Centre for General Practice, East Region, NHS Education for Scotland. Online. Available: http://www.dundee.ac.uk/generalpractice/postgraduate/summative/Annual%2OReport%202002-2003.doc

Stecher B 1998 The local benefits and burdens of large-scale portfolio assessment. Assessment in Education 5(3):335–351

Stockhausen L J 1996 The clinical portfolio. Australian Electronic Journal of Nursing Education 2:1–11

Webb C, Endacott R, Gray M et al 2002 Models of portfolios. Medical Education 36:897–898

Further reading

GMC 2000 Revalidating doctors: ensuring standards, securing the future. General Medical Council, London

Harden R M, Crosby J R, Davis M H et al 2000 Task-based learning: the answer to integration and problem-based learning in the clinical years. Medical Education 34:391–397

Chapter 38
External examiners

C. D. Forbes

Introduction

No matter what course of education is undertaken, it is critical for the candidate to be assessed or examined in some shape or form. In medicine, it has long been agreed that external examiners are required as assessors from outside the medical school to ensure that a common national standard is reached. This chapter will explore a variety of aspects of the role of external examiners and the problems associated with their use (Walters et al 1995). It is also clear that it is not just within countries that external examiners are required; they are needed to compare standards across Europe and internationally.

The alternative to having external examiners is to have external examinations and this has become the norm in the USA and Canada where various National Boards have been constituted. These include the national board of Medical Examiners (NBME), the Federal License Examinations (FLEX), the Educational Commission for Foreign Medical Graduates (ECFMG) and the Board Examinations in most specialties. These national examinations are an attempt to impose a standard at national level while allowing individual schools to develop their own curricula and to draw on their own strengths. By their very nature they consist of paper-based questions. To introduce a standardised objective structured clinical examination (OSCE) raises major logistical problems which still require to be overcome. The strength of such examinations is that they can act as a comparator, comparing the end results of a course in medical education delivered by a variety of means in different schools. In addition a national examination would allow comparison of the achievements of the teaching process in different schools as part of the recent Teaching Quality Assessment (TQA) exercise seen in the United Kingdom.

What is an external examiner?

Most universities in the UK accept the Committee of Vice Chancellors and Principals' Code of Practice for external examining in universities at first degree and taught master's level (CVCP 1985). This has since been extensively modified but sets down the rules for the appointment of external examiners. They should be of high regard within their profession and should be acknowledged leaders academically, clinically and as teachers in their medical subjects. They have to be objective in their assessment of the school they are visiting and remain impartial and dedicated to the setting and maintenance of national medical standards. They must also understand that as well as a global role in the examination

"we make the examination the end of education, not an accessory in its acquisition"

Osler 1913

"The concept of the external examiner appeals to notions of the universality of educational standards and justice for the individual student"

Walters et al 1995

"A major guarantee of quality and equality in higher education"

Piper 1985

"would promote higher quality medical education across the Continent"

Nystrup & Mårtenson 1992

The external examining experience consists of six steps:
1. appointment
2. contract
3. review of curriculum and examination materials
4. on-site visit
5. consolidating internal and external assessments
6. preliminary and final reports.

(Karuhije & Ruff 2002)

"a visiting assessor of high academic standing and possessed of absolute integrity and objectivity"

Walters et al 1995

system they have a responsibility to ensure that individual students are also looked at objectively, especially if there have been previous problems of discipline or performance in any individual.

Appointment

External examiners are appointed by the university court on the recommendation of the appropriate department, and the appointment is endorsed by the relevant dean. It is usual for the head of department to have already approached the potential external examiner to ensure that he or she is willing and able to undertake the duties which are set out below and therefore willing to serve as and when required for the appropriate duration.

The usual duration of appointment is 3 years in the first instance and may be extended to 4 years. It is not usual for the external examiner to be reappointed after that time for another period of office. It is also not usual for previous staff members to be appointed as external examiners to their previous department until a period of 3 years has elapsed.

An external examiner should not usually hold more than two other external examinerships for undergraduate courses. Care must be taken that the external examiner is not from a department in another institution in which a member of staff of the home department is currently serving as an external examiner. This is to avoid the possibility of a 'quid pro quo' situation. It is important that external examiners feel no pressure is brought to bear on them to provide a report other than a totally objective assessment of the quality of the course and it is usual that the report goes directly to the principal of the university and not directly to the department.

Duties of the external examiner

Duties of the external examiner will vary with the different phases of the curriculum. In the first year of the course, where the emphasis is on the scientific background of disease, it is difficult to find a single external examiner who is sufficiently knowledgeable in anatomy, biochemistry and physiology to cover all these requirements. It is therefore usual to have a panel of people with specialist knowledge. The middle years consist of mechanisms of disease and the start of the clinical curriculum. These are now totally integrated and a small panel of examiners overview the various subjects. By the last 2 years the curriculum is wholly clinical, covering the specialties of medicine, surgery, obstetrics, gynaecology, child health, psychiatry and general practice. Appropriate external examiners with the required clinical skills are appointed in each of these subjects, even though some of the examinations are now coordinated.

Special study modules present rather different problems because of their diverse nature and content and examiners for these must be chosen with special care.

Requirements for an external examiner

There is much more to being an external examiner than just to be present at the medical school on a few days per year (Sheehan 1994) (Fig. 38.1).

They must now expect to fulfil a contract with the other medical school which requires them to:

- have time to do the job
- have a broad range of knowledge
- be an established teacher
- be intimately aware of the curriculum to be examined before starting the examinations; prior briefing is required or better still a 'dry run' as an observer
- accept a firm brief or job description of the particular task
- be prepared to do the job for 3 years with the option of a further year
- be prepared to attend several times for the one examination which may be in different parts, and also to attend the meeting of the board of examiners and provide detailed discussion on students who fail to meet the standards.

It is important to note that external examiners are not to be appointed to rubber-stamp the processes of an individual school, subject or the internal examiner and preferably should not be appointed because they are old friends of the head of department.

They must have neutral attitudes to:

- gender
- race
- colour
- creed.

Approval of examination papers

All examination papers for a particular part of the course must be approved by the external examiners of the course. External examiners should contribute to the questions and ensure that their contribution is actually added to the examination paper. It would then be usual for an external examiner to be asked to mark that particular question, having provided an optimal outline answer. The external examiner should see the final format of the paper to check it for errors of omission or commission. There is now a requirement for papers to be marked by two examiners and to be marked anonymously. It is the duty of the external examiner to see that this is carried out.

It is also usual for the external examiner to look at a range of approximately 10% of all the candidates' answers, once marked, to ensure that an appropriate standard is met. If there is to be an oral examination after the written examination, then this survey should be done before the oral examination takes place. The external examiner should look at the better students in the year if there is a question of grading their marks as a 'merit' or 'distinction', as well as looking at all the borderline candidates. At the oral examination, external examiners should identify themselves to the candidate (wear a name badge) and clearly indicate that they are from outside that school and hence 'neutral'.

In addition, external examiners should look at all other pieces of work which are part of the assessment system, and in particular at

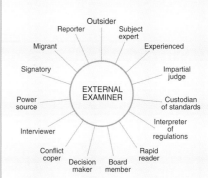

Fig. 38.1 Fifteen facets of the role of external examiner (redrawn from Sheehan J 1994 Journal of Advanced Nursing 20:943–949)

Choose a respected senior from another university:
- who has a reputation for ability in teaching/assessment and clinical care/research
- who can give the time commitment
- who has been involved in curriculum development
- who has a robust personality.

On appointment external examiners should be given:
- a detailed briefing on the curriculum with a focus on the part they are to examine
- a 'job description' of what is expected of them
- an agreement which they sign to indicate their willingness to attend as required over the period of the appointment.

course work which may include essays, projects and posters. It is more difficult for external examiners to come regularly to a distant university to look at presentations and attend seminars and so on, and probably this should not be required of them, but they should be in a position to make comments about the content of the course and the assessment system. The alternative is for course work to be sent in bulk to the external examiner.

Clinical examinations

External examiners should be prepared to give up enough time, often 2 or 3 days, to take part in the clinical examinations of a particular part of the course. This now tends to be done at the end of each teaching block so it may involve three or four visits to the school each year.

Normally they would be paired with an internal examiner of equivalent seniority and, once again, they should see the top and bottom ends of the spectrum of students. The profile of marks in previous internal examinations of the same course should be made available to them. It is particularly important that external examiners be involved with students who are likely to be deficient and at risk of not passing the diet of examinations. They should make available sufficient time to attend the board of examiners when each of these candidates is discussed in detail, especially if there is compensation in terms of other marks which might allow a candidate's work to be upgraded. External examiners report directly to the principal of the university and not to the head of department, the dean or the faculty.

Their report should follow the recommendations of the Committee of Vice Chancellors and Principals' Code of Practice (1985). The following questions are based on the requirements of the Academic Standards Committee, University of Dundee (1996):

- Was the information supplied on the course structure, content and methods of assessment adequate?
- Was the administration of the external process satisfactory?
- Was the assessment process appropriate to the subject matter and to the students?
- Were the examinations sufficiently comprehensive with regard to the course examined?
- Were the facilities and material for practical and/or clinical examinations adequate?
- Was there adequate opportunity to see scripts of borderline candidates and also of students at the top end of the scale?
- Was there access to a sufficient number and range of papers to enable a view to be formed as to whether internal marking was appropriate and consistent?
- Was there sufficient access to course work to enable the exercise of effective external judgement?
- Were the procedures followed by the board of examiners impartial and equitable?

- Were course objectives sufficiently well defined and appropriate to the subject matter and to the students?
- Was the course structure and content appropriate to the level at which it was taught?
- Were the quality of teaching and the methods used, as revealed in examinations, effective and appropriate?
- Was the general quality of candidates' work satisfactory?
- Was the failure rate acceptable?
- Was the distribution of final honours, merit or distinction comparable with other institutions?
- Were the standards achieved by students consistent with standards elsewhere in UK universities?

It is to be noted that the payment of the external examiner's fee is only authorised under receipt of this report and that this ensures almost 100% compliance!

Examination exemption and curriculum development

External examiners should also be involved in exemption schemes and should be consulted by departmental boards if new courses are to be introduced or if there are substantial changes to existing courses. As a result of the General Medical Council's drive to change the curriculum, it is also appropriate now to involve external examiners in curriculum development. The above information applies to the United Kingdom currently but in countries such as Canada, the United States and Australia there is movement towards a national curriculum with accreditation of medical schools and courses and centralisation of the examination system. The British system continues to be used in many former colonies and it is common for external examiners to be required for these medical schools. Indeed it is common for the General Medical Council to employ experienced examiners in this role for their own purposes abroad and in the UK for the examination of the Professional and Linguistic Assessment Board (PLAB).

The cost of external examination

There is little doubt that universities will continue to want objective assessment of their courses and require external reviews despite the costs for travel and accommodation plus fees. Thus it is important that the system does not degenerate into a 'freebie' for academic chums. Care must be taken also to offer hospitality during the stay which is commensurate with the job but which does not attract criticism as being too lavish or having any other motivation.

"against retention of the external examiner system is its high cost"

Walters et al 1995

Summary

The role of the external examiner remains critical to universities to ensure the maintenance of educational standards both nationally and internationally. Careful selection of the individual examiner is necessary.

As considerable abilities are required in the development of innovative curricula, the external examiner is often involved with contributing to the oversight of the whole course and not just of the written papers, clinical examinations and vivas. It must be recognised that such a position brings kudos to the home university and consequently appropriate time and resources should be given to enable the role to be filled adequately.

References

Academic Standards Committee 1996 External examiners for undergraduate and postgraduate courses. University of Dundee, Dundee

CVCP (Committee of Vice Chancellors and Principals) 1985 The external examiner system for first degree and taught masters courses. Revised code of practice. CVCP, London

Karuhije H F, Ruff C 2002 External examiners: international collaboration in nursing education. ABNF Journal 13:110–113

Nystrup J, Mårtenson D 1992 Reflections on possible virtues of European medical education. Medical Education 26:350–353

Osler W 1913 An introductory address on examinations, examiners and examinees. Lancet 11:1047–1050

Piper W D 1985 Enquiry into the role of the external examiners. Study on Higher Education 10:331–342

Sheehan J 1994 External examiners: roles and issues. Journal of Advanced Nursing 20:943–949

Walters W A, Sivanesaratnam V, Hamilton J D 1995 External examiners. Lancet 345:1093–1095

SECTION 7
STAFF AND STUDENTS

Chapter 39
Student selection

I. C. McManus

"For a man to be truly suited to the practice of medicine, he must be possessed of a natural disposition for it, the necessary instruction, favourable circumstances, education, industry and time. The first requisite is a natural disposition, for a reluctant student renders every effort vain"

Hippocrates

"Selection is of key importance to medical education. What sort of students are recruited at the beginning is a major determination of what kind of doctors come out at the end"

Downie & Charlton 1992

"although there are reasons for being anxious about medical school selection, not all of the blame can be laid at the door of the selectors. Self-selection and preselection out of the applicant pool is extensive"

Johnson 1971

Introduction

Selection seems deceptively easy; with more applicants than places, one simply selects the best applicants. In practice the process is much more complicated and may be:

- of dubious validity
- statistically unreliable
- a vulnerable process within the medical school
- open to legal challenge on grounds such as discrimination
- criticised by society at large
- under-resourced, particularly when compared with a medical school's implicit expectations of what it can do.

Why select?

A selection programme must clearly state the reasons for selection. If the *only* reason is reduction of numbers, a lottery-type process would suffice. In reality selection is a complex process with several different stages.

Selection of students by the medical school
The straightforward reason is to choose the best students. Although seemingly simple, this contains many complexities.

Selection by applicants of medicine as a career
The pool of applicants for medical schools to choose from consists only of those who have selected medicine as a career. The majority of the population who did not apply cannot be selected, even if they might make excellent doctors.

Initial selection of the medical school by applicants
Applicants study all medical schools and then choose which to apply to. There is no point in running a good selection system if most good applicants have already applied elsewhere. An effective selection system must encourage the best students to apply to a school.

Explicit selection of medical schools by applicants
Applicants receiving offers from several medical schools make an explicit choice and select one from those on offer. McManus and colleagues (1999) have shown that schools which interview are twice as likely to be preferred to schools which do not.

Selection for a particular course

Increasingly medical schools are developing courses with different emphases. A course, for example, with a large component of problem-based learning in small groups might choose to select students who can work together in a cooperative rather than a competitive fashion.

Selection by staff

If staff have been actively involved in the selection process and have met the students as applicants, a relationship can develop which can enhance the educational process. Staff feel ownership of selection and students feel membership of the institution.

The limits of selection

There is a fundamental misconception that medical schools receive numerous applications. In practice the ratio in the UK is now less than two applicants for every place (McManus 2002), although from the perspective of admissions officers it may seem much more than that because each candidate makes multiple applications. The power of selection depends to a large extent on the 'selection ratio', the number of applicants for each place. As the ratio grows, so selection can be more effective.

The limits of selection can be shown in a straightforward mathematical model. For example, if selecting on a single criterion (such as intellectual ability), assuming that this ability has a normal distribution and that the selection ratio is two applicants for every place, the optimal selection is as shown in Figure 39.1. One places the candidates in rank order and takes those above the median.

The limits of selection appear when two or more criteria are introduced. For example, if selecting on two independent ('orthogonal') criteria, for example intellectual ability and communication skills, there will now be a bivariate normal distribution (see Fig. 39.2) and the aim is to take the best 50% of candidates on the joint criteria. The dashed lines indicate the means of the distributions, which would be the thresholds if there were only one characteristic.

There are several ways to select the best 50%, according to the extent to which high ability on one criterion can compensate for poorer performance on the other, though all have similar effects (McManus & Vincent 1993). If selected candidates have to be above a certain threshold on *both* criteria they must be in the top right-hand corner of the figure. The important thing is that the threshold on either criterion must be substantially below the median. In fact, with two independent criteria, candidates selected are only in the top 71% of the ability range, rather than the top 50%. Therefore they are less able on average on either criterion than if it had been the sole criterion.

So, if one selects principally on just one attribute, and wishes to select also on a second attribute, it is necessary to reduce one's criterion on the first attribute. In the UK, medical student selection is currently based predominantly on academic achievement. If it is felt desirable to take nonacademic factors into account then current academic standards will have to be lowered.

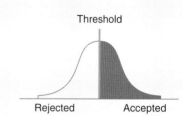

"The aim is not to pick men and women for specific tasks but to train wise, bright, humane, multipotential individuals who will find their niche somewhere in medicine"

Richards & Stockill 1997

Fig. 39.1 A simple model of selection when there is a single characteristic on which selection is taking place. Those above the threshold are accepted, those below are rejected

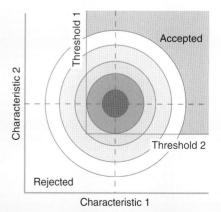

Fig. 39.2 Example showing two criteria

Once medical schools begin to consider nonacademic attributes for selection then they rapidly develop a long list. Even if these are not all statistically independent, one soon ends up with a system with 5, 10, 20 or even 50 statistical dimensions. Extending the selection process (see Figure 39.2) to three, four or five criteria and so on shows how the limits of selection rapidly appear. In Table 39.1 the proportion of candidates eliminated on a single criterion (shown in the second column) becomes smaller as the number of criteria rise. The criteria are assumed to be independent, and the selection ratio to be two (i.e. 50% of candidates are selected). To summarise it pithily, 'if one selects on everything one selects on nothing.'

Therefore:

- Selection should aim at a relatively small number of what we will call 'canonical traits'; the three or four characteristics which are likely to be predictive of future professional behaviour and can be assessed reliably at the time of application to medical school.
- Schools where selection is currently based almost entirely on academic ability will have to reduce those academic standards if they wish also to select effectively on nonacademic criteria.
- Selection should be recognised as being very limited in its power. The really powerful implements for effecting change are education and training (McManus & Vincent 1993).

Table 39.1 The effects of selection on the basis of multiple criteria (assuming two applicants for every place) (McManus & Vincent 1993)

Number of independent selection criteria	Proportion of applicants rejected on any single criterion
1	Bottom 50%
2	Bottom 29.3%
3	Bottom 20.6%
4	Bottom 15.9%
5	Bottom 12.9%
6	Bottom 10.9%
10	Bottom 6.7%
20	Bottom 3.4%
50	Bottom 1.4%
N*	Bottom 100. $(1- N\sqrt{1/r})$%

* N = number of criteria; r = selection ratio (i.e. 1/r is the proportion of applicants accepted).

What are the canonical traits that should be selected for?

Four principal canonical traits for selection have been identified (McManus & Vincent 1993).

Intelligence

Doctors probably cannot be too intelligent. Meta-analyses of selection across a wide range of different occupations at all social levels show that the best predictor of both job performance and the ability to be trained is intelligence (Schmidt & Hunter 1998).

Learning style and motivation

University students in general are motivated to study for different reasons and adopt different study habits and learning styles which are consistent with that motivation. Table 39.2 summarises the typology of Biggs (Biggs 1987, Newble & Entwistle 1986). Deep and strategic learning (but not surface learning) are both compatible with a self-directed, self-motivated approach to learning which is likely to result in the lifelong learning necessary of modern practitioners.

Communicative ability

The majority of complaints about doctors involve problems in communication so it makes some sense to include it in selection. Although communication skills should have been developing during life they can be further refined. However, individuals who are communicating poorly at age 17 are less likely to respond well to training. Assessment is not straightforward but questionnaires are available (McManus et al 1997).

" 'A' levels tell us nothing about some of the most desirable attributes of the doctor. The four desiderata are technical competence, human sympathy, wisdom and experience"

McKeown 1986

Table 39.2 Summary of the differences in motivation and study process of the surface, deep and strategic approaches to study (based on the work of Biggs 1978, 1985, 1987, 1993, 2003)

Style	Motivation	Process
Surface	Completion of the course	Rote learning of facts and ideas Focusing on task components in isolation
	Fear of failure	Little real interest in content
Deep	Interest in the subject Vocational relevance	Relation of ideas to evidence Integration of material across courses
	Personal understanding	Identification of general principles
Strategic	Achieving high grades	Use of techniques that achieve highest grades
	Competing with others	Level of understanding patchy and variable
	Being successful	

"Many claim that conscientiousness ...is a valid predictor [of outcome] across organisations, jobs and situations...Based on the...definition of conscientiousness as conformity and socially prescribed impulse control, conscientiousness would not likely predict performance across organisations, jobs, or situations in which creativity or innovation is important"

Hough & Oswald 2000

"A multitude of ad hoc policies implemented by miscellaneous admissions officers of various medical schools cannot be properly evaluated or criticized, and is open to considerable abuse. Selection itself is problematic enough, without trying to make it a panacea for the world's ills. If selectors are trying to do too much too well, they will end by failing to do anything properly"

Downie & Charlton 1992

Conscientiousness

The meta-analysis of Schmidt & Hunter (1998) showed clearly that the best predictor of job performance and trainability, after taking intellectual ability into account, was integrity or conscientiousness. Conscientiousness is one of the five personality dimensions assessed in the 'Big Five', which together account for the majority of important variations in personality (Matthews & Deary 1998), the other four being extroversion, neuroticism, agreeableness and open-mindedness. Conscientiousness probably gains a large part of its impact through the simple fact that highly conscientious people tend to work harder and be more efficient, and thereby gain more and better experience. There is however a worry that conscientiousness does not predict achievement where creativity or innovation is important (Hough & Oswald 2000), such as in the research productivity of doctors (McManus et al 2003).

Surrogates for selection

Although intelligence, learning style and motivation, communicative ability and conscientiousness should probably form the basis of selection, it is sufficient to select on other measures which correlate highly with them. Selection on school-leaving examinations is one surrogate as high grades correlate to some extent with level of intelligence, appropriate learning styles and a conscientious approach to study (and hence school-leaving exams predict career outcomes better than do pure psychometric tests of intelligence; McManus et al 2003). Of course a person of lower intellect may pass exams by prodigious rote learning, conscientiously carried out, but it is relatively unlikely. Playing in an orchestra or for a sports team can imply conscientiousness at practising, an ability to communicate well with other individuals when collaborating on an enterprise, and perhaps a certain interest in the deeper aspects of a skill (intrinsic motivation). Good selection processes should not use such surrogates uncritically, but should ask what underlying psychological traits this biographical data (biodata) is purporting to assess.

Methods and process of selection

The process of selection and the methods used to carry it out are entirely separate (Powis 1998). Medical schools should have a selection policy which clearly states how selection takes place, how appropriate information is collected, and how a decision will be made based on that information. Once the information has been acquired the selection policy can be implemented and a decision made. This decision making should be an entirely administrative process. Although seemingly absurd at first sight, this ensures good practice and avoids suggestions of discrimination or unfairness, or apparent inconsistencies in selection. The academic and educational input to the system should be in deciding the protocol and, where necessary, making subtle judgements about the information (such as evaluating aspects of the application form or interviewing). A corollary of the principle is that the separate items of information should be assessed separately. If interviewers are asked to judge a candidate's knowledge of medicine as a career then that is what they should do; they do not need information about interviewees' GCSE or 'A' level results, hobbies or so on, as this information can result in a 'halo effect' on the judgment interviewers are required to make.

Assessing methods of selection

There are many methods of selection, each of which has its strengths and weaknesses. Each may be assessed in terms of:

- *Validity*. All assessments in selection are implicit predictions of the future behaviour of a candidate. If there is no correlation with those future behaviours then they are not useful, however much assessors may agree about them.
- *Reliability*. If selectors disagree about a characteristic, or reassessment gives different answers, then the information is unlikely to be useful.
- *Feasibility*. Assessments can usually be made more reliable and more valid by extending them. The result is greater cost, financially or in staff time, the gain from which may not be worth the resource expended.
- *Acceptability*. Candidates and their teachers, friends and relations must feel that selection methods are appropriate.

Different methods of selection

Administrative methods

A method typically used by office staff, processing information from application forms is relatively objective and is mostly used for rejecting candidates.

It is usually reliable, cheap and acceptable but of uncertain validity.

Assessment of application forms

Application forms often contain unstructured personal statements and referees' reports, which must be assessed by a shortlister who attempts to determine a candidate's motivation and experience of medicine as a career.

Like interviewing, it is subjective and often of moderate or even poor reliability and of uncertain validity. It is, however, cost-effective and acceptable to applicants. Reliability can undoubtedly be improved by training and the use of structured assessment protocols, clear criterion referencing and carefully constructed descriptors of the various characteristics to be identified.

Biographical data (biodata)

This can be assessed either indirectly from an open-ended application form (e.g. the 'personal statement') or more reliably from a specially designed structured or semistructured questionnaire. It derives its usefulness from the psychological principle that the best predictor of future behaviour is past behaviour. It is usually reliable, valid (Cook 1990), cost-effective and acceptable to applicants.

"We have found dissatisfaction in many quarters with the basis on which applicants are selected for admission to the undergraduate medical course. Many headmasters and headmistresses believe, for example, that in at least some universities the selection of medical students is not based on clearly equitable criteria"

Royal Commission on Medical Education 1968

"There is a most odd tendency on the part of the British selectors to accept the headmaster's report as 'extraordinarily accurate', except in some particular instances, which the selectors seem to assume they can always recognise. This is part of a general delusion of selectors; that they are able to use imperfect materials such as other people's opinions (or, in the case of some headmasters' reports, other people's opinions of other people's opinion) but somehow, miraculously, in their hands, these base metals are transmuted into the finest gold"

Simpson 1972

"the personal character, the very nature, the will, of each student had far greater force in determining his career than any helps or hindrances whatever. . . . The time and the place, the work to be done, and its responsibilities, will change; but the man will be the same, except in so far as he may change himself"

Sir James Paget 1869

"Prolonged observation of candidates in different situations by trained selectors makes the final...decision relatively easy. This contrasts with the brief interviews done by ...medical schools where dubious decisions are often based on inadequate evidence. The experience of assessment centres is that early opinions may be suspect...The time has come to establish on an experimental basis a Medical Selection Board along the lines of the assessment centres of the Army, Civil Service and British Airways"

Roberts & Porter 1989

Referees' reports

These can be useful if they are totally honest, but referees often feel a loyalty to the candidate rather than the medical school. Experienced headteachers will say that they expect medical schools to 'read between the lines', so that it is not what is said that matters, but what is left unsaid or understated. Such an approach inevitably means reliability is low, validity very dubious and acceptability ambiguous. They are expensive in terms of referees' time but not the medical school's.

Interviewing

Not all UK medical schools hold interviews, suggesting genuine uncertainty about their usefulness, although in recent years noninterviewing schools have returned to interviewing candidates. Interviews can, however, be more reliable than suspected. Marchese & Muchinsky (1993) report that reliability and validity are mostly dependent on training of interviewers and on a clear structure. Behavioural interviewing, where the emphasis is upon how the candidate has behaved in concrete situations in the past, is usually more effective than interviews asking about hypothetical situations in the remote future. Although expensive in terms of staff time, interviews are highly acceptable to the general public who are not happy with doctors being selected purely on academic grounds. However, they are often criticised after the event by candidates, parents and teachers.

Psychometric testing

Typically this involves questionnaires for assessing motivation and personality, timed assessments of intellectual ability or psychomotor tests of manual dexterity. The validity of these tests has often been formally assessed with regard to jobs in general and undoubtedly they are very reliable if well developed. However, they are time-consuming to administer and may be unpopular with candidates, who may feel that there are 'trick' questions and that the characteristics being assessed are not necessarily relevant to a career in medicine. Many tests have been developed only for research purposes, and are vulnerable to training, leakage, or 'faking good' if used in real selection. Nevertheless psychometric tests may predict career outcomes in doctors (Ferguson et al 2002).

Assessment centres

Candidates are brought together in groups of 4–12, over a period of 1–3 days, and are asked to carry out a series of novel exercises, often involving group work (Roberts & Porter 1989). This is the core approach of the army, civil service and major companies. Assessment centres are particularly appropriate if the emphasis is upon assessing ability under competitive time stress or upon collaborating in group activities. Their reliability is good since assessors are highly trained but they are very time-consuming for staff and applicants and also expensive.

The cost(s) of selection

The direct costs of selection for a medical school are difficult to assess, but are probably about £1000 per entrant, mostly accounted for by staff time. The implicit criterion of success is that graduates will practise high-quality medicine in the National Health Service from graduation until retirement, perhaps 40 years later. This contrasts with the £50 000 or so spent by British companies whose criterion of success is that the graduate stays with the company for five years.

There are two reasons why so little is spent on medical student selection. At present student selection is an 'open-loop' system, without feedback. A bad doctor may cost society very large amounts of money, but none of that cost comes back to the medical school. Selection costs are therefore seen as of little benefit to an institution and the temptation is to minimise them. If lifelong medical practice were a closed-loop system, with graduates incurring costs and providing rewards to their medical school throughout their career, then selection and undergraduate training would be at the core of a medical school's activities, instead of being marginalised.

Routine monitoring of selection

Because selection is so vulnerable to criticism and possibly even to legal challenge, it is essential not only that clear policies are in place, but that routine data are collected for the monitoring of the process. Monitoring should look at the overall pattern of selection, assessing whether particular groups of applicants (women, ethnic minorities, students with disabilities etc.) are being systematically advantaged or disadvantaged. A simple head count is not sufficient for this purpose, since groups may also differ in a range of relevant background factors; multivariate analysis is the appropriate procedure, both for identifying possible disadvantage and understanding its locus (McManus 1998).

Studying selection and learning from research

Medicine can be notoriously insular. Research and experience outside of medicine are often ignored, and there are medical schools which will not even consider experience gained at other medical schools, never mind in industry, commerce and the public sectors in general. Personnel selection has been much studied and there is a vast literature. A good place to start is the regular series of articles in the *Annual Review of Psychology*, which are frequently updated (Borman et al 1997; Hough & Oswald 2000).

Evidence-based medicine and the scientific study of selection

Evidence-based medicine is the current dogma in all areas of medicine. Student selection and medical education should be no different. However the limitations of an overly pure evidence-based approach should be recognised. If only 'gold-standard' randomised controlled trials were accepted as the criterion of evidence then the vast majority of medical education would not be valid – with the inevitable result that opinion, prejudice and anecdote would end up as the bases for action.

"It is impossible to separate selection from training...In this country the only case I know of a thoroughly validated selection procedure from first to last was one in which selection and training were treated as a single problem"

Sir Frederick Bartlett 1946

"We hope that research will in the course of time lead to the establishment of reasonably objective criteria of professional performance, valid in the many different fields and kinds of medical practice, and thereby make possible an objective evaluation of student selection. This is a long-term aspiration however"

Royal Commission on Medical Education 1968

Observational studies and the powerful methods of epidemiology are also useful, particularly when embedded in robust theories based in psychology, sociology and other basic sciences. A frequently encountered error when discussing, say, a prospective study of selection is the use of both of the following arguments simultaneously:

- 'These students have only been followed up for 5 years, but our selection process was assessing who would become good practising doctors in the future. These results do not look far enough into the future.'
- 'This study was carried out over 5 years ago, and since then we have changed our selection process and our undergraduate curriculum, and the doctors will be working in a medical system that has also changed. These results are only of historical interest.'

When put like this the sophistry is immediately apparent – prospective, longitudinal studies for N years must, of necessity, have been started more than N years ago. Of course, the same arguments are not used in medical practice: chemotherapeutic regimes looking at 5-year survival must be subject to the same problems, but these trials are still done.

A further problem with studying selection is that it is very vulnerable, as are the egos of the individuals carrying it out. No one likes to think that their actions have been wasted or that their best-considered schemes are worthless. Neither does any institution like to see results published suggesting that it has not been doing a perfect job, particularly when its rivals' results are not publicly displayed. A common reflex response is to demand an unreasonably high criterion of evidence, which is a paragon of perfection. However, the best is the enemy of the good. The scientific study of selection is no different from any other science. One is not searching for proof of absolute truth, but identifying working explanatory hypotheses, compatible with evidence, which have acceptable methodology, take known problems into account, and are therefore robust against straightforward refutation and make useful predictions. That is then a basis for practical action and further research.

Summary

Selection is an important yet usually under-resourced aspect of medical school activity.

Applicants may select medical schools because of their particular courses or their invitation to attend an interview. Medical schools may select applicants by their intelligence, their learning style and motivation, their ability to communicate and by evidence that they are conscientious.

A variety of methods of selection may be used by schools, ranging from a purely administrative review of application form details, through assessment of personal biodata, to psychometric testing of candidates.

Whatever process is used it is likely to be costly and should be routinely monitored, evaluated and compared with examples of best evidence-based practice.

References

Bartlett F C 1946 Selection of medical students. British Medical Journal iii:665–666

Biggs J B 1978 Individual and group differences in study processes. British Journal of Educational Psychology 48:266–279

Biggs J B 1985 The role of meta-learning in study processes. British Journal of Educational Psychology 55:185–212

Biggs J B 1987 Study process questionnaire: manual. Australian Council for Educational Research, Melbourne

Biggs J S 1993 What do inventories of students' learning processes really measure? A theoretical review and classification. British Journal of Educational Psychology 63:3–19

Biggs J S 2003 Teaching for quality learning at university. SRHE Open University Press, Milton Keynes

Borman W C, Hanson M A, Hedge J W 1997 Personnel selection. Annual Review of Psychology 48:299–337

Cook M 1990 Personnel selection and productivity: John Wiley, Chichester

Downie R S, Charlton B 1992 The making of a doctor: medical education in theory and practice. Oxford University Press, Oxford

Ferguson E, James D, Madeley L 2002 Factors associated with success in medical school and in a medical career: systematic review of the literature. British Medical Journal 324:952–957

Hough L M, Oswald F L 2000 Personnel selection: looking toward the future – remembering the past. Annual Review of Psychology 51:631–664

Johnson M L 1971 Non-academic factors in medical school selection: a report on rejected applicants. British Journal of Medical Education 5:264–268

Marchese M C, Muchinsky P M 1993 The validity of the employment interview: a meta-analysis. International Journal of Selection and Assessment 1:18–26

Matthews G, Deary I J 1998 Personality traits. Cambridge University Press, Cambridge

McKeown T 1986 Personal view. British Medical Journal 298:200

McManus I C 1998 Factors affecting likelihood of applicants being offered a place in medical schools in the United Kingdom in 1996 and 1997: retrospective study. British Medical Journal 317:1111–1116

McManus I C 2002 Medical school applications – a critical situation. British Medical Journal 325:786–787

McManus I C, Vincent C A 1993 Selecting and educating safer doctors. In: Vincent C A, Ennis M, Audley R J (eds) Medical accidents. Oxford University Press, Oxford. pp 80–105

McManus I C, Kidd J M, Aldous I R 1997 Self-perception of communicative ability: evaluation of a questionnaire completed by medical students and general practitioners. British Journal of Health Psychology 2:301–315

McManus I C, Richards P, Winder B C, Sproston K A 1999 Do UK medical school applicants prefer interviewing to non-interviewing schools? Advances in Health Sciences Education 4:155–165

McManus I C, Smithers E, Partridge P et al 2003 A levels and intelligence as predictors of medical careers in UK doctors: 20 year prospective study. British Medical Journal 327:139–142

Newble D I, Entwistle N J 1986 Learning styles and approaches: implications for medical education. Medical Education 20:162–175

Paget J 1869 What becomes of medical students. Saint Bartholomew's Hospital Reports 5:238–242

Powis D 1998 How to do it: select medical students. British Medical Journal 317:1149–1150

Richards P, Stockill S 1997 The new learning medicine, 14th edn. BMJ Publishing, London

Roberts G D, Porter A M W 1989 Medical student selection – time for change: discussion paper. Journal of the Royal Society of Medicine 82:288–291

Royal Commission on Medical Education 1968 Royal Commission on Medical Education (The Todd Report), Cmnd 3569. HMSO, London

Schmidt F L, Hunter J E 1998 The validity and utility of selection methods in personnel psychology: practical and theoretical implications of 85 years of research findings. Psychological Bulletin 124:262–274

Simpson M A 1972 Medical education: a critical approach. Butterworths, London

Chapter 40
Student support
J. A. Dent, S. Rennie

"Medical students enrolled today have greater expectations for student personal services than previously and a high attrition rate in medical education is not tolerated"

Heins et al 1980

"Appropriate intervention may be required to reduce student stress in revised curricula"

Moffat et al 2004

"the psychological well-being of students needs to be more carefully addressed and closer attention paid to the styles of medical teaching that may provoke avoidable distress"

Guthrie et al 1995

Introduction: why is student support necessary?

Medical students are exposed to a variety of pressures, many of which may cause stress. These 'stresses', examinations, competition, information overload, time management, financial difficulties, relationship problems and career decisions, are similar to the pressures encountered by all students. In addition, however, it is recognised that medical students face other stressful issues particularly associated with medical training, including relating to professionals in their workplace, dealing with death and dying, making mistakes, facing uncertainty and lack of time for recreation, relationships and family (Folse et al 1985). Guthrie and colleagues (1995) reported that even in the early years at medical school up to 50% of students related stress to aspects of the course work and Moffat and colleagues (2004) found the recent introduction of curriculum change in some medical schools to be a further source of student stress.

Medical students spend most of their time studying away from the university campus and are periodically at peripheral hospitals or in general practice placements. This, combined with unsociable hours of study, means that they are often away from their familiar social contacts and the support services provided by the university. In addition university services may not be able to provide help for problems specific to medical students such as careers advice on medical specialties.

Problems experienced by medical students commonly fall into five categories:

- academic
- careers
- professional
- personal
- administrative.

Academic support may include identifying and helping students in academic difficulty, providing feedback and advice after exams, study skills advice or guidance on the selection of elective components of the course including student-selected components, projects and elective periods of study.

Careers counselling may include advice about the early years of post-graduate training as well as future career paths. It may involve help in preparing curricula vitae, writing references for students and giving advice about interview technique.

Professional counselling may be required to help students develop attitudes and behaviour appropriate for a doctor or to consider professional conduct and ethical issues. Patients expect to be treated politely and considerately and expect their doctor to be honest and trustworthy. It is important for students to develop a professional approach to patients early in their undergraduate career. Some students require support from a tutor in these areas as they develop a capacity for self audit and an awareness of personal limitations.

Personal problems experienced by students include adjustment to medical school, relationship concerns, financial difficulties and accommodation worries.

Administrative problems deal mainly with the 'how', 'where', 'who', 'what' and 'when' questions that students have about the organisation of the course and university administration. These questions may seem trivial but can often cause students unnecessary concern and stress.

However, it is important not to view a student support system as a scheme primarily for students in trouble but as a stress-management system available for all to sustain academic performance (Stewart et al 1999). Stress is a central component of a doctor's job and learning to cope with stress is an important part of the training of a doctor. The ways in which medical students cope with stress often provides a blueprint for how they deal with future professional and personal stress.

The aim of a student support system should therefore be to facilitate medical students' development, to ensure that their education is a positive experience and to create relationships which may be beneficial in the future. The support system can help the student adjust to medical school, learn stress-management strategies and develop competencies for future use as a doctor. In addition, the scheme can provide a forum for feedback, advice and enhanced communications between faculty and students.

How can students be supported?

Students can be supported in a number of different ways through:

- tutor schemes
- student advisory office
- university and external support services
- peer support systems
- email and the internet.

These strategies may be used individually in isolation or in combination by faculties to provide a support system tailored to the needs of the students and the resources of the faculty.

Tutor schemes

This involves the allocation of staff from within the faculty to act as tutors to students on either a one-to-one or a group basis. Groups may be

"Medical educators and those with responsibility for curricular development should be more aware of the stresses of medical life and take prophylactic action for the prevention of short- and long-term stress-related problems for medical students"

Stewart et al 1995

"Physicians must view the mentor/student relationship as a valuable opportunity to nurture the total growth of a young physician rather than merely to focus on the student's academic or personal problems"

Flach et al 1982

"if students who have important personal qualities in caring for patients are also the ones for whom medical training is the most stressful, then they must be provided with extra support"

Stewart et al 1999

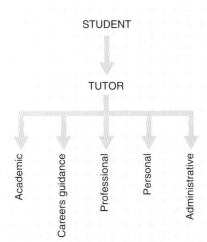

STUDENT

TUTOR

Academic

Careers guidance

Professional

Personal

Administrative

Fig. 40.1 Referral pathways for particular questions

horizontal, with students drawn entirely from one year, or vertical with a mix of students from all years. Tutors may meet with students individually to discuss specific problems. On occasions students may develop a relationship with another staff member who may become an 'unofficial tutor'.

There are advantages to a group system. In this age of increasing numbers of medical students, it reduces the number of tutors needed to provide a support scheme. It also enables peer support within the group. Peer support within horizontal systems often comes from identifying common problems and concerns, whereas a vertical system enables senior students to give empathy and advice to more junior students.

The tutor generally follows the students through the course, ensuring the continuity which can lead to the development of a solid relationship with them. This relationship can be strengthened by engaging in social as well as educational activities. A tutor can help students with problems which may be academic, career-related, professional, personal or administrative by either providing that help personally or by referring them on to other resources (see Fig. 40.1). A tutor may also be required to act as an advocate for students in particular difficulties by making representations to appropriate faculty or senate committees.

Student advisory office

A student advisory office staffed by a small number of full-time advisers with an extensive knowledge of the medical course and its administration may be used as an initial contact point for students with queries or problems. These advisers can act as a filter for medical students dealing with their academic, career, professional, personal and administrative concerns or directing them to the most appropriate person within the faculty, the university services or outside agencies. An advantage of this system is that advisers for students are readily available and accessible. This office may also be responsible for coordinating the tutor scheme and providing staff support and training.

The advisers may include nonmedical staff members who are perceived as having the advantage of being separate from the staff members students may subsequently see, either during assessment or in their future career. One such member is a study skills tutor who works with students on an individual or group basis to help with the development of study methods, time-management skills and revision and exam techniques. It is also useful to have a list of specialty advisers who are willing to speak to students about careers in their field of medicine.

University and external support services

Most universities have a variety of student welfare services including financial advisers, accommodation offices, disability support, legal advice, a health service and a counselling service. The finance officer is able to help students to budget, manage debt and find grants. Accommodation offices provide lists of landlords and of accommodation to let. The university counselling service provides independent trained counsellors who are able to assist students with emotional and practical problems.

There is also a wide range of external advice agencies available such as the Citizens' Advice Bureau and the Samaritans. Students may access these services directly or be referred by their tutor. It may be useful in some cases for the tutor to act as an advocate for a student approaching any of these services.

Peer support systems

'Senior–junior', 'big sibs', or 'parenting' schemes provide great benefits to junior students if they are organised effectively. They involve the pairing of first-year students with a second- or third-year student, either on a one-to-one basis or in groups. These schemes have mixed success and usually work better when the senior students are volunteers. Senior students are often a good source of advice to junior students as they have personal experience of many of the problems students may face. Junior doctors may also provide excellent advice to medical students about the medical course, electives and securing jobs. Most universities have a wide range of student interest or affinity' groups (sports, music, religious and social activities groups), which can all contribute to student support.

Medical student councils or associations should be encouraged and supported by faculty. They can provide a focus for student support through academic, recreational and social events. They often produce newsletters and information leaflets which deal with concerns and enhance communication. A 'medical student survival guide' can provide information, advice and useful tips on a whole range of issues, such as which books to buy, how to study for exams, where to look for grants and information specific to the medical school. A student guide is especially useful in helping first-year students orientate themselves and in providing answers to many of their questions.

E-mail and the internet

Computers have rapidly become an essential part of medicine, and most medical students now have email and internet access. Email provides an ideal interface for dealing with administrative queries and concerns. An email address to which concerns can be directed should be given to students and administered directly by the faculty's administrative staff. Most medical schools have internet websites which can also be utilised to provide 'bulletin boards' or talkshops, where problems and concerns can be aired and advice given by other students or staff.

How to organise a tutor scheme

What makes an effective tutor?

The most effective tutors are volunteers who are committed, enthusiastic, self-motivated and accessible to students. They must be sensitive to the stresses and needs of medical students and have a genuine desire to help them grow into well rounded doctors. Tutors, if they are to be successful, must, from the outset, be perceived as credible by the student body. Good tutors must be effective listeners as often this is all that the

"The value of peer-group relationships in providing support and growth during the educational process should not be underestimated"

Adsett 1968

A 'tutor support pack' can be devised that provides information about
- how to be a tutor
- sources of specialist support
- staff development opportunities.

"the best advisers are individuals who are warm, empathetic and spontaneous, who have constructive, sound judgement, and who get satisfaction out of watching medical students grow into mature adults as well as competent physicians"

Eckenfels et al 1984

Tutors are not required to:
- have a specialist knowledge of the content of each part of the course
- have first-hand experience of the training requirements of all specialties
- be a health, financial or marital counsellor
- have a degree in psychotherapy
- understand the administrative details of the medical school.

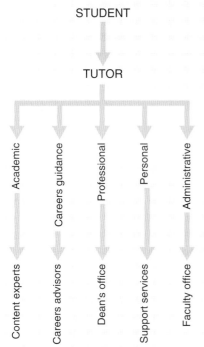

Fig. 40.2 Examples of referral pathways for particular questions

A 'Getting started pack' can be circulated to tutors and should include:
- suggestions on possible times and nonthreatening venues for the first meeting
- names and email addresses of the group
- list of key people in the medical school
- outline of other support services
- list of specialty advisors
- how to contact the scheme coordinator
- a model invitation to send out prior to the first meeting
- instructions for the content and frequency of meetings.

student requires. It is expected of course that a tutor will be trustworthy and will handle any confidential information appropriately. Tutors must be aware that students may view them as a role model, confidant, friend and advocate.

What does a tutor need?

Basic requirements

Tutors need to understand the faculty's chosen student support scheme and know where they fit into it. It is important that they understand that their role is initially to provide a point of contact and support for all students (not just those with problems) and subsequently to be able to direct them to any of the five specialist areas of support described previously:

- *Academic*. Tutors may be able to help with questions about study technique or with questions of a general nature on the content. They should have a working knowledge of the structure and content of the curriculum and be familiar with its objectives and with the range of options available for elective components of the course.
- *Career*. They should have some knowledge of the range of junior training posts available in the area.
- *Professionalism*. Tutors should be able to give advice and guidance about standards of professional behaviour, and be aware that they are often seen as a role model.
- *Personal*. Active listening and the ability to empathise is probably all that is required for the majority of personal problems.
- *Administrative*. Tutors should know the basics of the organisation of the curriculum and the names of key people in it, such as medical school office bearers, curriculum administrators and course secretaries.

Additional resources

Tutors need to have access to information which will help them direct students to sources of specialist information (see Fig. 40.2).

- *Academic/educational*. Tutors require lists of names of the systems teachers, and other content experts for the course, and the names of block or phase coordinators.
- *Career*. Specific questions regarding entry requirements to training programmes are best referred to specialty career advisors. Questions about junior postgraduate training posts and how to apply for them should be referred to the postgraduate dean's office.
- *Professional*. Persisting problems with a student's professional behaviour, for example if there is a problem of plagiarism, are best referred to the dean, or faculty secretary for appropriate action.
- *Personal*. Accommodation, financial or health problems should be referred to the appropriate university support services. More serious personal or emotional problems probably require the help of the professional counselling services which may be available in the university.

- *Administrative*. Specific details pertaining to the administration of the course are best referred to the medical school office secretaries and phase coordinators.

Student information

Tutors need to know the names of the students allocated to them and the best method to get in touch with them quickly. Available information about their students should be provided for the tutors but previous counselling information from meetings with other members of staff should only be passed between tutors with the student's consent. A note of the student's academic progress to date is valuable, and competency profiles should be made available for post-assessment discussion and feedback. Knowledge of the student's performance may be of help if the tutor is called on for any advocacy role. However, it must be emphasised that all such information must be handled according to the university's policy on confidentiality.

What does the scheme need?

Recognition

To be a success the scheme must be valued, tutors must be appreciated, their efforts must be recognised, and events aimed to raise the profile of the scheme must be appropriately promoted and supported by the dean and faculty.

Similarly, it is important that the student body understand and participate appropriately in the scheme if they are to benefit by it. Student involvement with the scheme can be enhanced by inviting them, or a representative group, to meetings with faculty members for discussion on the development of the scheme or for feedback.

Flexibility

Not all students require the same extent of contact with their tutors and most are content to know that they have one available if necessary. The scheme should recognise that, whatever the system, there are three levels of student–tutor interactions which will develop (see Fig. 40.3):

- Close relationship – one third of students establish a personal relationship with their tutor; this follows meetings to discuss personal or academic problems or simply because they naturally get on well together.
- Contractual relationship – about half of the students see their tutor only as requested and would rarely initiate contact.
- Constrained relationship – a small peripheral group choose not to participate and are only seen when important information is being disseminated or when they perceive that it is to their advantage to be present.

The last group probably represents a variety of personalities, including those who are very self-sufficient or independent students, those who are reserved or intimidated and those who have chosen not to participate in any aspect of medical school life. It is important for

"Despite the heavy load of responsibilities they carry, faculty must show interest in the students and their activities to the degree that they do not let other responsibilities always crowd out their attending student functions or having informal chats with students"

Adsett 1968

"serving as a mentor is included as one of the recognized criteria for faculty promotions"

Flach et al 1982

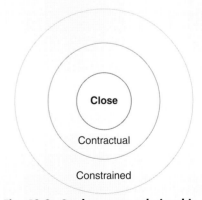

Fig. 40.3 Student–tutor relationships

The university year can begin with a social evening for all tutors and peer supporters to meet their new students.

"Meet the person who will get you your first PRHO job"

Quote from a tutor's invitation to second-year student group

"Graduating seniors...have expressed regret that they did not put more effort into the mentor relationship"

Flach et al 1982

tutors to seek to reduce the size of this group and to recognise and address the problems and needs which they present. However, some students in this group may have developed relationships with other faculty members who act as unofficial tutors.

Not all tutors are able to relate with equal effectiveness to students and a flexible rather than a rigidly applied scheme is more likely to be successful. Individual tutors can then adapt the scheme to their own style while still following the main principles of providing support as required. Some tutors use academic exercises, such as discussion of a learning styles questionnaire, to facilitate their initial interaction with the group. Others are comfortable with an informal meeting in a coffee-shop venue. Whatever ploys are adopted, the scheme should aim to be social as well as educational so that students are encouraged to move from the outer towards the inner circles of interaction.

Administration

An enthusiastic coordinator should be appointed who will identify the most appropriate scheme for the medical school, invite suitable members of staff to become tutors and gain the support and recognition of the faculty so that the initiating momentum of the scheme is maintained.

The coordinator will have to act as a resource back-up for tutors and be able to supply additional information to them as required. For this to be possible (or tolerable!) appropriate secretarial assistance is necessary to provide a filter for inquiries from tutors and students. Secretarial assistance is also required for compiling the 'Tutor support pack'. An information pack for students is also necessary to explain the purpose and benefits of the scheme and what can be expected from it.

Staff development programmes are also required. These are best structured as informal meetings to provide feedback, discussion and training opportunities which are especially important for first-time tutors. A newsletter can be used to follow up these sessions, expand on issues raised in discussion and remind tutors of impending events which may have a bearing on student wellbeing, such as forthcoming examinations.

Information for both students and tutors should be available in the library and on the university website.

Finally, internal audit and review of participants' perceptions of the student support scheme may be helpful in identifying deficiencies and in indicating appropriate changes (Malik 2000).

Summary

Student support is required in relation to five areas of potential stress: academic problems, careers advice, personal worries, professional issues and administrative questions. Support can be provided in a variety of ways by tutor schemes, students' advisory offices, university and external support services, peer support groups or via the internet. Successful tutors are required to be good listeners and set a good example as role models. They should be able to provide first-line help in each of the areas of student concern but need additional resources which will help them direct students as required to further sources of expert help.

For their part, students should participate appropriately in the scheme and realise that it is not just for students in trouble but may help all students to develop stress-management strategies that will be useful in their later career. The scheme must be appropriately resourced, administered and recognised as important by faculty. Individual medical schools can make a selection of an appropriate mixture of several of the methods described and the final scheme should be administered with some flexibility so that all students and tutors involved can participate in it to the extent that they require.

"The relationship that is formed between students and tutors is the most important factor contributing to the success of the scheme"

Malik 2000

References

Adsett C A 1968 Psychological health of medical students in relation to the medical education process. Journal of Medical Education 43:728–734.

Eckenfels E J, Blacklow R S and Gotterer G S 1984 Medical student counseling: the Rush medical college adviser program. Journal of Medical Education 59:573–581

Flach D H, Smith M F, Smith W G, Glasser M L et al 1982 Faculty mentors for medical students. Journal of Medical Education 57:514–520.

Folse M L, DaRosa D A, Folse R 1985 The relationship between stress and attitudes towards leisure among first-year medical students. Journal of Medical Education 60:610–617

Guthrie E A, Black D, Shaw C M et al 1995 Embarking upon a medical career: psychological morbidity in first-year medical students. Medical Education 29:337–341

Heins M, Clifton R, Simmons J et al 1980 Expansion of services for medical students. Journal of Medical Education 55:428–433

Malik S 2000 Students, tutors and relationships: the ingredients of a successful student support scheme. Medical Education 34:635–641

Moffat K J, McConnachie A, Ross S, Morrison J M 2004 First-year medical students' stress and coping in a problem-based learning medical curriculum. Medical Education 38:482–491

Stewart S M, Betson C, Marshall I et al 1995 Stress and vulnerability in medical students. Medical Education 29:119–127

Stewart S M, Lam T H, Betson CL et al 1999 A prospective analysis of stress and academic performance in the first two years of medical school. Medical Education 33:243–250

Further reading

Coombs R H and Virshup B B 1994 Enhancing the psychological health of medical students: the student well-being committee. Medical Education 28:47–54

Cotterel D J, McCrorie P and Perrin F 1994 The personal tutor system: an evaluation. Medical Education 28:544–549

Michie S, and Sandhu S 1994 Stress management for clinical medical students. Medical Education 28:528–533.

Plaut S M, Walker-Bastnick L, Helman L et al 1980 Improving staff–student relations: effects of a humanistic medicine programme. Medical Teacher 2:32–39

Rathburn J 1995 Helping medical students develop lifelong strategies to cope with stress. Academic Medicine 70:955–956

Weston J A, Paterson C A 1980 A medical student support system at the University of Colorado school of medicine. Journal of Medical Education 55:624–626

Chapter 41
Study skills
R. C. Bandaranayake

"Scientific knowledge grows exponentially, with a doubling time of fifteen years"

Unattributed

"Departmental allegiance often takes precedence over institutional allegiance, as academicians train the medical student to be a clone of their own speciality or sub-speciality"

Bandaranayake 1999

Constantly encourage students to recall the basic science concepts underlying the clinical knowledge and skills they encounter.

Introduction

Learning for life
In most areas of science knowledge grows exponentially, and medicine is no exception. With increasing knowledge it is imperative for medical students to develop sound learning habits which will stand them in good stead throughout their professional life. Such habits include the selection of what is learnt as well as how it is learnt. The latter is one factor which determines whether what is learnt will be remembered long enough to become part of the student's repertoire of knowledge (long-term memory) or will be discarded as soon as it ceases to be of immediate use (short-term memory).

Growth of knowledge
Knowledge in every discipline has grown to such an extent that subdisciplines have grown out of erstwhile disciplines and departments have split into subdepartments. The daunting task facing today's medical student is often compounded by the discipline specialist who has expectations of the student far beyond those required for basic medical practice.

In facing this challenge the average student resorts to the most expedient strategy of studying to satisfy immediate concerns of assessment. After the examination much of what is learnt is forgotten and only that which is used in the period immediately following is remembered. Students and clinical teachers frequently complain of the futility of forgotten preclinical anatomy and biochemistry. Preclinical teachers argue that such learning is more easily recalled if required during the postgraduate phase.

Can students study these subjects in a way which enables the retention of learning essential for professional practice so that re-learning does not become a major endeavour but is seen as part of the continuum of learning?

The continuum of learning
Learning is continuous, with new learning built on what has already been learned. Medical education is a continuum which starts at entry to medical school and ends with cessation of professional practice. Only a relatively small, though important, part of this continuum takes place in the undergraduate medical school. However, both the content of what is learnt and the process of learning make a significant impact on the remaining phases of the continuum.

Most medical students have not decided, during their undergraduate training, which specialty they will follow, partly because they have not yet experienced those specialties. Thus selection of what is to be learnt to be a sound specialist in any field becomes critical.

Component study skills

Many important process skills must be developed in the medical student:

- self-directed learning
- learning with understanding (deep learning), leading to long-term retention, rather than through rote (surface) learning, which is likely to result in short-term retention
- seeking and retrieving information from an increasing variety of sources
- critically reviewing what is read, rather than blindly accepting the written word
- integrating new learning with existing knowledge by seeking links between them, and dealing with dissonance
- assessing oneself on learning that has occurred to ensure that it can be remembered and applied to the situations likely to be encountered in professional practice.

Study plan

The medical student, constantly faced with new areas for learning across a spectrum of subjects, must develop a study plan for each significant period of time, such as a week. Often subjects are not organised in a way that enables the student to see the links between them. In some curricula, integration among subjects is achieved through themes, such as organ systems or clinical problems. Yet the student must learn to establish priorities for study, based not on expediency but on *importance*, *difficulty* and *timeliness*.

Importance must be judged in terms of:

- usefulness for professional practice
- the degree of understanding required for further learning
- the place of new learning in the unfolding of a continuing story.

Difficulty depends on:

- the existence of prerequisite learning
- the predilection of the individual for the subject
- the level of abstraction of the subject
- the degree and nature of the initial exposure to the subject.

Each student has to learn to identify areas of individual difficulty and plan study in such a way as to devote more time to such areas.

Timeliness relates to a number of factors, which include:

- readiness for the next phase of study, i.e. what is about to be learnt is considered prerequisite to what is to follow

"Systematic methods of learning may require more effort and patience in the beginning, but soon they become habitual and effective"

Smith et al 1951

"the most significant and common factors hindering academic growth result from the lack of adequate secondary school preparation in the basic skills of language"

Wilcox 1958

Avoid requiring students to provide lists from memory, such as investigations, without providing the reason for each item in the list.

Encourage the student to link the subject you teach with related learning outside your specialty.

"Learning may be enhanced if a variety of presentation methods is used with students. . . . Learning occurs when students use a combination of senses"

Lock 1981

- synchronisation among different subject areas related to a common integrating theme
- assessment points during the course of study which drive the student to concentrate on certain areas.

Readiness for learning depends on intrinsic motivation, an inner urge to learn, as well as the acquisition of prerequisite learning on which new learning is built. This includes the basic skills of language and communication and the ability of the learner to identify discrepancies between what he or she knows and does not know.

In developing a study plan, the student must:

- identify the focus of study
- determine the depth to which study of a particular topic is to be undertaken
- understand the interrelationships of topics by designing a logical sequence of topics for study.

Focus of study is determined by learning objectives. However, a student confronted with a daunting array of objectives must determine priorities among them, based on their relative importance for progressive learning and for future application, and on perceived gaps in knowledge which hinder further learning.

Depth of study is that which is required for understanding and depends on the complexity of the subject matter. As this cannot often be judged prior to actually undertaking study, the student must build into the plan study time in proportion to the relative difficulty of each subject area as experienced previously. The temptation to memorise without understanding should be resisted.

Learning occurs as new material is related to previously learned material. If the steps are properly sequenced and studies undertaken accordingly, both horizontal and vertical integration will be facilitated. In other words, the learner will be able to see the links in progressive learning as well as among parallel learning in related areas. Often, lack of synchronisation across disciplines hinders horizontal integration between them. The student must learn to develop a study plan which brings these relationships to the fore, even if it may not correspond to the school's formal timetable.

Resources for study

For the individual student, multiple stimuli aid learning as long as there is no dissonance among them. For example, when concepts are presented as descriptive text, graphs and three-dimensional models, students are better able to grasp them. Learning which is reinforced by multiple stimuli is likely to be retained longer.

At the same time, individual students may learn best in different ways. For example, in anatomy, learning may best occur through:

- dissection
- prosected specimens

- projected images
- two-dimensional pictures, or
- printed text.

Teachers should help students identify the method(s) of study by which they learn best. Methods are determined by:

- type of learning objective
- individual preferences and style
- practicalities of a given situation
- priorities in the purpose of learning
- time available for learning.

A skill of paramount importance to the medical student during a lifetime of continuing education is the ability to seek, retrieve and store information. Students must learn to undertake this task efficiently early in their medical education. Many, not having acquired these skills during secondary education, need training in them. While orientation courses at entry to medical school include visits to libraries, relatively few include training in these skills. Locating information from different sources includes the skills of using library filing systems, referring to indices, scanning reading material to determine relevance and importance, and referencing for subsequent easy retrieval (Saunders et al 1984).

The tendency to accumulate photocopied material for later use without adequate discrimination should be avoided. Immediate study of the material, highlighting important points and noting them on index cards, would save hours of wading through piles of accumulated material subsequently.

Learning style

A considerable body of literature now exists in the field of medical education on the approaches to learning adopted by students. A learning approach does not describe a particular attribute of the student, but a relationship between the learner and the learning task (Ramsden 1987). In other words, a given student may adopt a particular learning approach for one learning task and a different approach for another.

Three approaches, related to the student's motivation and purpose for study, have been described:

- surface learning
- deep learning
- strategic learning

(see chapter 39, Student selection, Table 39.2, page 367).

Study skill courses should focus on developing students' awareness of these approaches so that they could select that which is most suited to a given learning task.

Superficial reading of text does not guarantee that what is read, and even understood, will be retained in the long-term memory. Students must develop the practice of reflecting on the subject matter, connecting

Provide a variety of learning experiences for your students when you help them learn a given topic.

"in many of the problem-based medical schools the ability of the student to identify and utilize appropriate learning resources is an established component of student assessment"

Saunders et al 1984

Give your students assignments which require them to study beyond their textbooks and class notes.

"The (anatomy) student (who learns) to reason anatomically ... will find the acquisition of new and related facts an easier task"

Grant 1937

In clinical teaching, challenge students with problem-solving exercises based not only on what they already know, but also on what they should but do not know.

"The best way to learn to appreciate and understand scientific method is to practice until it becomes habitual"

Smith et al 1951

When you have demonstrated a clinical skill to your students, let each in turn practise it under your supervision and then encourage them to practise it by themselves.

it with what they already know and summarising new learning in their own words.

Few would disagree that the attributes and study skills we would desire in a medical student are those embedded in the deep approach to learning. However, many curricula are planned and implemented in ways that promote surface or strategic approaches (Stiernborg & Bandaranayake 1996). The surge of curricula adopting problem-based learning to varying extents favours the deep approach (Newble & Clarke 1987). There is no reason, however, for not inculcating such an approach even in the more conventional curricula.

While the most *efficient* reader may be the 'one who can gather the most amount of information from the printed page in the least amount of time' (Wilcox 1958), he or she may not be the most *effective* learner, as much of that information may be retained for only a short time. The reflective process involved in the deep approach to learning may, ostensibly, be more time-consuming. However, longer retention of learning makes this approach more effective in the long term. One reason why students complain of the tedious nature of basic science courses may be the lack of time and opportunity for reflection.

The key to the development of any skill is practice until perfection is achieved. This applies to both cognitive and psychomotor skills. Students accustomed to surface learning may have initial difficulty adopting a deep approach. Effective ways of reflecting on newly learned material are writing essays, discussion with peers, teaching others and entertaining questions.

Teachers have an important role to play in this process, as they must devise assignments which compel students to reflect on their learning. Such reflection is encouraged by requiring students to apply their new learning to problems and situations which they have not encountered hitherto. Teachers must also help students relate such learning to their personal goals to enhance motivation.

Practice of psychomotor skills is a three-stage process of:

1. observation of a demonstration
2. practice under supervision
3. independent practice until perfect.

In the clinical situation the last step depends on the student's initiative and industry. Recent development of clinical skills laboratories has contributed to expansion of the opportunities available to students to hone their clinical skills.

Review of learning

Review and application of new learning must take place periodically if it is to be built into the student's cognitive framework. Memory is enhanced not only by actively seeking links between new learning and previous learning and experience, but also by deriving logical associations among areas of new learning. For example, the student who is learning about renal function for the first time should seek relationships, on the one hand, with the circulatory system (which may have been learnt earlier) and, on the other, with the microscopic structure of the nephron (which may be introduced at the same time). This helps in acquisition of the new learning as well as review of the old.

In reviewing learning, the student is often confronted with the problem of deciding what topics are important for review. Importance is a matter of perception: to the practitioner, that which is applicable to practice is important; to the teacher, that which is essential for understanding the subject; to the student, that which is likely to be examined.

In a course which aims to prepare future professionals, rationality dictates that importance be related to practice. However, preparation for practice without understanding the basis of that practice merely results in a technician rather than a professional. Hence emphasis should be placed on understanding the basic sciences rather than memorising that which is applicable.

Many problem-centred curricula adopt the concept of the spiral problem. The same problem is introduced at increasingly complex levels during successive phases of the curriculum. This helps the student identify content which is considered important for review. When the same content is required for different problems, opportunities are provided for students to review and practise its application in different situations.

A useful technique for review is to organise information that has been learnt into chunks, around certain principles, generalisations or cues. These form pegs on which more detailed information may be hung. Such organisation aids easy retrieval of the information, as the pegs are more easily recalled. Thus the student learning about the joints of the body may remember a few principles which govern classification of joints in relation to movement. Even if the details pertaining to a particular joint may be forgotten, recalling the principles would facilitate their retrieval.

Assessment of learning

Assessing oneself is perhaps the most difficult, yet most important, skill that must be undertaken for effective study. Active participation in the process of learning requires insight into one's strengths and weaknesses through self-analysis. Development takes place through capitalising on strengths and eliminating weaknesses. To identify deficiencies one must not only be a good judge of oneself, but also be aware that a deficiency exists. Students who are coached by a teacher have these deficiencies pointed out to them; those studying in groups are often helped thus by their peers; the individual learner, however, has to depend on certain cues, such as an inability to understand a difficult topic, to identify deficiencies in prior learning. A sound practice is to test oneself on what one has just read using pre-designed questions or exercises. Frequent reviews help students follow their progress.

Formative assessment is now a regular feature of many medical curricula. Unfortunately, it is often misused in that feedback from such assessment is not provided to students in a way which helps them identify

"Of two men with the same outward experiences and the same amount of mere native tenacity, the one who thinks over his experiences most, and weaves them into systematic relations with each other, will be the one with the best memory"

W James, in Smith et al 1951

"Boiling down ideas to a few words is a practical test of your understanding of the material"

Crawford, in Smith et al 1951

When you teach, question your students regularly, but react to their responses in such a way that they feel comfortable to display, rather than hide, deficiencies. Only then will they be able to take remedial action.

deficiencies. In many instances, formative assessment consists of a series of summative exercises, which contribute to a final grade on which pass–fail decisions are based. While such a practice has the advantage of increased sampling of topics tested, it fails to serve a formative purpose. The problem is compounded by students attempting to hide rather than display their weaknesses, as they are aware of the important decisions that are based on the results.

If student assessment is to play a role in helping students learn, class tests conducted before and during a unit should provide feedback detailed enough to point out areas or skills where deficiencies in learning exist.

It is well known that assessment is the strongest motivator of student learning. While this is unfortunate, teachers should capitalise on this fact and set tests which call upon the students' higher cognitive skills, rather than on the ability to reproduce what is learnt. Assessment should encourage students to search for application of what they learn both in their personal lives and in the context of their future practice, and test their ability to discriminate between fact and opinion, between assumption and established truth. The critical appraisal of ideas should be an essential ingredient of the total assessment package, as should the ability to gather information pertaining to a given problem.

Unfortunately most tests in medical education call upon the lower cognitive skills of recall and recognition. We fail to harness the greatest motivator of student learning to bring about desirable learning habits in our medical students. Most study skill courses aim at helping students pass these types of examinations rather than pursue learning which would arm them with the skills and attributes for a lifetime of continuing education.

Summary

In facing the challenges created by the explosion of medical knowledge, students resort to the expedient strategy of acquiring knowledge to satisfy immediate concerns of assessment, with much of it forgotten thereafter. This chapter provides suggestions for teachers to help students learn with understanding that which is essential for professional practice, while minimising the amount forgotten. The component study skills which are emphasised in this chapter are those of self-directed learning, learning with understanding and reflection, seeking and retrieving information, critical review, integration of new learning with old and the use of feedback.

A weekly plan of study designed by the student should be based on priorities determined by the importance of the topic for both understanding and application, its relative difficulty and its timeliness. The student should be helped to make decisions with regard to the focus of study as determined by objectives, its depth for understanding and its sequence. While teachers should ensure that students are exposed to a variety of sources for studying a given topic, the individual nature of learning determines which of these is optimal for a given student. Study skill courses should utilise recent findings on the relationship between the learner and the learning task to inform students of the different approaches to learning, and help each of them select that which is best suited for a given task.

Opportunities for repeated independent practice of both cognitive and psychomotor skills should be provided, the former through assignments, which call upon the student to apply learning to unfamiliar situations, and the latter through such facilities as skill laboratories. Review of learning should emphasise links between concurrently and progressively learnt topics, thereby promoting horizontal and vertical integration. Formative assessment by teachers, peers and students themselves should be geared to providing feedback on individual strengths and weaknesses. The powerful effect summative assessment has on driving student learning should be capitalised on to promote desirable learning habits by testing higher cognitive skills in examinations.

References

Bandaranayake R C 1999 Basic sciences in the undergraduate medical curriculum: relevance and motivation. In: Medical Education in GCC Countries, First GCC Conference of Faculties of Medicine, Kuwait University

Grant J C B 1937 Grant's method of anatomy. Williams & Wilkins, Baltimore

Lock C 1981 Study skills. Kappa Delta Pi Northeastern University Publishing Group

Newble D, Clarke R 1987 Approaches to learning in a traditional and an innovative medical school In: Richardson J T E, Eysenck M W, Piper D W (eds) Student learning: research in education and cognitive psychology. Society for Research into Higher Education and Open University, Milton Keynes

Ramsden P 1987 Improving teaching and learning in higher education: the case for a relational perspective. Studies in Higher Education 12:275–286

Saunders K, Northup D E, Mennin S P 1984 The library in a problem-based curriculum. In: Kaufman A (ed.) Implementing problem-based medical education. Springer, New York

Smith S, Shores L, Brittain R 1951 An outline of best methods of study, 2nd edn. Barnes & Noble, New York

Stiernborg M, Bandaranayake R C 1996 Medical students' approaches to studying. Medical Teacher 18:229–236

Wilcox G W 1958 Basic study skills. Allyn & Bacon, Boston

Chapter 42
Staff development

Y. Steinert

Introduction

Staff development, or faculty development as it is often called, has become an increasingly important component of medical education. Staff development activities have been designed to improve teacher effectiveness at all levels of the educational continuum (e.g. undergraduate, postgraduate and continuing medical education) and diverse programmes have been offered to healthcare professionals in many settings.

For the purpose of this discussion, staff development will refer to that broad range of activities that institutions use to renew or assist faculty in their roles (Centra 1978). That is, staff development is a planned programme designed to *prepare* institutions and faculty members for their various roles (Bland et al 1990) and to *improve* an individual's knowledge and skills in the areas of teaching, research and administration (Sheets & Schwenk 1990). The goal of staff development is to teach faculty members the skills relevant to their institutional and faculty position, and to sustain their vitality, both now and in the future.

Although a comprehensive staff development programme includes attention to all faculty roles, including research, writing and administration, the focus of this chapter will be on staff development for teaching improvement. More specifically, the first section will review common practices and challenges; the second section will provide some practical guidelines for individuals interested in the design, delivery and evaluation of staff development programmes.

Common practices and challenges

Knowledge of the following common practices and challenges will help guide the design and delivery of innovative staff development programmes.

Key content areas

The majority of staff development programmes focus on teaching improvement. That is, they aim to improve teachers' skills in clinical teaching, small-group facilitation, lecturing, feedback and evaluation, and teaching in the ambulatory setting. In fact, many of the chapters in this book are – and can be – the focus of staff development programmes.

In looking at the literature on teaching improvement, minimal attention has been paid to the personal development of healthcare professionals, educational leadership, or organisational development and change.

"It goes without saying that no man can teach successfully who is not at the same time a student"

Sir William Osler

"The one task that is distinctively related to being a faculty member is teaching; all other tasks can be pursued in other settings; and yet, paradoxically, the central responsibility of faculty members is typically the one for which they are least prepared"

Jason & Westberg 1978

In addition, the teaching of specific content areas (e.g. interprofessionalism, communication skills, evidence-based medicine) as well as curriculum design and development have been frequently ignored. Although instructional effectiveness at the individual level is critically important, a more comprehensive approach should be considered. We need to develop individuals who will be able to provide leadership to educational programmes, act as educational mentors, and design and deliver innovative educational programmes. As Cusimano & David (1998) have said, there is an enormous need for more healthcare professionals trained in methods of educating others so that medical education will continue to be responsive to driving forces of change. Staff development has an important role to play in promoting teaching as a scholarly activity and in creating an educational climate that encourages and rewards educational leadership, innovation and excellence.

Target population

To date, the majority of staff development programmes focus on the medical teacher. Staff development initiatives should also target curriculum planners responsible for the design and delivery of educational programmes, administrators responsible for education and practice, and all healthcare professionals involved in teaching and learning. Teachers in different settings, including the university, the hospital, and the community, should be included in all activities.

Staff development also needs to target the organisation that supports teaching and learning. Organisational staff development strategies include the provision of resources that address faculty needs, changing systems through which faculty are evaluated and rewarded, and fostering mentoring and professional networks for faculty (Ullian & Stritter 1997). Clearly, in order to be successful we need to target the organisational climate and culture in which teachers work.

Educational formats

The most common staff development formats have included workshops and seminars, short courses, sabbaticals and fellowships. Workshops are one of the most popular formats because of their inherent flexibility and promotion of active learning. In fact, faculty members value a variety of teaching methods within this format, including interactive lectures, small-group discussions and exercises, role plays and simulations, and experiential learning. However, given the changing needs and priorities of medical schools and healthcare professionals, we should consider alternative formats for staff development that include integrated longitudinal programmes, decentralised activities, peer coaching, mentoring, self-directed learning, and computer-aided instruction.

Integrated longitudinal programmes

Integrated longitudinal programmes have been developed as an alternative to fellowship programmes. These programmes, in which faculty commit 10–20% of their time over 1–2 years, allow healthcare professionals to maintain most of their clinical, research, and administrative

"The greatest difficulty in life is to make knowledge effective, to convert it into practical wisdom"

Sir William Osler

responsibilities while furthering their own professional development. Programme components typically consist of a variety of methods, including university courses, monthly seminars, independent research projects, and involvement in a variety of staff development activities. Integrated longitudinal programmes such as the Teaching Scholars Program (Steinert et al 2003) have particular appeal because teachers can continue to practise and teach while improving their educational knowledge and skills. As well, these programmes allow for the development of educational leadership and scholarly activity in medical education.

Decentralised activities

Staff development programmes are often departmentally based or centrally organised (i.e. faculty-wide). Given the increasing use of community preceptors and ambulatory sites for teaching, staff development programmes should be 'exported' outside of the university setting. Decentralised, site-specific activities have the added advantage of reaching individuals who may not otherwise attend staff development activities and can help to develop a departmental or programme-based culture of self-improvement (Baxley el al 1999).

Peer coaching

Peer coaching as a method of faculty development has been described extensively in the educational literature. Key elements of peer coaching include the identification of individual learning goals (e.g. improving specific teaching skills), focused observation of teaching by colleagues, and the provision of feedback, analysis and support (Flynn et al 1994). This underutilised approach, sometimes called 'co-teaching', has particular appeal because it occurs in the teacher's own practice setting, enables individualised learning, and fosters collaboration. It also allows healthcare professionals to learn about each other as they teach together.

Mentorship

Mentoring is a common strategy to promote the socialisation, development, and maturation of academic medical faculty (Bland et al 1990). It is also a valuable, but underutilised, staff development strategy. Daloz (1986) has described a mentorship model that balances three key elements: support, challenge, and a vision of the individual's future career. This model can serve as a helpful framework in staff development. The value of role models and mentors has been highlighted since Osler's time, and we should not forget the benefits of this method of professional development despite new technologies and methodologies.

Self-directed learning

Self-directed learning initiatives are not frequently described in the staff development literature. However, there is clearly a place for self-directed learning that promotes 'reflection-in-action' and 'reflection-on-action', skills that are critical to effective teaching and learning. As Ullian & Stritter (1997) have said, teachers should be encouraged to determine their own needs through self-reflection, evaluation by students, and peer feedback, and they should learn to design their own development activities. Self-directed learning activities have been used extensively in continuing

"Mentoring is vital to create new leaders and new kinds of leadership"

Anderson 1999

medical education (CME) and staff development programmes should build on these experiences.

Computer-aided instruction

Computer-aided instruction is closely tied to self-directed learning initiatives. As time for professional development is limited, and the technology to create interactive instructional programmes is now in place, the use of computer-based staff development should be explored. Web-based learning can allow for individualised programmes targeted to specific needs and the sharing of resources, as long as we do not lose sight of the value and importance of working in context, with our colleagues.

Frequently encountered challenges

Staff development programmes cannot be designed or delivered in isolation from other factors that include institutional support, organisational goals and priorities, resources for programme planning and individual needs and expectations. These very same factors can be challenges as well. Common challenges faced by faculty developers include: defining goals and priorities; balancing individual and organisational needs; motivating faculty to participate in staff development initiatives; obtaining institutional support and 'buy-in'; promoting a 'culture change' that reflects renewed interest in teaching and learning; and overcoming limited human and financial resources. As motivating faculty to participate in staff development is one of the key challenges, it will be discussed in greater detail.

Teachers differ from students and residents in a number of ways. They have more life experiences, more self-entrenched behaviours, and may see change as a greater threat. In addition, motivation for learning cannot be assumed and time for learning is not routinely allocated. Staff development programmes must address these challenges. Teachers do not participate in staff development activities for a variety of reasons. Some do not view teaching – or teaching improvement – as important; others do not perceive a need for improvement or feel that their institution does not support or value these activities. Many are not aware of the benefits (or availability) of staff development programmes and activities. We must be cognisant of all these factors in programme planning.

To motivate faculty we need to develop a culture that promotes and encourages professional development; consider multiple approaches to achieving the same goal; tailor programmes to meet individual and organisational needs; and ensure relevant and 'high quality' activities. We must also build a network of interested individuals; encourage the dissemination of information; utilise student feedback to illustrate need; recognise participation in staff development; and if possible, provide 'release time'. Whenever possible, it is also helpful to link staff development activities with ongoing programmes (e.g. hospital rounds; CME events); to provide a range of activities and methods; and to offer free and flexible programming. Organisational support for these initiatives is also critical, as are staff development strategies that target organisational norms and values (e.g. recognising the importance of teaching and learning).

"We must find new ways to help faculty adapt to their new roles and responsibilities while coping with the day-to-day demands that these changes bring"

Ullian & Stritter 1996

"The goal of faculty development is to empower faculty members to excel in their role as educators and, in so doing, to create organisations that encourage and reward continual learning"

Wilkerson & Irby 1998

"My view of myself as a teacher has changed, from an information provider to a 'director' of learning"

McGill Teaching Scholar

"I leave rejuvenated and ready to go out and teach a thousand students again!"

McGill Teaching Scholar

Programme effectiveness

Despite numerous descriptions of staff development programmes, there has been a paucity of research demonstrating the effectiveness of most faculty development activities (Sheets & Schwenk 1990; Steinert 2000). Few programmes have included comprehensive evaluations to ascertain what effect the programme is having on faculty, and data to support the efficacy of these initiatives have been lacking. Of the studies that have been conducted in this area, most have relied on the assessment of participant satisfaction; some have assessed the impact on cognitive learning or performance; and several have examined the long-term impact of these interventions. In addition, most of the research has relied on self-report rather than objective outcome measures or observations of change. More specifically, methods to evaluate staff development programmes have included end-of-session evaluations; follow-up survey questionnaires; pre- and post-assessments of cognitive or attitudinal change; direct observations of teaching behaviour; and student evaluations and faculty self-ratings of post-training performance. Common problems have included a lack of control or comparison groups, heavy reliance on self-report measures of change, and small sample sizes.

Despite these limitations, we do know that staff development activities have been rated highly by participants and that teachers rate the experience as useful, recommending participation to their colleagues (Skeff et al 1997). A number of studies have also demonstrated an impact on teachers' knowledge, skills, and attitudes, and several have shown change in student behaviour as a result of staff participation in faculty development programmes. Other benefits have included increased personal interest and enthusiasm, improved self-confidence, a greater sense of belonging to a community, and educational leadership and innovation (Steinert et al 2003).

The challenge in this area is to conduct more rigorous evaluations of staff development initiatives from the outset, to consider other models of programme evaluation, to make use of qualitative research methods, and to broaden the focus of the evaluation itself. In no other area is the need to collaborate or transcend disciplinary boundaries greater. We should also reassess the importance of participant satisfaction. Although researchers often question the value of this data source, participant satisfaction remains important if faculty members are to be motivated to learn and recommend staff development initiatives to their colleagues. Participant satisfaction also gives valuable feedback to programme planners.

Designing a staff development programme

The following guidelines are intended to help individuals design and deliver effective staff development programmes.

Understand the institutional/organisational culture

Staff development programmes take place within the context of a specific institution or organisation. It is imperative to understand the culture of that institution and to be responsive to its needs. Staff development programmes should capitalise on the organisation's strengths and work with the leadership to ensure success. In many ways, the cultural context can be used to promote or enhance staff development efforts. For example, staff development during times of educational or curricular reform can take on added importance (Rubeck & Witzke 1998). It is also important to assess institutional support for staff development activities, ascertain available resources, and lobby effectively. Clearly, staff development cannot occur in a vacuum.

Determine appropriate goals and priorities

As with the design of any other programme, it is important to clearly define goals and priorities. What are you trying to achieve – and why is it important to do so? It is imperative to carefully determine goals – and objectives – as they will influence your target audience, choice of programme, content and methodology. Determining priorities is not always easy. However, it is essential to balance individual and organisational needs.

Conduct needs assessments to ensure relevant programming

As stated earlier, staff development programmes should base themselves on the needs of the individual as well as the institution. Student needs, patient needs, and societal needs may also help to direct relevant activities. Assessing needs is necessary to refine goals, determine content, identify preferred learning formats, and assure relevance. It is also a way of promoting early 'buy-in'. Common methods include: written questionnaires or surveys; interviews or focus groups with key informants (e.g. participants, students, educational leaders); observations of teachers 'in action'; literature reviews; and environmental scans of available programmes and resources. Whenever possible, we should try to gain information from multiple sources and distinguish between 'needs' and 'wants'. Clearly, an individual teacher's perceived needs may differ from those expressed by their students or peers. Needs assessments can also help to further translate goals into objectives, which will serve as the basis for programme planning and evaluation of outcome.

Develop different programmes to accommodate diverse needs

Different educational formats have been described in an earlier section. Clearly, we must design programmes that accommodate diverse goals and objectives, content areas, and the needs of the individual and the organisation. For example, if your goal is to improve lecturing skills, a half-day workshop on interactive lecturing might be your programme of choice. On the other hand, if you wish to promote educational leadership and scholarly activity among your peers, a teaching scholars programme or educational fellowship might be the preferred method. In this context, it is also helpful to remember that 'staff development' can include development, orientation, recognition, and support, and different programmes will be required to accommodate diverse objectives. Programme content and methods will also need to change over time to adapt to evolving needs.

Capitalise on the institution's strengths, and promote organisational change and development.

Assess needs to refine goals, determine content, identify preferred learning formats and promote 'buy-in'.

Incorporate principles of adult learning and instructional design

Adults come to learning situations with a variety of motivations and expectations about teaching methods and goals. Key principles of adult learning (e.g. Knowles 1988) include the following:

- Adults are independent
- Adults come to learning situations with a variety of motivations and definite expectations about particular learning goals and teaching methods
- Adults demonstrate different learning styles
- Much of adult learning is 'relearning' rather than new learning
- Adult learning often involves changes in attitudes as well as skills
- Most adults prefer to learn through experience
- Incentives for adult learning usually come from within the individual
- Feedback is usually more important than tests and evaluations.

Incorporation of these principles into the design of a staff development programme can enhance receptivity, relevance and engagement. In fact, these principles should guide the development of all programmes, irrespective of their focus or format, as physicians demonstrate a high degree of self-direction and possess numerous experiences that should serve as the basis for learning.

Principles of instructional design should also be followed. For example, it is important to develop clear learning goals and objectives, identify key content areas, design appropriate teaching and learning strategies, and create appropriate methods of evaluation of both the students and the curriculum (see Fig. 42.1). It is equally important to integrate theory with practice (e.g. Kaufman et al 2000), and to ensure that the learning is perceived as relevant to the work setting and to the profession. Learning should be interactive, participatory, and experientially based, using the participants' previous learning and experience as a starting point. Detailed planning and organisation involving all stakeholders is critical, as is the creation of a positive learning environment. However, although theory should inform practice, staff development initiatives must remain relevant and practical.

Offer a diversity of educational methods

In line with principles of adult learning, staff development programmes should try to offer a variety of educational methods that promote experiential learning, reflection, feedback, and immediacy of application. Common learning methods include interactive lectures, case presentations, small-group exercises and discussions, role plays and simulations, videotape reviews, and live demonstrations. (Many of these methods are described in an earlier section of this book.) Practice with feedback is also key, as is the opportunity to reflect on personal values and attitudes. Computer-aided instruction, debates and reaction panels, journal clubs and self-directed readings are additional methods to con-

Incorporate principles of adult learning to enhance receptivity, relevance and engagement.

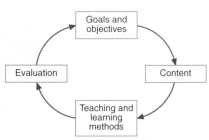

Fig. 42.1 The educational cycle

Promote experiential learning, reflection, feedback and immediacy of application.

sider. In line with our previous example, a workshop on interactive lecturing might include interactive plenaries, small-group discussions and exercises, and opportunities for practice and feedback. A fellowship programme might include group seminars, independent projects and structured readings. Whatever the method, the needs and learning preferences of the participants should be respected, and the method should match the objective. Healthcare professionals learn best 'by doing', so experiential learning should be promoted whenever possible.

Promote 'buy-in' and market effectively

The decision to participate in a staff development programme or activity is not as simple as it might at first appear. It involves the individual's reaction to a particular offering, motivation to develop or enhance a specific skill, being available at the time of the session, and overcoming the psychological barrier of admitting need (Rubeck & Witzke 1998). As faculty developers, it is our challenge to overcome reluctance, and to market our 'product' in such a way that resistance becomes a resource to learning. In our context, we have seen the value of targeted mailings, professionally designed brochures, and 'branding' of our product to promote interest. Continuing education credits as well as free and flexible programming can also help to facilitate motivation and attendance. 'Buy-in' involves agreement on importance, widespread support, and dedication of time and resources at both the individual and the systems level, and must be considered in all programming initiatives.

Work to overcome commonly encountered challenges

Common implementation problems, such as a lack of institutional support, limited resources, and limited faculty time, have been discussed in an earlier section. Faculty developers must work to overcome these problems through creative programming, skilled marketing, targeted fundraising, and the delivery of high quality programmes. Flexible scheduling and collaborative programming, which address clearly identified needs, will also help to ensure success at a systems level.

Prepare staff developers

The recruitment and preparation of staff developers is rarely reported. However, it is important to recruit carefully, train effectively, partner creatively, and build on previous experiences. Faculty members can be involved in a number of ways: as co-facilitators, programme planners or consultants. In our own setting, we try to involve new faculty members in each staff development activity and conduct a preparatory meeting (or 'dry run') to review content and process, solicit feedback and promote 'ownership'. We also conclude each activity with a 'debriefing' session, to discuss lessons learned and plan for the future. Whenever possible, staff developers should be individuals who are well-respected by their peers and have some educational expertise and experience in facilitating groups. It has been said that 'to teach is to

"I was given new tools to teach. Not only were they described to me in words, but they were also used in front of me and I was part and parcel of the demonstration"

McGill Teaching Scholar

learn twice'; this principle is clearly one of the main motivating factors for staff developers.

Evaluate – and demonstrate – effectiveness

The need to evaluate staff development programmes and activities is clear. In fact, we must remember that the evaluation of staff development is more than an academic exercise; our findings must be used in the design, delivery and marketing of our programmes. It has been stated earlier that staff development must strive to promote education as a scholarly activity; we must role model this approach in all that we do (Steinert 2000).

In preparing to evaluate a staff development programme or activity, we should consider the goal of the evaluation (e.g. programme planning vs. decision making; policy formation vs. academic inquiry), available data sources (e.g. participants, peers, students, or residents), common methods of evaluation (e.g. questionnaires, focus groups, objective tests, observations), resources to support assessment (e.g. institutional support, research grants), and models of programme evaluation (e.g. goal attainment, decision facilitation). Kirkpatrick's levels of evaluation are also helpful in conceptualising and framing the assessment of outcome (Kirkpatrick 1994). They include the following:

- *Reaction* – participants' views on the learning experience
- *Learning* – change in participants' attitudes, knowledge or skills
- *Behaviour* – change in participants' behaviour
- *Results* – changes in the organisational system, the patient, or the learner.

At a minimum, a practical and feasible evaluation should include an assessment of utility and relevance, content, teaching and learning methods, and intent to change. Moreover, as evaluation is an integral part of programme planning, it should be conceptualised at the beginning of any programme. It should also include qualitative and quantitative assessments of learning and behaviour change, using a variety of methods and data sources.

Summary

Academic vitality is dependent upon faculty members' interest and expertise. Staff development has a critical role to play in promoting academic excellence and innovation. In looking to the future, we should: focus on content areas that go beyond the improvement of specific teaching skills (e.g. educational leadership, or the teaching of specific content areas); adopt diverse educational formats, such as integrated longitudinal programmes, decentralised activities, and self-directed learning; use staff development programmes and activities to promote organisational change; and evaluate the effectiveness of all that we do so that practice informs research and research can inform practice. We should also remain innovative and flexible so that we can accommodate the ever-changing needs of our teachers, our institutions and the healthcare systems in which we work.

Evaluate effectively – and ensure that research will inform practice.

"A medical school's most important asset is its faculty"

Whitcomb 2003

References

Anderson P C 1999 Mentoring. Academic Medicine 74:4–5

Baxley E G, Probst J C, Shell B J, Bogdewic S P, Cleghorn G D 1999 Program-centred education: a new model for faculty development. Teaching and Learning in Medicine 11:94–99

Bland C, Schmitz C, Stritter F et al 1990 Successful faculty in academic medicine. Springer-Verlag, New York

Centra J A 1978 Types of faculty development programs. Journal of Higher Education 49 (2):151–162

Cusimano M D, David M A 1998 A compendium of higher education opportunities in health professions education. Academic Medicine 73:1255–1259

Daloz L A 1986 Effective teaching and mentorship: realizing the transformational power of adult learning experiences. Jossey-Bass, San Francisco

Flynn S P, Bedinghaus J, Snyder C, Hekelman, F 1994 Peer coaching in clinical teaching: a case report. Educational Research and Methods 26:569–570

Jason H, Westberg J 1978 Teachers and teaching in US medical schools. Appleton-Century-Crofts, Norwalk CT

Kaufman D M, Mann K, Jennett P A 2000 Teaching and learning in medical education: how theory can inform practice. Association for the Study of Medical Education, Edinburgh, Scotland

Kirkpatrick D L 1994 Evaluating teaching program. Berret-Koehler Publishers, San Francisco

Knowles M S 1988 The modern practice of adult education: from pedagogy to androgogy. Cambridge Books, New York

Rubeck R F, Witzke D B 1998 Faculty development: a field of dreams. Academic Medicine 73:S33–S37

Sheets K J, Schwenk T L 1990 Faculty development for family medicine educators: an agenda for future activities. Teaching and Learning in Medicine 2:141–148

Skeff K M, Stratos G A, Mygdal W et al 1997 Faculty development: a resource for clinical teachers. Journal of General Internal Medicine 12:S56–S63

Steinert Y 2000 Faculty development in the new millennium: key challenges and future directions. Medical Teacher 22:44–50

Steinert Y, Nasmith L, McLeod P, Conochie L 2003 A teaching scholars' program to develop leaders in medical education. Academic Medicine 78:142–149

Ullian A J, Stritter F T 1997 Types of faculty development programs. Family Medicine 29(4):237–241

Whitcomb M 2003 The medical school's faculty is its most important asset. Academic Medicine 78(2):117–118

Wilkerson L, Irby D 1998 Strategies for improving teaching practices: a comprehensive approach to faculty development. Academic Medicine 73:387–396

Chapter 43
Academic standards

S. P. Mennin

Introduction

More is known today than ever before about how people learn and develop expertise. Knowledge and technology continue to mushroom and none of us can keep up. Fed by an information explosion, unprecedented attention is focused on a global scale on medical and health professions' education. Everywhere there are calls for change and innovation in medical education, to modernise curricula, incorporate new pedagogies, introduce or enhance early clinical experiences, foster community-based education and improve the health of the public. At the same time, the pressures on faculty and staff in academia to do more with less are greater than ever before. In the United States, monetary pressures have pushed leaders at academic medical centres to adopt values and fiscal policies more attuned to the entrepreneurial world of business than to the primary goals of scholarship, learning and the health of the public. A real danger exists that universities are on the way to becoming 'busiversities' in which core values are shifting from learning and scholarship to those more prevalent in business.

Education, and by extension scholarship, is not neutral. It is political, social and historical (Freire 1993) and involves choices about setting the agenda for what and how future health professionals will learn. In the US, for example, there are now national requirements for the implementation of core (standard) competencies for postgraduate medical education as well as enhanced attention to professionalism in medical education. At the same time, one observes in medical curricula much less attention and time devoted to discussion and problem-solving related to its failed healthcare system. This is characterised by 42 million people with no healthcare insurance, rapidly rising healthcare costs and lower indices of health outcomes compared with other industrialised countries that spend significantly less money on healthcare.

From this confluence emerges a mandate for global standards for medical education (Hamilton 2000, WFME 2000, Schwarz 2001, Wojtczak & Schwarz 2000). This evolving landscape directly affects the roles and responsibilities of academia and the professoriate at medical schools. Thus it is not surprising that recent literature heralds a call for standards that can be applied to the individual teacher (Fincher et al 2000, GMC 1999, Purcell & Lloyd-Jones 2003). It is, after all, the faculty and staff, one by one, who will be called upon to transform contemporary visions of standards for medical education into tangible outcomes.

Standards for teaching in medical schools

Standards may also be conceptualised in the form of competencies defined as outcomes expected of teachers and graduates (Harden et al 1999). Clear, well-established rules, expectations and standards exist for the conduct of research and patient care. Academic status and political power in medical centres in the US are based on expertise and performance within a specialty. The ability to generate outside funding from research and/or clinical care confers influence and standing in the academic and political processes of US medical schools. The culture of research and patient care endeavours is highly developed and almost universally accepted. Not so for education. A double standard exists: one for research and patient care and another for education (Mennin 1999).

Unlike research and patient care activities, teachers of medical students rarely receive formal training or preparation in teaching, education or assessment of learners. Chairs of departments often fail to distinguish between teaching as a scholarly activity and teaching as a routine service. Poor teaching performance is tolerated, whereas poor quality in research or substandard patient care is not. While peer review is well established for research and patient care activities, it is as yet relatively undeveloped in education at most medical schools. Teachers at medical schools are well aware that the rewards and recognition for research and patient care are substantive; those for teaching and education suffer by comparison. Faculty speak to each other about teaching and education without a shared vocabulary or language. It is a disturbing observation that those who are entrusted with the care and preparation of their successors are ill informed about the latest methods and knowledge about teaching and education.

Professionalising teaching

Few teachers could accurately describe how people learn, what is known about the development of expertise or different approaches to assessing learners. Educationally, we profess but we are not professional. It is time to professionalise teaching and education, to have agreed standards for teaching that are part of, rather than separate from, scholarly work and to hold teaching to the same high standards as research and patient care. Imagine that each faculty member meets annually with the chair of his or her department to review evidence of performance in teaching and education according to agreed standards and criteria. The absence of a common language and shared values represents a major barrier to the coherent integration of teaching, research and patient care. By broadening the definition of scholarship to include the scholarship of discovery, application, integration and teaching (Boyer 1990), it becomes feasible to hold ourselves accountable to high standards of excellence and give form and function to a much needed culture for education and teaching in medical schools.

"standards operate as benchmarks against which performance may be judged and they crucially determine professional practice in either health care delivery or educational contexts"

Purcell & Lloyd-Jones 2003

"Broaden the definition of scholarship to include the scholarship of discovery, application, integration and teaching"

Boyer 1990

"We believe that it is time to move beyond the tired old 'teaching versus research' debate and give the familiar and honorable term 'scholarship,' a broader, more capacious meaning, one that brings legitimacy to the full scope of academic work. Surely, scholarship means engaging in original research. But the work of the scholar also means stepping back from one's investigation, looking for connections, building bridges between theory and practice, and communicating one's knowledge effectively to students"

Boyer 1990

"What we urgently need today is a more inclusive view of what it means to be a scholar – a recognition that knowledge is acquired through research, through synthesis, through practice and through teaching"

Boyer 1990

"inspired teaching keeps the flame of scholarship alive. Almost all successful academics give credit to creative teachers – those mentors who defined their work so compellingly that it became, for them, a lifetime challenge. Without the teaching function, the continuity of knowledge will be broken and the store of human knowledge dangerously diminished"

Boyer 1990

"Academics feel relatively confident about their ability to assess specialized research, but they are less certain about what qualities to look for in other kinds of scholarship, and how to document and reward that work"

Glassick et al 1997

In this way, we can move forward to meet the challenges of preparing future health professionals to engage health issues vital to the health of the public.

Broadening the definition of scholarship

Scholarship, a cornerstone of university life, is inextricably linked to the future of medical education. The definition of scholarship generally applied by medical schools is limited and excludes areas of legitimate academic activity and productivity vital to fulfilling the educational mission and challenges inherent in contemporary educational changes. Such a limited definition holds that scholarship is demonstrated only by research and the dissemination of new knowledge in peer reviewed journals. Thus, faculty essential to the success of innovations, educational changes, and the ongoing core educational mission of their medical schools are at risk of not being promoted because they do not engage in accepted forms of scholarship. A broadening of the definition of scholarship and its more inclusive application in medical schools for recognition and promotion is particularly relevant at this time.

The classic work of Boyer at the Carnegie Foundation for the Advancement of Teaching (1990) proposed and delineated four arenas of scholarship:

- discovery
- integration
- application
- teaching.

Scholarly teaching is marked by the same discipline and habits of mind as other types of scholarly work. Characteristics of scholarly teaching are that it is open and accessible to the public; subject to peer review, critique and evaluation; informed by both the latest ideas in the subject field and the most current ideas in the field of teaching; and in a form upon which others can build (Hutchings & Shulman 1999). By this definition, scholarly work in education includes the discovery of new knowledge as well as the integration, application and teaching of knowledge. It is also reflected in the transmission and transformation of knowledge with learners. Products of scholarly teaching may consist of syllabi, web-based instructional materials, fellowship programmes, continuing medical education programmes, performance data about learners, accomplishments of advisees, and educational leadership programmes.

Criteria for scholarly teaching

What vocabulary could define the common dimensions of scholarship? Are general standards for judging scholarly performance already available? An inquiry by the Ernest L. Boyer Project of the Carnegie Foundation for the Advancement of Teaching analysed information about hiring, promotion and tenure practices from dozens of colleges and universities, and information about the standards used to decide the scholarly merit of proposals and manuscripts from 51 granting agencies and the editors and directors of 31 scholarly journals and 58 university presses. What emerged as key was the process of scholarship itself. Scholarly works of discovery, integration, application and teaching shared and were guided by the 'common sequence of unfolding stages' listed in Table 43.1 (Glassick et al 1997). These criteria are remarkably similar to those that define quality teaching.

It is helpful to remind ourselves periodically that the call for innovations and changes in medical education, the broadening of the definition of scholarship, and the development of the means to assess it are directed toward improving the healthcare systems and the public they serve.

Assessing scholarly teaching

Promotion committees often lack the criteria and related tools to assess the scholarship of teaching. One approach to this problem can be found in the answers to a set of questions based on the six criteria of scholarship. Responses to these questions can provide evidence of scholarly teaching for four different roles of educators: lecturing, teaching in the clinical setting, teaching in small groups, and educational administration (Fincher et al 2000). Table 43.2 provides some examples of how these criteria can be applied to teaching by someone presenting a lecture. A more complete set of questions for other modalities of teaching can be found in Fincher et al (2000).

Institutional support for scholarly teaching

Faculty and staff cannot elevate teaching to the level of scholarly work without the support of departments, medical schools, universities and

"The effort to broaden the meaning of scholarship simply cannot succeed until the academy has clear standards for evaluating this wider range of scholarly work. After all, administrators and professors accord full academic value only to work they can confidently judge"

Glassick et al 1997

Table 43.1 Comparison of criteria for assessing scholarship and quality teaching

Six criteria for scholarship (Glassick et al 1990)	Criteria for quality teaching (Fincher et al 2000)
Clear, achievable goals that are important to the field	Establish clear, achievable, measurable, relevant objectives
Adequate preparation, including an understanding of existing work in the field	Identify and organise key materials appropriate to audience level and objectives
Appropriate methods relative to goals	Select teaching methods and assessment measures to achieve and measure objectives
Significant results that contribute to the field	Assess learner performance
Effective communication of work to intended audiences	Assess quality of presentation/ instruction
Reflective critique to improve quality of future work	Critical analysis of teaching that results in changes to improve it

Table 43.2 Questions to be answered to provide evidence of scholarly teaching as a lecturer (see Fincher et al 2000 for more complete discussion)

Criteria	To what extent does the lecturer...
Clear goals	• Articulate clear, realistic, achievable goals/objectives that relate to the course/clerkship expectations and level of the learners? • Appropriately sequence goals and objectives, and state them in the context of basic knowledge and/or important/current questions in the field?
Adequate preparation	• Use accurate, current resources to develop the content of lectures? • Select, synthesise, and interpret material matched to the level of the learners? • Demonstrate command of basic concepts and current thinking?
Appropriate methods	• Use methods that reveal the logic, organisation, and relevance of the material? • Match the quantity of material to audience level and allotted time? • Use images, metaphors, analogies, and examples that connect the subject matter to the students' experience and knowledge? • Demonstrate responsiveness to learners' reactions during the presentation?
Significant results	• Link the topic to health outcomes? • Use learners' narrative comments and ratings to determine the extent to which the lecturer achieved the goals and objectives of the presentation? • Analyse learners' performance on comprehensive, cumulative examinations and demonstrate achievement of objectives? • Model teaching techniques that are adopted/adapted by other faculty members?
Effective presentation	• Integrate relevance of the topic with local and regional health issues? • Communicate to learners evidence of systematic application of intellect? • Demonstrate enthusiasm and interest in the topic? • Deliver the message with clarity and organisation? • Provide handout material matched to the goals and objectives of the presentation? • Capitalise on the spontaneous occurrence of 'teachable moments' during the presentation? • Present difficult topics in ways that help students learn?
Reflective critique	• Enhance his or her teaching skills through reading, discussion with colleagues and/or participation in workshops? • Seek and respond to feedback regarding his or her teaching?

professional organisations. Specific infrastructure is required to support the creation, critical review and dissemination of educational scholars' works. Local, national and international institutions or organisations are needed to provide resources equivalent to those that support traditional basic and applied research. For example, abundant mechanisms exist to support peer-reviewed research, but similar mechanisms for teaching are variable and intermittent. Fincher et al (2000) proposed a modification of the four 'frames' from the work of Bolman & Deal (1997), which is useful to assess an organisation's infrastructure related to the scholarship of teaching and education. Highlights of that model are presented in Table 43.3. A more complete presentation is found in Fincher et al (2000).

The change process and the scholarship of teaching

Insight into the nature of the change process and specifically into its application to the sociopolitical and economic interactions related to academic life, teaching/learning, healthcare and health are essential if the scholarship of teaching is to be adopted as part of the structural and cultural reality in medical schools. Many models have been proposed for understanding the change process. Levine (1980) describes four stages:

1. *Recognising the need* – it is realised that some organisational need is not being satisfied.
2. *Planning* – a concrete plan is developed.
3. *Implementing* – the plan is put into operation on a trial basis.
4. *Institutionalisation* or *termination* – either the operating plan becomes routine and is integrated into the organisation or it is ended.

In this model, the scholarship of teaching, for most medical schools, is largely at stage one, of recognition of the need for change (in some cases, the need is yet to be recognised). Some institutions may be in the planning stage. The first stage is essentially an information-seeking and information-processing phase in which individuals are motivated to reduce uncertainty about the relative advantages and disadvantages of the scholarship of teaching (Rogers 2003). Important strategies at this stage deal with providing information, having formal and informal discussions, informing leadership and opinion leaders and clarifying issues by posing questions such as:

- 'What is it?'
- 'How does it work?'
- 'Why do we need it?'
- 'What's wrong with the way things are now?'
- 'What will the advantages and disadvantages be in my situation?'

The adoption of a change in curriculum at a given medical school, or the adoption of global standards in medical education, or the implementation of scholarship in teaching as a way to professionalise teaching will not happen unless the leadership and faculty feel that it will resolve some crisis or uncertainty that affects them directly. Another way to look at

Table 43.3 Key infrastructure features of medical schools and professional organisations supportive of the scholarship of teaching/education (from Fincher et al 2000)

Department/medical school	Professional organisation
[Frame 1: Structural]	
Educational leadership positions listed on organisational chart	Formal affiliation opportunities for medical educators
• Equivalent to research and/or clinical practice positions	• Committees, sections, special interest groups, leadership positions related to education
School-wide medical education office, committee, or individual	Peer review committees/panels
Medical school library/website to access literature and websites specific to medical education	Society publishes peer-reviewed education papers
Education facilities and support personnel	Education clearinghouse/bookstore
[Frame 2: Human resources]	
Orientation programmes about medical education	Fellowships in medical education
• For new faculty, course directors, clerkship directors, committee members	• Teaching-career advancement fellowships
Education handbooks/web-based materials	Educational resource materials
• 'How-tos' for course and programme directors; relevant skills, resources, policies for education programmes	• Society-supported guidelines and materials for education-based work • How to document activities for promotion
Faculty development programmes/ workshops	Faculty development workshops/ programmes
• Curriculum development, teaching skills, preparation of promotion materials as educational scholarship, mentoring from senior faculty	• Annual skills workshops, refresher courses related to educational skills
Hiring process for educational positions	
[Frame 3: Politics]	
Selection/election/appointment process for key positions and committees	Selection/election/appointment process for key positions
Educators in leadership positions	Educators in leadership positions
• Chairs of key committees, working groups, promotion and tenure groups, budget process	• Key decision-making positions, resource allocation, policy and by-law decisions

Table 43.3   Key infrastructure features of medical schools and professional organisations supportive of the scholarship of teaching/education (from Fincher et al 2000)—Cont'd

Department/medical school	Professional organisation
Educator coalitions to influence decisions • Influence resource allocation for education	Educator coalitions to influence decisions • Resource allocation, presence on organisation website
[Frame 4: Symbolic]	
Public documents • Department/medical school committee agendas have a standing education line item	Public documents • Education is featured in multiple venues
Rituals/traditions/ceremonies • Awards, recognition for education scholarship	Rituals/traditions/ceremonies
Department/medical school-wide public forums • Visiting or distinguished lectureship on education attended by leaders • Education periodic focus of grand rounds or conferences	Public forums • Annual lectureship • Listserves for educators

moving the process along is to create a sense of urgency (Kotter 1996). Leaders or early adopters often assemble a group of like-minded people to create a guiding coalition. This group develops a vision and strategy and then sets out to communicate it to others as they seek to broaden understanding and ownership of the change. To do this they need to query the perceived attributes of the innovation.

Some important strategic approaches at this stage are linking the scholarship of teaching with a larger perceived need (for example, the call for global standards for medical education, or the desire by a rector or dean to change the way a curriculum is structured, or a plan to introduce community-based medical education in service of regional health needs). In addition, it is important to interact with a wide representation of faculty to build a broad base of support and participation (Mennin & Kaufman 1989).

Academic organisations guard themselves against disruptive forces within the organisation and from the outside by establishing boundaries based on norms, values and institutional history. This helps to define the organisation's environment and functions, retaining a limited set of activities and a stable pattern for operating within the larger environment. The primary function of boundaries in a medical school is to maintain norms and values, which often means the status quo. Thus, in a bounded organisation, change is more likely to occur when an environmental change makes living within the current boundaries unworkable, when the institution fails to achieve its stated and desired goals, or when it is thought that the goals can be better satisfied in another way (Levine 1980). The University of Kentucky School of Medicine can illuminate these issues. An internal review of the school revealed that its faculty recruitment, development, retention and promotion processes were not working optimally, particularly in the clinical departments (Nora et al 2000). A task force, including a broad representation of senior basic and clinical scientists as well as nontenured faculty and others, collected data, developed procedures, examined policies and perceptions, kept in close contact with the larger faculty community, the university administration and governing bodies and reported findings publicly to the general faculty. These activities represent normal academic processes. Although the mission of the school embraced all four areas of scholarship outlined by Boyer, the majority of the faculty perceived that only the scholarship of discovery mattered in the promotion process. Subsequently the University clarified promotion guidelines and implemented new mechanisms to support faculty in all forms of scholarly work. They also reaffirmed their support for the basic values in all forms of scholarship, including teaching.

The implementation of the scholarship of teaching will require careful attention to how it is perceived by individual faculty. Rogers (2003) describes five characteristics to consider about the perception of innovations by potential adopters:

The Eight-Step model for change (Kotter 1996)

Step 1: Establish a sense of urgency.
Step 2: Create the guiding coalition.
Step 3: Develop a vision and strategy.
Step 4: Communicate the change vision.
Step 5: Empower broad-based action.
Step 6: Generate short-term wins.
Step 7: Consolidate gains and produce more change.
Step 8: Anchor new approaches in the culture.

- *Relative advantage.* To what degree is the scholarship of teaching perceived as better than the status quo? Does it have an economic advantage? Is it socially prestigious? Is it more or less convenient or more satisfying? One advantage of introducing a broader definition of scholarship and recognising it as part of the promotion process is that it could facilitate the promotion and retention of faculty vital to the success of a schools education mission in a rapidly changing world.
- *Compatibility.* Is the scholarship of teaching consistent with existing values, past experiences and the needs of potential adopters? Scholarship is clearly an academic value and norm. Expanding the definition of scholarship to include application, integration and teaching in addition to discovery creates a more inclusive environment without lowering the standards of scholarship. It could fit well with faculty who produce educational products and innovations and who could receive recognition for that work if it met the criteria of scholarship. At the Medical College of Wisconsin, promotion criteria based on a narrow interpretation of scholarship (publications, grants and awards) were inconsistent with the rising demands of clinical productivity (earning money), resulting in the loss of outstanding clinicians and educators (Simpson et al 2000). Following an eight-step model of change (Kotter 1996) the College embraced the educator's portfolio (Simpson et al 1994) as a tool for promotion of clinical faculty; provided institutional support; drew on Boyer's expanded concept of scholarship of teaching; and modified the criteria for promotion and the forms of acceptable evidence for scholarship in teaching (Simpson et al 2000).

- *Complexity*. How difficult is it to grasp the idea of the scholarship of teaching and implement it? For some faculty, education is a foreign language that is not the most important part of their day-to-day activities. Few people give their best effort to activities for which they are insufficiently prepared or do not fully understand, and for which they receive insufficient recognition. The University of Louisville, also caught in the economic crunch of having to earn more clinical dollars to support faculty and to subsidise other activities, found itself using a research-focused promotion and reward system to evaluate clinician educators (Schweitzer 2000). Further, structural changes requiring post-tenure review stimulated a reconsideration of the best way to maximise faculty resources and talent. The University adopted the Boyer approach, broadening the definition of scholarship to include the scholarship of teaching. However, the faculty had difficulty in understanding how scholarship applied to a variety of faculty activities, as did the promotion and tenure committee in seeing how the model could be adapted to their school. The model was too complex and burdensome and was not adopted by the faculty (Schweitzer 2000).
- *Trialability*. To what degree can faculty or institutions experiment with the scholarship of teaching on a limited basis? Educational approaches that can be pilot tested have a much better chance of succeeding than those for which a small-scale trial is not possible. The Uniformed Services University of the Health Sciences School of Medicine adopted the Boyer model of scholarship in order to find a more inclusive way to recognise the diversity of faculty activities and to clarify further the definition of scholarship for its promotion process (Marks 2000). Teaching was seen as not being appropriately rewarded and some faculty chose not to pursue their interests in the educational process. Criteria for scholarship were adopted that were designed to be applied universally without regard to the forum in which the activity occurred or the subject. The critical step was when the faculty gained a shared understanding of scholarly acts. A new dean supportive of this process was important to their success.
- *Observability*. To what extent will the results of the scholarship of teaching be observable? If faculty can see it working in a department or with someone they respect (opinion leader), they are more likely to adopt it. Visibility stimulates peer discussion and helps disseminate the innovation to others.

Adaptive leadership for scholarly teaching

The role of leadership is critical for change and innovation in medical education (Mennin & Kaufman 1989). Change in academic medical centres is a complex mixture of the norms, values, history, social conditions, and institutional culture; the real and perceived constraints and pressures on those in the organisation; the distribution and allocation of available resources; and human creativity, capability and talent. Effective leaders, those with and those without authority, engage in activities that are adaptive.

"The scholarship of teaching communicates understanding. It challenges, extends, and transforms the knowledge of discovery into something students can comprehend. The scholarly enterprise of teaching includes the creative development of innovative pedagogic practices and course materials, and aims to encourage independent learning and critical thinking. Scholarly teaching requires enthusiastic, intellectually engaged faculty who are well informed about the latest advances in their disciplines"

Marks 2000

"most individuals do not evaluate an innovation on the basis of scientific studies of its consequences...instead, most people depend mainly upon a subjective evaluation...conveyed to them from other individuals like themselves who have already adopted the innovation"

Rogers 2003

"Adaptive work consists of the learning required to address conflicts in the values people hold, or to diminish the gap between the values people stand for and the reality they face. Adaptive work requires a change in values, beliefs, or behavior. The exposure and orchestration of conflict – internal contradictions – within individuals and constituencies provide the leverage for mobilizing people to learn new ways"

Heifitz 1994

It is not unreasonable to expect resistance to a proposal to expand the definition of scholarship to include the teaching, application and integration of knowledge in addition to the discovery of knowledge.

Summary

Scholarship is clearly understood within a defined set of behaviours. The challenge is to broaden the acceptable definition of scholarship to encompass education and establish criteria for its measurement and structures to recognise and reward it. Linking the scholarship of teaching to the norms of the institution is an important strategy for change. Norms are the established behaviour patterns for the members of a social system. They define a range of tolerable behaviour, serving as a guide or standard for the members of a social system. They tell the individuals what behaviour they are expected to perform (Rogers 2003) and what outcomes are expected (Harden et al 1999).

It is still too early to say whether or not the scholarship of teaching has been permanently institutionalised at the University of Kentucky, the Medical College of Wisconsin and the Uniformed Services University of the Health Sciences School of Medicine. Clearly, they have created and activated interpersonal networks that have served to provide a critical mass of adopters using an expanded definition of scholarship as part of their institutions' promotion process. The University of Louisville encountered problems with relative advantage, compatibility, complexity, and trialability and did not fully adopt the innovation.

Successful movements and campaigns in medical education to broaden the definition of scholarship and its application to the norms and values of academic life, will depend largely on an understanding of the theoretical and practical aspects of the change process and adaptive leadership. They will require dedicated staff and faculty capable of expanding the boundaries of education, together with a system capable of recognising and supporting those who do so. Academic health science centres, medical education, and healthcare systems are part of a complex ecology that emerges from the individual dialogues that we have with one another. It is up to each of us to put knowledge into motion so that understanding can emerge.

References

Bolman L, Deal T 1997 Reframing organizations. Jossey-Bass, San Francisco

Boyer E L 1990 Scholarship reconsidered: priorities of the professoriate. The Carnegie Foundation for the Advancement of Teaching. Jossey-Bass, San Francisco

Fincher R M E, Simpson D E, Mennin S P et al 2000 Scholarship as teaching: an imperative for the 21st century. Academic Medicine 75:887–894

Freire P 1993 Pedagogy of the oppressed. The Continuum International Publishing Company, New York

General Medical Council 1999 The doctor as teacher. General Medical Council, London

Glassick C E, Huber M T, Maeroff G I 1997 Scholarship assessed: evaluation of the professoriate. Jossey-Bass, San Francisco

Hamilton J D 2000 International standards of medical education: a global responsibility. Medical Teacher 22:547–548

Harden R M, Crosby J R, Davis M H 1999 AMEE guide no. 14. Outcome-based education: Part 1. An introduction to outcome-based education. Medical Teacher 21:7–14

Heifitz R A 1994 Leadership without easy answers. Belknap Press of Harvard University Press, Cambridge MA

Hutchings P, Shulman L S 1999 The scholarship of teaching: new elaborations, new developments. Change September/October:11–15

Kotter J P 1996 Leading change. Harvard Business School Press, Boston

Levine A 1980 Why innovation fails. State University of New York Press

Marks E S 2000 Defining scholarship at the Uniformed Services University of the Health Sciences School of Medicine: a study in cultures. Academic Medicine 75:935–939

Mennin S P 1999 Standards for teaching in medical schools: double or nothing. Medical Teacher 21:543–545

Mennin S P, Kaufman A 1989 The change process and medical education. Medical Teacher 11 (1):9–16

Nora L M, Pomeroy C, Curry Jr T E et al 2000 Revising appointment, promotion, and tenure procedures to incorporate an expanded definition of scholarship: The University of Kentucky College of Medicine experience. Academic Medicine 75:913–924

Purcell N, Lloyd-Jones G 2003 Standards for medical educators. Medical Education 37:149–154

Rogers E M 2003 The diffusion of innovations, 5th edn. Free Press, New York

Schweitzer L 2000 Adoption and failure of the 'Boyer Model' in the University of Louisville. Academic Medicine 75:925–929

Simpson D, Morzinski J, Beecher A, Lindemann J 1994 Meeting the challenge to document teaching accomplishments: the educator's portfolio. Teaching and Learning in Medicine 6:203–206

Simpson D E, Wendelberger Marcdante K, Duthie Jr E H et al 2000 Valuing educational scholarship at the Medical College of Wisconsin. Academic Medicine 75:930–934

Schwarz M R 2001 Globalization and medical education. Medical Teacher 23:533–534

WFME (World Federation for Medical Education) 2000 Defining international standards in basic medical education. Medical Education 34:665–675

Wojtczak A, Schwarz 2000 Minimum essential requirements and standards in medical education. Medical Teacher 22:555–559

Chapter 44
Research and publication

J. Bligh, J. Brice

"The capacity of human beings to bore one another seems to be vastly greater than that of any other animal"

H. L. Mencken (1880–1956)

Introduction

There are many ways in which success in your career as a clinical teacher may be measured and you may choose to specialise in any of a number of paths to progression. Your strengths may, for example, lie in teaching, counselling and student support, or you may become expert in innovative and effective curriculum design and evaluation; you may excel in the development of good assessment methods; you could be an excellent manager or have particular success in attracting grant funding, or you might have special skills in educational technology. The outputs of any of these activities can be used to support your claim for career development. Increasingly, however, universities require proof of peer reviewed publication and many clinical teachers are therefore looking to medical education journals to provide them with the evidence they need to make a case for advancement.

Journals are naturally biased towards research. What most journal editors are hoping, frequently in vain, to see when they approach a pile of new submissions is innovative, ground-breaking research which will be frequently read and widely cited. Although, as we have said, there are many valid products of excellence in medical education, the majority of journals cannot provide space for people to display their skills in clinical teaching unless the work they have submitted is:

- *Original*. It should be an addition to the literature that has already been published on the subject. It needs to add to, and develop, what is known already about the topic.
- *Educationally important*. It should offer some insight from which other clinical teachers can benefit.
- *Academically rigorous*. High quality medical education research uses an increasingly wide variety of quantitative and qualitative methods. Whatever the methodology chosen, it must be scrupulously clear and unambiguous in its planning, application and reporting.

This chapter is aimed mainly at the clinical teacher who is interested in publishing the results of education research in an academic journal, although many of the principles described will apply equally to other products of medical education development and innovation.

Planning a research project

Think carefully about what you want to achieve

You may have many reasons for conducting research, but if your ultimate intention is to get your work published in an academic journal you need to make this a priority right from the very beginning. Even at the planning stage you should be thinking carefully about the questions that editors, reviewers and readers will want to be answered when they come to read the results.

There are six fundamental questions which you should ask yourself, and keep asking, throughout your project. As we have already said, publication may not be your main intention in conducting medical education research, but even if you don't intend to submit your work to a journal, these questions are still worth asking. They will help you to clarify your ultimate goals and to communicate them clearly to the people who will be reading your research.

- *What am I trying to find out?* What are my research questions and why are they important now?
- *Why am I doing it?* What is the background to my thinking on this question – practical or theoretical?
- *Am I doing this in the best way?* Do I need professional advice in designing my project and data collection and analysis methods?
- *Who will care about the results?* Who will be my audience and which journals do they read? What will they do with the information once they have it?
- *What did I find in my research?* Select a maximum of three key messages that you want to put across.
- *What does it mean?* Remind yourself that readers will want to understand the implications of what you have found out. You will need to make this clear in the text.

If you want to get published – do your homework

There are hundreds of authors out there

Academic publishing is a difficult market and journals need to be competitive in order to survive. An increasing number of editors these days are professional or semiprofessional with training, and they take their responsibilities seriously – rejection decisions are not made on a whim.

Whilst editors are, by the very nature of their role, dedicated to serving the academic community in which they work, they have to set priorities. Chief among these is survival of the journal so that it can continue to advance the academic discipline it serves. Put simply, editors have to care more about their readers than about you as an author. This means you need to sell your story – to make the piece stand out amongst the hundreds or even thousands of other manuscripts being read by the journal each year.

Learn how peer review actually works

Although it may feel as if your manuscript vanishes into a black hole when you submit it, a great deal in fact happens to it once it has left your hands and entered the editorial process. Each journal has its own style and requirements, but the basic procedures for handling, processing, selecting and publishing papers are broadly similar. Once you understand how your manuscript will be assessed for publication, then you will find the process of submitting it and waiting for a result much easier to bear.

Editors usually base their decisions on advice from other people working in the same field. In most journals, your work will be assessed by one or more editors and it is also likely to be sent for external peer review to colleagues in other departments and universities. These reviewers usually work for no fee, although some large journals may offer a small token payment. Reviewers tend to see their work in helping and advising colleagues as a professional responsibility and an opportunity for learning.

The review process may be done with varying degrees of anonymity – you may be told the reviewers' names, they may know yours, or peer review may be carried out 'double-blinded' so that neither side is aware of the other's identity. The process of peer review may take anything from a few days to a couple of months depending on the speed with which the reviewers respond. The reviewers' reports will be assessed, sometimes by an editorial committee, and a decision letter containing varying amounts of feedback will be prepared.

You can see from this that the process is highly formalised, involving many individuals. When preparing a manuscript for publication, you will have to please more people than just your research director; you need to impress the editor, the reviewers and, ultimately, the readers of the journal.

Read your target journal

We can't stress this strongly enough. Ideally you should do this before you start to write up your research although this is not always possible. Editors can always tell when someone has not bothered to read their journal before submitting a paper. This is not very flattering, of course, but, much more importantly, it indicates that the author is out of touch with the current debates.

Ensure your paper is appropriate for the journal

Choose your journal carefully. Editors know what their readers want and don't like to waste their – or your – time on assessing a paper which is outside the scope of their journal. Reading several recent issues is the only way to get a good idea of what your target journal is publishing. You can see what debates are going on in its pages, and editorials and mission statements in particular can sometimes give you a clue as to what the editor is looking for. Look at the other papers in the issue; what do they have in common? Would your paper look out of place among them? Will it add anything to what has already been published on the subject?

There is no point in submitting papers of a type that the journal does not publish. For example, some journals do not accept case reports, others are explicit in refusing to consider reports of work in progress or pilot studies. Check the journal's Guidelines for Authors to make sure.

Occasionally journals publish 'Calls for Papers' where the editor asks for submissions on particular topics for a theme issue. Look out for these. If your paper's subject matter is appropriate for a 'Call for Papers', it probably stands a better than average chance of being accepted since the editor has already set aside the space in a future issue and wants to fill it.

A word of caution: some authors try to hedge their bets by contacting the journal in advance of submission, but this can waste time. The Guidelines for Authors, mission statement and content of the journal are usually perfectly adequate guides as to whether your paper's subject matter will be suitable. You are unlikely to get much more in the way of guidance from the editorial office on whether your paper is going to be acceptable, nor on how to modify it if it isn't. Editors don't like to give summative judgements on papers they haven't read.

Check the journal for quality

Big, high-impact international journals may give a less personal service and your risk of rejection is almost certainly higher but the prestige of being published in one is considerable and, if it gets accepted, your paper is more likely to be extensively cited. You therefore need to think carefully and objectively about the subject matter of your paper and to ask yourself how far you are prepared to risk rejection in order to get it published in the best possible journal.

Journals vary considerably in their scope and in the quality of the research they publish. One indicator of quality is the *impact factor* and most high-prestige journals are ranked by this. Put simply, the impact factor is a measure of how often the 'average article' in a journal has been cited in a particular year. The higher a journal's impact factor, the more frequently cited are its contents. The impact factor is calculated by dividing the number of current citations to articles published in the two previous years by the total number of articles published in the two previous years. A variation of the impact factor is the *immediacy index*, which will tell you how often articles published in a journal are cited within the same year. A good immediacy index shows that the journal is publishing a lot of 'cutting-edge' articles which are read and cited quickly by other authors in the field.

Some questions to ask about a journal's quality

- What are its impact factor and immediacy index and how do they compare with other journals in the field? Are they rising or falling?
- What is its readership?
- Is it indexed and by which indexes?
- Is it peer-reviewed? Open or blinded review?
- Who is the editor; who is on the editorial board?
- Is it the journal of an academic association? If so, which one?
- Does it declare its ethical standards? Has it got a policy of openness and is it clear about its processes?

Beware of very slow journals

Feel free to ask the editorial office what review times, publication lag and acceptance rates are like – a good journal should have this information readily to hand. Some journals publish submission, review and acceptance dates at the end of papers so you can see for yourself how quick they are. A nine-month delay between acceptance and publication is not unusual

Dr G's paper, which dealt with a small study in one university in Turkey, had been rejected by three different high-impact international journals in a row. Although there was nothing technically wrong with her paper, the editors knew that their readers would not be able to use the findings in their own context because the study was too local and particular and it didn't tell them anything they did not already know. Dr G then submitted her manuscript to a Turkish journal and it was accepted at once.

You can find out more about impact factors from your library or by looking at Thomson ISI's website: http://www.isinet.com

"Writing is easy. All you do is stare at a blank sheet of paper until drops of blood form on your forehead"

Gene Fowler (1890–1960)

Professor E was very annoyed when his paper was returned to him for reformatting ten days after he mailed it. But the journal uses blinded review and he had put his name on every page of the manuscript, revealing his identity to everyone who read his paper. He had also forgotten to supply an abstract and his references were incomplete. The editorial office could not send his paper out to reviewers until it was properly formatted. Five minutes spent reading the Guidelines to Authors before he submitted would have saved him a lot of time.

but 18 months is unacceptable and you may risk your work becoming out of date before it even appears in print.

Start writing

Having selected your journal, read the Guidelines for Authors

Guidelines for Authors are usually published in the journal, at the back or front, and they will also be available on the journal's website. Read them carefully. Then read them again. If something's not clear, don't guess, ask the editorial office. The Guidelines are there for a reason, and a little time spent getting the formatting of your paper correct in the initial stages may save you a great deal of time later. Guidelines vary from journal to journal, and they can be very boring and difficult to understand, but it's unwise to ignore them and it wastes your own and the editorial office's time if you get it wrong.

Choose a format

Research papers are not the only way to get your message across. Ask yourself if your work would be better presented in one of the other formats offered by your target journal. These may include commentaries, case reports, letters to the editor, short communications, discussion papers, review articles and personal accounts. The Guidelines for Authors will tell you which of these the journal is willing to consider and what the word lengths and formats are.

Tips for writing good English

There are many books giving advice on how to write clear and precise English, and several very good ones are mentioned in the Further reading list at the end of this chapter. The most important piece of advice we can offer is to write simply and keep what you have to say brief and to the point.

Writing simply is hard. It is much easier to repeat the type of ready-prepared phrases which can be found in any biomedical journal, such as 'A study was undertaken', 'Further research is indicated', 'The subjects were invited to participate in the study' and so on, rather than to express yourself using your own words and a more conversational style. There is always a temptation when you are writing for publication to write in order to impress readers with your scholarship by using long and complicated words where short ones will do. In addition, many writers make the mistake of thinking that because scientific research is supposed to be impartial, they need to write themselves out of the paper entirely. They do this by writing passively ('a questionnaire was designed' instead of 'we designed a questionnaire') and by being very tentative in their discussion ('the tendency of the results is to indicate' as opposed to 'the results show'). Although we are not proposing that you should 'dumb down' your key messages, there is no point in making your paper unnecessarily difficult for the reader.

Here is a brief list of simple ways in which you can make your writing more accessible for readers.

- Use the active, rather than the passive voice. Say 'we did this' rather than 'this was done'.
- Avoid unnecessarily complex words, such as 'indicate' for 'show'; 'initiate' for 'start' and so on.
- Avoid redundancies; for example, 'the resultant observational findings indicated' can be more simply expressed as 'the findings showed'.
- Keep your sentences short. 15–20 words are usually enough to express an idea.
- Keep your paragraphs short. Four or five sentences are usually long enough to close your point and take your argument on to the next paragraph.
- Consider using bullet points, subheadings and diagrams to break up the text.
- Be brave and keep to the point. If you have something positive to say, don't hedge it about with unnecessary qualifications and meanderings. On the other hand, be equally forthright about your study's shortcomings.

Keep within the word limit or you may be wasting your time

Pressure on journal space is enormous and editors have to be ruthless in allocating it, so ask yourself why your paper deserves to be given the extra page or two. If you really have to go over the word limit, be prepared to justify this in your covering letter.

Get a colleague or three to read your paper

It is very important that they are honest with you. If they think it's boring or difficult to follow, the likelihood is that the editor and reviewers won't like it either. From whom would you rather hear the bad news?

Get someone who is not an expert in the field to look at your paper for readability

Remember that not all of your readers will be fully conversant with your field of research. A substantial number will be 'interested amateurs'. Your work needs to be accessible to as wide a range of people as possible, so try it out on a non-expert who may be better able to point out areas where concepts and technical terms need clarification.

If English is not your first language

It is becoming increasingly important to write and to publish in English whatever your country of origin. This puts writers whose first language is not English at an unfair disadvantage in a highly competitive market. While editors may be sympathetic to the difficulties faced by non-English speaking authors, however, most do not have the resources to spend time deciphering and rewriting a paper written in very poor English. It is therefore essential, if you don't have English as a first language, to get your manuscript read by someone who does. If that person is not an expert in the field in which you are working, you will also need the advice of someone with excellent English who has a good grasp of the technical complexities of your paper.

"Say all you have to say in the fewest possible words, or your reader will be sure to skip them; and in the plainest possible words or he will certainly misunderstand them"

John Ruskin (1819–1900)

"Read over your compositions, and wherever you meet with a passage which you think is particularly fine, strike it out"

Samuel Johnson (1709–1784), from Boswell's *Life of Johnson*

Give your manuscript a good title

The title of your manuscript is the first thing that the editor and reviewers will read. If it is published, researchers will be searching for papers by title and comparing yours with others they have found in their search results. If the title of your paper is boring, wordy, vague or unoriginal, it may give an unfairly bad impression of the content. Keep it as short as you can while making sure it gives a good idea of what readers can expect to find in the paper.

Write the covering letter

A good covering letter is vital. Spend time on preparing it. If you have pre-planned your research and targeted your journal carefully it should be easy to write a really good letter. Tell the editor what your paper adds to the literature in the field and – most importantly – why you think readers *of his or her journal* will want to read it. The editor wants to know why you think readers and reviewers will be more interested in your paper than in all the others they see. One small but critical point: get the editor's name and title right. A letter directed to the editor of another journal, or to an editor who retired years ago, will create a bad impression; it will be obvious that you haven't been reading the journal.

Once you have submitted

As we have said, editors don't select papers for publication haphazardly. Most editors ask for advice from a variety of experts including peer reviewers. This process takes time.

Be realistic about timescales

You should have been told how long a decision will take so don't worry that nothing's happening if you don't hear during that period. But once the deadline for a decision is past, feel free to ask what is happening. Delays are almost always due to slow referees. Before you send that righteously indignant email, however, you should remember that referees are giving up their time to review your paper and many of them are busy senior academics and internationally acknowledged experts. Good referees are as valuable and hard to find as Périgord truffles and editors can only put a certain amount of pressure on them to review quickly.

The final decision

Don't get mad

When you receive a final decision, there is a high probability that you will be disappointed. Remember that in most journals more papers are rejected than accepted. In some specialist and high-prestige journals such as *JAMA*, the *British Medical Journal* and *Medical Education*, the rejection rate can be as high as 90%. You may wish to challenge the decision, but it is wise to wait until you have calmed down before writing a letter of appeal. Editors don't usually mind being asked for further details and will try to help where they can – but they do not have time to spare on soothing bruised egos.

Don't delay

If you are asked for revisions, don't hang around. Every day you put off revising and resubmitting your paper, someone else is being given a print slot ahead of you.

Don't give up

It is tempting to go into a terminal sulk if your paper is rejected by your first choice of journal. A more constructive course of behaviour is to take on board the reasons for rejection and make amendments before resubmitting to a more appropriate journal. But keep a list of the journals you have tried so you don't accidentally resubmit and make sure you revise your paper between submissions so that it is kept up to date. You may need to reformat it too, so that it conforms to the new journal's guidelines for authors. For example, journals use different reference systems, such as Harvard and Vancouver – or Ciba, which is used in this book. A new journal may want you to revise your references, prepare your summary in a particular way or it may require you to supply particular information, such as a statement concerning conflicts of interest or details of ethical approval. If you don't check the Guidelines for Authors before submitting to a new journal your paper will be bounced back and you will waste time.

You may have to submit your work to several journals before it is accepted. Keep trying, working your way down your list of suitable journals and, sooner or later, you will have the very satisfying experience of seeing your paper in print. It is an exciting moment and a great achievement. Enjoy it.

Summary

Clinical teachers work in a wide range of fields and produce work in a variety of formats. Some choose to specialise in education research. If they do this, they will want and need to publish their findings in academic journals.

Academic publishing is a highly competitive field, so in order to write a paper which will be acceptable to the most highly regarded journals, experienced and successful authors take the time to organise themselves carefully before they even begin their research. They think carefully about their aims and objectives in conducting the research and keep their goals constantly under review. They select and target the most appropriate journal, checking its quality and performance against that of other journals in the field. They make themselves familiar with the editorial system of peer-reviewed academic journals. By doing this they can begin to understand the priorities of the editor and reviewers and ways in which they can respond to these in order to make their manuscript as acceptable as possible. They study their target journal, reading both the content and the Guidelines for Authors to make sure that their work will fit comfortably within the scope and format of the journal.

"You must keep sending work out; you must never let a manuscript do nothing but eat its head off in a drawer. You send that work out again and again, while you're working on another one. If you have talent, you will receive some measure of success – but only if you persist"

Isaac Asimov (1920–1992)

For a crash course in how journals do things, why not contact journals in your field to see if they would like you to review for them? You don't have to wait to be asked. Journals are always looking out for new reviewers, and you can learn a lot about the process by participating in this way.

Having written the paper, wise authors will get a range of opinions from colleagues, both expert and nonspecialist, on the readability of the paper. Successful authors are good writers; they understand that their aim is to communicate a clear message to their readers, so they cultivate a simple and direct style. A plain style is perfectly capable of conveying complex and abstract concepts but to write in this way is sometimes difficult. Less experienced writers tend to adopt the 'scientific' style, which is superficially impressive but can obscure the message and will make the paper less acceptable to the editor.

Once a final decision is made, it can be very discouraging to receive a rejection, but successful authors don't give up; they revise and reformat their papers and carry on submitting. Sooner or later their paper will be accepted if they persist.

Further reading

Albert T 1997 Winning the publications game. Radcliffe Medical Press, Oxford

Albert T 2004 Why are medical journals so badly written? Medical Education 38:6–8

Barrass R 2002 Scientists must write: a guide to better writing for scientists, engineers and students (Routledge Study Guides) Routledge, London

Bligh J 1998 What happens to manuscripts submitted to the journal? Medical Education; 32:567–570

Greenhalgh T 1997 How to read a paper: the basics of evidence-based medicine. BMJ Publishing Group, London

Hall G M 1994 How to write a paper. BMJ Publishing Group, London

Matthews J, Bowen J M, Matthews R W 2000 Successful scientific writing: a step-by-step guide for the biological and medical sciences. Cambridge University Press, Cambridge

Orwell G 2000 Politics and the English Lanuage. In Orwell; Essays. Penguin, London

Parsell G, Bligh J 1999 AMEE Education Guide no 17. Writing for journal publication. Medical Teacher 21:457–468

Uniform requirements for manuscripts submitted to biomedical journals 1999 Medical Education 33:67–68. Online. Available: http://www.icmje.org/

Useful link

Thomson ISI. http://www.isinet.com

INDEX